Clinical Manual of
Cultural Psychiatry

Clinical Manual of Cultural Psychiatry

Edited by

Russell F. Lim, M.D.

Associate Clinical Professor and
Director of Diversity Education and Training,
Department of Psychiatry and Behavioral Sciences
University of California, Davis, School of Medicine,
Sacramento, California

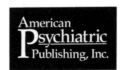
American Psychiatric Publishing, Inc.

Washington, DC
London, England

Copyright © 2006 American Psychiatric Publishing, Inc.
ALL RIGHTS RESERVED
Manufactured in the United States of America on acid-free paper
10 09 08 07 06   5 4 3 2 1
First Edition

Typeset in Adobe's Formata and AGaramond.

American Psychiatric Publishing, Inc.
1000 Wilson Boulevard
Arlington, VA 22209-3901
www.appi.org

To buy 25–99 copies of any APPI title at a 20% discount, please contact APPI Customer Service at appi@psych.org or 800-368-5777. To buy 100 or more copies of the same title, please e-mail bulksales@psych.org for a price quote.

Library of Congress Cataloging-in-Publication Data
Clinical manual of cultural psychiatry / edited by Russell F. Lim.
    p. ; cm.
  Includes bibliographical references and index.
  ISBN 1-58562-256-7 (pbk. : alk. paper)
  1. Cultural psychiatry--United States--Handbooks, manuals, etc. 2. Psychiatry, Transcultural--United States--Handbooks, manuals, etc.
  [DNLM: 1. Mental Disorders--ethnology. 2. Community Psychiatry. 3. Cross-Cultural Comparison. WM 31 641 2006] I. Lim, Russell F., 1961-
  RC455.4.E8C577 2006
  362.2089--dc22

                                                                        2006002768

British Library Cataloguing in Publication Data
A CIP record is available from the British Library.

To Francis Lu, who led the way, and Liz Kramer, who got us there.

Contents

PART I

Culture and Psychiatric Assessment

1 The Assessment of Culturally Diverse Individuals 3

Hendry Ton, M.D., M.S.
Russell F. Lim, M.D.

PART II

Cultural Issues in Assessment and Treatment

2 African American Patients 35

Annelle B. Primm, M.D., M.P.H.

PART III

Culture, Psychopharmacological Treatment, and Case Formulation

Appendix A: A Resident's Guide to the Cultural Formulation 243

Angel Caraballo, M.D., Hamada Hamid, D.O.,
Jennifer Robin Lee, M.D., Joy D. McQuery, M.D.,
Yanni Rho, M.D., M.P.H., Elizabeth J. Kramer, Sc.M.,
Russell F. Lim, M.D., Francis G. Lu, M.D.

Appendix B: Annotated Bibliography of Cultural Psychiatry and Other Topics 271

Francis G. Lu, M.D.

Appendix C: Glossary of Culture-Bound Syndromes 291

Contributors

Angel Caraballo, M.D.
APA/AstraZeneca Minority Fellow, Stony Brook University Hospital, Stony Brook, New York

Nang Du, M.D.
Clinical Professor of Psychiatry, Department of Psychiatry, University of California, San Francisco, School of Medicine; Unit Chief, Asian Focus Unit, San Francisco General Hospital, San Francisco, California

Candace M. Fleming, Ph.D.
Associate Professor, University of Colorado at Denver and Health Sciences Center, and Associate Director of Training, National Center for American Indian and Alaska Native Mental Health Research, Denver, Colorado

Hamada Hamid, D.O.
APA/AstraZeneca Minority Fellow, Department of Psychiatry, New York University School of Medicine, New York, New York

Elizabeth J. Kramer, Sc.M.
Research Assistant Professor, Department of Psychiatry, New York University School of Medicine; Special Projects Consultant, New York Coalition for Asian American Health, New York, New York

Amaro J. Laria, Ph.D.
Lecturer, Department of Social Medicine, Harvard Medical School, Boston, Massachusetts; Faculty and Director, Latino Mental Health Program, Massachusetts School of Professional Psychology, Boston, Massachusetts

Jennifer Robin Lee, M.D.
APA/AstraZeneca Minority Fellow, New York-Presbyterian Hospital, New York, New York

Roberto Lewis-Fernández, M.D.
Associate Professor of Clinical Psychiatry, Columbia University School of Medicine, New York, New York; Lecturer on Social Medicine, Harvard University, Boston, Massachusetts; and Director, Hispanic Treatment Program, New York State Psychiatric Institute, New York, New York

Russell F. Lim, M.D.
Associate Clinical Professor and Director of Diversity Education and Training, Department of Psychiatry and Behavioral Sciences, University of California, Davis, School of Medicine, Sacramento, California

Francis G. Lu, M.D.
Professor of Clinical Psychiatry and Director, Cultural Competence and Diversity Program, San Francisco General Hospital Department of Psychiatry, University of California, San Francisco.

Joy D. McQuery, M.D.
APA/SAMHSA Minority Fellow, Cambridge Health Alliance, Harvard Medical School, Cambridge, Massachusetts

Annelle B. Primm, M.D., M.P.H.
Director of Minority and National Affairs, American Psychiatric Association, Arlington, Virginia; Associate Professor of Psychiatry, Department of Psychiatry and Behavioral Sciences, Johns Hopkins University School of Medicine, Baltimore, Maryland

Yanni C. Rho, M.D., M.P.H.
Child and Adolescent Psychiatry Fellow, APA/SAMHSA Minority Fellow, Cambridge Health Alliance, Harvard Medical School, Cambridge, Massachusetts

Michael W. Smith, M.D.
Associate Professor of Psychiatry, Department of Psychiatry, UCLA School of Medicine, Los Angeles, California; Director, Research Center on the Psychobiology of Ethnicity, Los Angeles Biomedical Research Institute at Harbor UCLA Medical Center, Torrance, California

Hendry Ton, M.D., M.S.
Assistant Clinical Professor, Department of Psychiatry and Behavioral Sciences, University of California, Davis, School of Medicine, Sacramento, California

Preface

The inspiration for this book was a continuing medical education (CME) course entitled "DSM-IV Cultural Formulation: Diagnosis and Treatment," first offered at the American Psychiatric Association's 149th annual meeting in New York in 1996. That course has since been revised, repeated 10 times, presented at three meetings of the Institute for Psychiatric Services, used as a model for a successful CME program at the University of California, Davis, Medical Center, and used as a faculty development course for Department of Psychiatry faculty and staff at University of California, Davis, and University of California, San Francisco. In first creating the course, I wanted to gather the experts in the four major nationally recognized ethnic minority groups and have them present cases that would demonstrate particular aspects of working with those groups. I also recruited experts in the area of cultural competence and ethnopsychopharmacology. I never imagined that I would be running the course 10 years later, or that I would edit a book distilling what we have learned after teaching the course almost 20 times.

As I do in the course, I invite you to see the United States from a different perspective, as an outsider from another country, as my father did when he came to this country in 1941. He taught me to understand the differences between his life in China and my life in America. Having the ability to see someone else's worldview is essential to working with ethnic minority and culturally diverse patients, even if diversity consists of being from the South, East, Midwest, or West regions of the United States. We all have our own "cultures," and the techniques and the information contained in this book will help you to understand all patients better, regardless of their background, nationality, or ethnicity.

The book contains an introductory chapter on how to apply the DSM-IV-TR Outline for Cultural Formulation. The next four chapters concern the four federally identified minority groups. Each chapter details the heterogeneity of a specific group as well as the commonalities among its members, offering practical advice and illustrative case examples. These chapters are supplemented by a review of ethnopsychopharmacology and a concluding chapter that presents a synthesis of the preceding chapters, organized by the DSM-IV-TR Outline for Cultural Formulation.

I hope this handbook will be useful to medical students, psychiatry residents, psychiatrists, psychologists, psychology graduate students, and trainees in social work and counseling, along with social workers, case managers, and other mental health practitioners, when they begin the evaluation of patients belonging to diverse minority groups. The chapters are meant to be an introduction to working with these groups. They are not intended to be a substitute for cultural consultation with a person familiar with a specific group. Nor are they meant to be stereotypical. I have always felt that I could trust my audience to use this type of cultural information as a reference point from which to ask the question, "Is what I am seeing in this patient normal behavior in his or her culture?" If readers feel they have learned when to ask this question, then their understanding of the interaction of culture and mental illness will have begun, and this book will have served its purpose.

There are many people without whom this book would not have been possible. First and foremost is my mentor and friend, Francis Lu, who suggested that I put the course together in 1995 and who has been one of my course speakers since the beginning. Elizabeth Kramer has been a friend, supporter, and editor without whose help I could not have completed the manuscript. Many thanks to Michelle Clark, Kenneth Gee, N. Charles Ndlela, Jessie Sanchez, Maria Oquendo, Silvia Olarte, Renato Alarcon, David Henderson, Linda Naluhu and, Frank Brown, who have all served as faculty in my course, as well as the authors of the chapters, many of whom were presenters as well. I thank my former supervisors in the residency program at the University of California, San Francisco, especially Francis Lu, Nang Du, and Frank Johnson, who opened up the world of cultural psychiatry for me and who taught me most of what I know about psychiatry. In addition, I would like to thank my wife, Sally, and my two children, Jackie and James, for putting up with my typing at odd hours of the night (and morning) and on weekends. Finally, I thank my greatest teachers—my course attendees, residents, and students, who have asked the important questions that caused me to revise my course and other presentations in helpful ways and who continue to show us that there still is a need to teach these skills to psychiatrists and trainees.

Russell F. Lim, M.D.
Davis, California

Foreword

Francis G. Lu, M.D.

The Outline for Cultural Formulation, first published in DSM-IV in 1994 and reprinted in DSM-IV-TR (American Psychiatric Association 1994, 2000), provides the starting point for this book. The Outline had been proposed by the National Institute on Mental Health Workgroup on Culture, Diagnosis and Care, which was initiated by Delores L. Parron, Ph.D., Director of the Office of Special Populations, and chaired by Juan Mezzich, M.D., a member of the American Psychiatric Association Task Force on DSM-IV (Mezzich et al. 1999). Although the Workgroup had recommended that the Outline and several cultural case examples be placed immediately after the introduction to DSM-IV to reiterate the importance of this topic, it was published as part of Appendix I, along with the Glossary of Culture-Bound Syndromes. This placement left the Outline in relative obscurity at first, but that situation has begun to change. In 1995, I, along with Drs. Lim and Mezzich, wrote one of the first explications of the Outline (Lu et al. 1995). In 1996, Dr. Lim initiated the first continuing medical education course on the Outline, and the course has been given continuously through 2006. This book represents the collected wisdom from the years of teaching these courses as well the professional experience of the authors in using and teaching about the Outline.

The publication of this book is very timely, coming after the release of *Mental Health: Culture, Race, and Ethnicity* (U.S. Department of Health and Human Services 2001), a supplement to the Surgeon General's report on mental health. That report documented mental health disparities for racial and ethnic minority groups and challenged the field to reduce those dispari-ties through culturally competent clinical care and training and through re-search to provide further evidence that culturally competent care would reduce mental health disparities. The Liaison Committee on Medical Educa-tion (LCME) (2005) and the Accreditation Council for Graduate Medical Education (2005) have added accreditation standards involving cultural com-petence. I believe this manual will be very helpful to teachers in medical stu-dent education and psychiatry residency programs as they plan to incorporate cultural competence issues into their curricula to meet these standards.

This book joins a small but growing body of work that helps clinicians and trainees bring culture into the clinical setting through the use of the Out-line as a concise clinical tool. Several teaching tools exist that explicate both the content and the process of using the Outline. First, the Cultural Psychi-atry Committee of the Group for the Advancement of Psychiatry published an important monograph on the Outline and illustrated its use in six clinical cases (Group for the Advancement of Psychiatry Committee on Cultural Psy-chiatry 2002). Second, Harriet Koskoff (2002), a filmmaker, created a 58-minute training videotape with 23 multicultural, multidisciplinary mental health professionals commenting on the five sections of the Outline (I served as the executive scientific advisor to the film). Third, approximately 17 clin-ical cases demonstrating the use of the Outline have been published since 1995 in the quarterly journal Culture, Medicine and Psychiatry; Roberto Lewis-Fernández, M.D., serves as the editor of this section of the journal. In addition, a search of PubMed and PsycINFO databases for "DSM-IV Out-line for Cultural Formulation" from 1994 to 2005 yielded 10 unduplicated citations (Christensen 2001; Dillard et al. 2000; Harper 2001; Hinman 2003; House 2002; Lu et al. 1995; Mezzich et al. 1999; Novins et al. 1997; Paniagua 2000; Takeuchi 2000) that described the Outline or illustrated its use with 1 to 4 cases.

Yet as Neighbors (2003) has pointed out, there is a need for further re-search studies on the usefulness of the Outline in the clinical setting. Studies are urgently needed to determine outcomes obtained by using or not using the Outline with culturally diverse populations broadly defined, in regard to effectiveness and appropriateness of care, patient and family satisfaction, and cost-effectiveness. To what extent can use of the Outline improve the thera-peutic alliance between clinician and individual and thereby improve the di-

PART I

Culture and Psychiatric Assessment

The Assessment of Culturally Diverse Individuals

Hendry Ton, M.D., M.S.

Russell F. Lim, M.D.

The United States is becoming increasingly diverse. Although non-Hispanic whites represent 69% of the population, minority groups are rapidly growing. Figure 1–1 illustrates the percentage growth of various ethnic/racial groups over the past several decades.

Ethnic minorities have grown at rates far greater than those of non-Hispanic whites over the past 20 years. Currently, there are more than 35 mil-

---

Portions of this chapter are based on Lu FG, Lim RF, Mezzich JE: "Issues in the Assessment and Diagnosis of Culturally Diverse Individuals," in *American Psychiatric Press Review of Psychiatry,* Vol. 14. Edited by Oldham JM, Riba MB. Washington, DC, American Psychiatric Press, 1995, pp. 477–510. Used with permission.

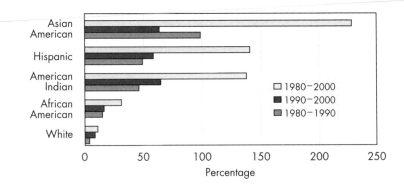

Figure 1–1.   U.S. population growth by race, 1980–2000.

Source.   U.S. Census Bureau 2000.

lion Hispanics and nearly the same number of African Americans. Asian Americans number about 10 million, and the Native American community is nearly 2 million in size. By the middle of the twenty-first century, it is estimated that the U.S. population will be 72.1% non-Hispanic white, 24.4% Hispanic (nonexclusive category, meaning that one can claim to be Hispanic *and* some other designation), 14.6% African American, 8% Asian, and 5.3% other ethnic groups (U.S. Census Bureau 2004). Ethnic variations reflect only a fraction of the diversity in our society, however. Tremendous diversity exists also in gender, sexual preference, age, occupational, and religious and spiritual affiliations. In addition, technological advances in communication and transportation have enabled the development of a global community comprising multitudes of languages, customs, and beliefs.

Our society will undoubtedly continue to be enriched by the ideas, perspectives, and contributions of the many groups of which it is composed. Mental health providers, however, face the particularly challenging task of providing culturally competent care to an increasingly diverse community. In 2001, the Office of the Surgeon General released a detailed supplement to its report on mental health entitled *Mental Health: Culture, Race, and Ethnicity* (U. S. Department of Health and Human Services 2001) about the growing crisis of inadequate mental health services for the country's ethnic minorities.

The report identifies several disparities in mental health care of racial and ethnic minorities compared with whites: 1) minorities have less access to, and availability of, mental health services; 2) they are less likely to receive needed mental health services; 3) those who are in treatment often receive poorer-quality mental health care; and 4) minorities are underrepresented as subjects in mental health research. However, the report also states that the recognition of these disparities brings hope that they can be addressed and remedied.

The purpose of this handbook is to help clinicians take steps to address these important issues. This chapter, specifically, will highlight the principles of cultural psychiatry used in the assessment and treatment of psychiatric conditions.

Historical Perspective

Work on cultural psychiatry dates back to more than 100 years ago, when unusual clinical syndromes seen in non-Western countries were examined using Western universalistic interpretations of the findings (Group for the Advancement of Psychiatry Committee on Cultural Psychiatry 2002). This ethnocentric approach tended to limit the focus of cultural inquiry to exotic or isolated locations and cultural groups, and thus it did little to incorporate cultural evaluation into mainstream psychiatry. By the latter half of the twentieth century, modern psychiatry came under criticism by sociologists and cultural anthropologists, who were concerned with the cultural relativity of mental disorders, believing that mental illness is socially defined (Kleinman 1988). This belief was in direct opposition to the perspective of scientific universalism held within mainstream psychiatry.

Psychiatry's initial response was to reaffirm its scientific foundations and to view culture as a set of confounding variables that distorted the ways in which the real psychiatric disorders manifested (Fabrega 2001). However, interest in investigating the interplay between psychiatric disorders and sociocultural factors continued to develop, culminating in the universal acceptance of Engel's biopsychosocial approach in the 1980s (Group for the Advancement of Psychiatry Committee on Cultural Psychiatry 2002). Subsequently there have been significant advances in our understanding of the impact of culture on psychopharmacology, psychotherapy, the application of treatment to ethnic minorities, and the development of mental health services. An example of this change can be seen in DSM-IV-TR, with its Outline for Cul-

Table 1–1.   Essential components of culture

- Culture is learned.
- Culture refers to a system of meanings.
- Culture acts as a shaping template.
- Culture is taught and reproduced.
- Culture exists in a constant state of change.
- Culture includes patterns of both subjective and objective components of human behavior.

Source.   Adapted from Gaw 2001.

tural Formulation and Glossary of Culture-bound Syndromes (American Psychiatric Association 2000). Consideration of cultural factors in the evaluation of patients with mental illness will result in improved access to care, an increased understanding of patients' illness experiences, more accurate diagnosis, and, ultimately, better treatment.

Critical Concepts

Culture has been defined in many different ways, an indication that even the most comprehensive definitions cannot encompass all of its attributed meanings. In this section we attempt to define culture in terms that are usable and relevant to the mental health clinician. Culture can be defined as a set of meanings, norms, beliefs, and values shared by a group of people. It is dynamic and evolves over time and with each generation (Matsumoto 1996). Gaw (2001) describes six essential components of culture (Table 1–1). Culture is learned, and therefore it can be taught and reproduced. The term *culture* refers to a system of meanings in which words, behaviors, events, and symbols have attached meanings that are agreed upon by the members within the cultural group. Hence, culture shapes how individuals make sense of the social and natural world. Culture also encompasses a body of learned behaviors and perspectives that serves as a template to shape and orient future behaviors and perspectives from generation to generation and as novel situations emerge. Finally, culture includes both the subjective components of human behavior (the shared ideas and meanings that exist within the minds of individuals within a group) and the objective components (the observable behaviors and interactions of these individuals).

Culture shapes what symptoms are expressed and how they are expressed (Mezzich et al. 2000; Rogler 1993). It influences the meaning that one attributes to symptoms. Culture also influences what a society regards as appropriate or inappropriate behavior. In other words, it influences the conceptualization and rationale of psychiatric diagnostic categories and groupings. In addition, culture provides the matrix for the clinician-patient exchange. It can operate as a pathogenic and pathoplastic agent (Alarcon et al. 1999). The association of war with posttraumatic stress disorder is one example of how historical events can cause or contribute to psychopathology (Du and Lu 1997; Kirmayer 2001). Likewise, culture exerts a protective influence on mental health. There is some evidence, for example, that the extended family systems in non-Western cultures mitigate the effects of schizophrenia (Kulhara and Chakrabarti 2001). Traditional healing approaches and spiritual/religious interventions can also provide meaningful benefits to patients (Kinzie 2000; Lee 1997a; Lukoff et al. 1995; Muskin 2000).

The terms *culture, ethnicity,* and *race* are often used interchangeably, but it is important to highlight the distinctions among the three concepts. Like culture, ethnicity and race have been defined in many ways. *Ethnicity* can be used to refer to an individual's sense of belonging to a group of people who have a common set of beliefs and customs (culture) and who share a common history and origin. It may imply nationality, geographic location, and religious beliefs. Examples of ethnicity include Vietnamese American, Russian Jewish, and Ethiopian. *Race* is often used to refer to a group of people who share biological similarities (Lu et al. 1995). Application of this concept has often meant grouping people according to physical appearance, such as skin color, with little attention to actual biological or genetic determinants. However, there is much disagreement about what the biological similarities attributed to a particular race are. In much of the history of the United States, the use of race has had the effect of furthering racial prejudices and inequalities. In psychiatry, race is a powerful influencing factor in the clinician-patient dyad. African Americans, for example, have often been misdiagnosed with schizophrenia (Adebimpe 1981), likely because of differences in interactional styles and values rather than any specific biological predisposition to psychosis (U.S. Department of Health and Human Services 2001). It is important to note, however, that although biological definitions of ethnicity and race may be problematic and difficult to validate, the concepts as they are described here do not exclude biological similarities between members of an ethnic group. Each individual's culture may encompass a sense of ethnicity and perhaps race, but there are many other affiliations, such as occupation, age, gender, sexual orientation, spirituality, and religion, that contribute to his or her overall cultural identity.

The Outline for Cultural Formulation

The publication of DSM-IV (American Psychiatric Association 1994) and its text revision in 2000, DSM-IV-TR, represented a turning point in the application of cultural psychiatry principles by introducing the Outline for Cultural Formulation. This tool gives clinicians a framework for assessing the impact of culture on psychiatric illness.

Because culture plays such a crucial role in all aspects of mental health and illness, it is important to incorporate cultural assessment as part of intervention. The astute clinician strives to gain knowledge about the cultural groups to which his or her patients belong. The complexity of the interplay between culture and illness can make this process potentially overwhelming. Factual knowledge about cultural groups, while essential, can have limited utility without a framework to organize and to make sense of the information. Further, the clinician will encounter many patients who are affiliated with one or more cultural groups of which the clinician may have inadequate knowledge. In these instances, an organizing framework is helpful to guide the clinician to areas of potentially important inquiry.

Historical Background

In 1990, the DSM-IV Task Force, chaired by Juan Mezzich, M.D., convened for the planning of DSM-IV. For the first time, serious consideration was given to incorporating cultural factors into diagnosis and evaluation of mental disorders (Mezzich et al. 2001). The Task Force formed the Culture and Diagnosis Work Group, composed of many of the leading clinical and scholarly experts on culture in the mental health disciplines, to address culture in DSM-IV. The Outline for Cultural Formulation was one of the Work Group's later contributions. It is based on an extensive review of the literature that identified five major areas in which culture had major influences on mental health and illness (Table 1–2). This finding was further substantiated by

Table 1–2. DSM-IV-TR Outline for Cultural Formulation

A. Cultural identity of the individual

B. Cultural explanations of the individual's illness

C. Cultural factors related to psychosocial environment and levels of functioning

D. Cultural elements of the relationship between the individual and the clinician

E. Overall cultural assessment for diagnosis and care

Note. In this volume, the sections of the Outline have been lettered for ease of reference.

Source. American Psychiatric Association 2000.

field trials (Mezzich et al. 2001). Although a significant portion of the Work Group's recommendations was omitted in the final text, the Outline for Cultural Formulation was included in Appendix I to DSM-IV, along with a glossary of culture-bound syndromes. These guidelines quickly became regarded as a crucial innovation in cultural psychiatry.

In the following section, we discuss the five major areas of the DSM-IV-TR Outline for Cultural Formulation with reference to a case example. We first present the patient's history, followed by a discussion of each of these five major areas. Drawn from an actual cultural evaluation, this case is meant to illustrate the practical application of the cultural formulation in clinical practice.

> X.W. is a 30-year-old Mandarin/English-speaking woman from Hong Kong who was hospitalized after jumping off a multistory building. She had immigrated to the United States 6 months earlier with her husband to work at an industrial company. She had left her 7-year-old daughter in Hong Kong because she felt that she was unable to care for her while she worked. Ms. W. reports that since the move, she had felt depressed because of isolation and work stress. She also felt unhappy about her relationship with her husband, who remained distant despite numerous overtures on her part to become more intimate. Her husband reports that their relationship was "good" but that she was overly dependent on him. Ms. W. found work very competitive, which she attributed to downsizing and to discrimination against non-U.S. citizens. One month prior to her hospitalization, she had become increasingly worried about the safety of her daughter, although she recognized that the worries were unfounded. Several days before her hospitalization, Ms. W. lost her job. Her husband encouraged her to return to Hong Kong for a break and visit with family. During a layover to Hong Kong, she encountered ticketing difficulties. She reportedly became overwhelmed and jumped off a multistory building. She later reported that this was due to the shame and stress of losing her job. X.W. was interviewed with a Mandarin-speaking interpreter.

Table 1–3.   Aspects of cultural identity

- Ethnicity
- Race
- Country of origin
- Language
- Gender
- Age
- Marital status
- Sexual orientation
- Religious/spiritual beliefs
- Socioeconomic status
- Education
- Other identified groups
- Migration history
- Level of acculturation
- Degree of affiliation with above

Source.   Adapted from Lu et al. 1995.

A. Cultural Identity of the Individual

Cultural identity can be understood as a multifaceted core set of identities that contributes to how an individual understands his or her environment. Ethnic identity is often a crucial facet of an individual's overall cultural identity, but many other facets may contribute to it as well. The greater the amount of detail a clinician is able to ascertain about the individual's cultural identity, the better understanding he or she will have of the individual's perspectives on health, illness, and the mental health system. Moreover, the clinician will more readily anticipate issues of cultural and identity conflict that may arise during the course of evaluation and treatment. Table 1–3 highlights the most common aspects of cultural identity.

Another important aspect of cultural and ethnic identity is the objective versus the subjective dimension of identity definition. In this respect, it is important to note the distinction between the terms *identity* and *identification;* the latter term refers to a subjective identification with a reference group, the former to a more solidly internalized individual core identity (Phinney 1995). Another relevant conceptual distinction, often obscured, is that between *culture* and *eth-*

nicity. These terms tend to be used interchangeably without much definitional clarity. *Ethnicity* typically refers to one's roots, ancestry, and heritage, whereas the concept of *culture* captures more active elements, such as values, understandings, behaviors, and practices. Based on this conceptual distinction, it would seem appropriate to claim a Latino *ethnic* identity based solely on Hispanic roots and heritage, but claiming a Latino *cultural* identity would necessitate participation in, for example, values and behaviors that have been shaped by Latino culture. In contrast to non-Western cultures, U.S. mainstream society is heavily influenced by Euro-American Protestant culture, which places a high value on independence, autonomy, and self-sufficiency, perhaps best reflected in the pioneer image of self-reliance and "rugged individualism" (Hsu 1983).

In considering cultural and ethnic identity it is important to remember that these identities emerge in particular social contexts and, as such, are fluid, multiple, and changing. Rather than viewing them as fixed traits of individuals or groups, it is best to regard them as "contextualized identities." New identities that did not formerly exist for a person may develop in response to migration. For example, a Latino immigrant may adopt a new "ethnic minority" identity after residing in the U.S. for several years, despite perhaps never having previously encountered that term in his or her country of origin. An immigrant woman from the Dominican Republic may have been familiar with the terms "Hispana" or "Latina" before migrating to the U.S. yet may come to experience these cultural descriptors as more relevant self-identifiers in the new sociocultural milieu. Similarly, old labels may lose salience, so that Mexican *chilangos* (natives of Mexico City) may gradually become more strongly identified as Mexican or Latino the longer they reside in the United States, only to find themselves readopting those previous identity labels upon traveling back to Mexico. In a sense, one may think of identities as having varying degrees of latency or manifest activation according to different situational and contextual factors. Of course, this process of contextual activation of identities is not unique to Latino cultures.

Ideally, the clinician should encourage the patients themselves to describe the aspects of identity that are important to them. In reviewing these aspects, the clinician should also note the degree of affiliation or involvement, negative or positive, that the patient has with each aspect, as this may highlight areas that strongly influence clinical care. The number of foreign-born residents in the United States is estimated to be over 30 million (U.S. Census

Table 1–4. Migration history

Pre-migration history

- Country of origin, family, education, socioeconomic status, community and family support, political issues, war, trauma

Experience of migration

- Migrant vs. refugee: Why did they leave? Who was left behind? Who paid for their trip?
- Means of escape, trauma

Degree of loss

- Loss of immediate family members, relatives, and friends
- Material losses: business, careers, properties
- Loss of cultural milieu, community, religious, and spiritual support

Traumatic experience

- Physical: torture, rape, starvation, imprisonment
- Psychological: rage, depression, guilt, grief, posttraumatic stress disorder

Work and financial history

- Original line of work, current occupation, socioeconomic status

Support systems

- Community support, religion, family

Medical history

- Beliefs in herbal medicine, somatic complaints

Family's concept of illness

- What do family members think the problem is? Its cause? What do they do for help?
- What result is expected?

Level of acculturation

- First or second generation

Impact on development

- Level of adjustment, assess developmental tasks

Source.   Adapted from Lee 1990.

Bureau 2000). Therefore, it is important to ask ethnic minority patients where they were born. Ascertaining a migration history is often crucial (Lee 1990) (see Table 1–4). Elements of the migration history that should be obtained include reason for migration, time spent in transit, and losses and trauma associated with migration, as well as traumatic events before and after migration.

Table 1–5. Cultural identity: advantages of assessment

- Identifies potential areas of strengths and supports that may enhance treatment planning or vulnerabilities that may impede treatment success.

- Identifies areas of cultural conflict that may need to be addressed. These conflicts can be between the various aspects of identity (e.g., parent vs. worker), or between traditional and mainstream expectations for a particular aspect (e.g., traditional parenting role vs. mainstream parenting role).

- Clinician becomes more informed about the patient's perspective on his or her illness and treatment by trying to understand who the patient is.

- Assists in building rapport because clinician is attempting to understand the individual as a "whole person" rather than an ill person.

The latter factors are particularly important to assess in refugee groups such as Southeast Asians and Eastern Europeans, whose migration history is often in the context of violence and war. Care must also be taken to explore the patient's level of acculturation. This includes the patient's prior experience with racism, and the degree to which he or she uses mainstream sociocultural resources (mainstream supermarkets, social networks, etc.). The evaluation of cultural identity helps to clarify a number of clinical issues. Table 1–5 lists some of the advantages of assessing cultural identity.

The prevailing view of acculturation encourages examination of the process on several levels (Escobar and Vega 2000). Is the process one in which the individual is actively or passively involved? Does the push for acculturation come from external sources or from within the individual? Is it a solitary endeavor, or do others participate with the individual? Is the process constant or intermittent? Is it subtle, dramatic, or somewhere in between? What are the individual's attitudes about acculturation in general, and specifically about an episode of acculturation? What vision does the individual hold about where the new mix of cultural elements will take him or her? A useful way of describing one's relationship to one's acquired culture (as opposed to one's inherited culture) was described by Berry (1997). The individuals who do not adopt the host country customs are described as "separated," while those who fully accept them are known as "assimilated." Individuals who successfully incorporate both acquired and inherited cultures are "integrated" or "bicultural," and those who reject both are "marginalized" or "deculturalized."

The following discussion of the case example illustrates how inquiry into cultural identity can enhance clinician understanding of the patient's problems:

When asked what she wanted most, Ms. W. responded, "All I want is to be with my daughter and husband, and to have a good job." Note that she clearly struggles between conflicting roles. Her identity as a working woman is clearly important to her. This may originate partly from China's post–Cultural Revolution expectations that women contribute equally with men economically. It also coincides with the values of more industrialized societies like Hong Kong. However, this priority conflicts with Ms. W.'s identity as a mother and a wife, which are roles that are traditionally considered important to women in Chinese culture. The patient has difficulty integrating these different identities. She seems unable to assume these roles simultaneously at important times, as shown when she immigrated to the U.S. to work but left her child behind. Although her extended family's role helps to lessen the conflict, X.W. nonetheless becomes anxious and depressed about it. This conflict will be further addressed in the section on treatment planning.

B. Cultural Explanations of the Individual's Illness

Patients' and providers' explanations of the illness represent an important part of clinical care. An explanatory model can have a number of components. It is an attempt to understand how and why one becomes ill. In addition, explanatory models define the culturally acceptable symptoms of the illness. These "idioms of distress" are strongly influenced by cultural values. In many Asian cultures, emotional symptoms of depression (such as depressed mood) are not as well accepted as somatic symptoms (such as poor energy and insomnia). The cultural explanations of illness also help define the behavior or role the sick individual is expected to assume. Finally, explanatory models contain elements of prognosis, which include ideas of the treatment options in addition to the general course of the illness.

Some patients' explanatory models are ill defined, whereas others are quite fixed. Many patients entertain multiple explanatory models for a particular illness as well. For example, many patients will seek spiritual/religious assistance or alternative treatments, such as acupuncture or herbal medicine, in addition to medical treatment for their condition.

Providers' explanatory models also have a varying degree of heterogeneity for any given illness. It is essential that the clinician elicit the patient's understanding of the cause of the illness while also explaining his or her own perspectives of illness to the patient. The following paragraphs illustrate the use of clinical methods and knowledge of the patient's cultural explanations of the illness to improve rapport with the patient.

Table 1–6. Consequences of conflicting explanatory models

Type of conflict	Consequences
Patient–provider	Diminished rapport, treatment nonadherence, treatment dropout
Patient–family	Lack of support, shame, family discord
Patient–community	Social isolation, stigmatization

Westermeyer (1989) discusses the usefulness of demonstrating interest, clarifying the patient's explanatory models, facilitating the patient's story, and ensuring that the patient understands the interviewer's questions by having him or her restate the question. Rapport with the patient is created by assessing the symptoms that the patient is most comfortable expressing. In many cases, these are the somatic symptoms; treating these idioms of distress with respect and appropriate concern often facilitates rapport with the patient and lays the groundwork necessary to address more difficult, yet clinically relevant issues. Patients who present with somatic complaints, for example, should be evaluated as if they were presenting for medical evaluation, with an exploration of precipitating, ameliorating, and aggravating factors. Next, the clinician should carefully review their complaints (review of symptoms), looking for the somatic symptoms of depression and anxiety such as sleep or appetite disturbances, decrease in energy level, weight change, tachycardia, shortness of breath, and tremors. As the patient is engaged, other, more sensitive topics can be broached, such as the psychological symptoms of irritability, fears, thoughts of a gloomy future, crying spells, nightmares, and then personal or family problems, as well as a history of trauma. Other psychological symptoms that also need to be assessed directly include problems with concentration and memory, hallucinations, feelings of mistrust, intrusive thoughts, and suicidal or homicidal ideas (Cheung 1987).

Successful treatment also requires the formation of a collaborative model that is acceptable to both provider and patient. This includes arriving at an agreed-upon set of symptoms to treat, treatment expectations, and general course of illness. It may also be helpful to involve members of the patient's primary support group as well. Difficulties arise when there are conflicts between explanatory models. Table 1–6 illustrates some potential consequences of these conflicts.

Although a full discussion of the types of explanatory models is beyond the scope of this chapter (see Ton 1996), a number of the more common types, including moral, spiritual, religious, magical, medical, and psychosocial stress, are described below. Clinicians should keep in mind that these are general descriptions. A patient's particular model may incorporate elements of one or more of these common types. Some patients have poorly defined explanatory models, whereas others may have very detailed explanations. Moreover, patients may use more than one explanatory model, and the different models may operate independently or even in conflict with each other. Efforts should therefore be taken to clarify the patient's models through cultural assessment.

The *moral model* asserts that the patient's condition is caused by a moral defect such as laziness, selfishness, or weak will. Family members can be seen operating with this model, although patients themselves may use this as well. Typical statements include "you just have to work harder and get over this," or "I was able to overcome this on my own, so why can't you?" Patients working under this model typically attempt to change their character flaws.

The *spiritual/religious model* maintains that illness is caused by spiritual or religious transgressions. As a result, the patient is punished by angered spirits or the patient's higher power(s). Typical interventions include atonement, ritual appeasement of the angered spirits, or efforts to more closely follow prescribed spiritual/religious practices. Often, a spiritual leader is enlisted to treat the affliction.

The *magical explanatory model* suggests that sorcery or witchcraft causes illness. Magic-based treatments vary from culture to culture and may include finding the person who has caused the illness or involving a sorcerer or shaman to counteract the spell.

Patients who attribute a biological etiology to the illness learn to use a *medical model.* This is not limited to traditional Western allopathic medicine, which is only one type of medical model. Others include traditional Chinese medicine, ayurvedic medicine, homeopathy, osteopathy, and various herbal medicine traditions. In a national survey, Eisenberg and colleagues (1993) estimated that one of every three Americans used non-Western allopathic medicine remedies. Given the growing number of patients who are using alternative medical therapies and the drug interactions that can result, it is important for the clinician to adequately assess for usage.

Individuals who use the *psychosocial stress* model may maintain that illness is caused by overwhelming psychosocial stressors. Treatment includes addressing the psychosocial stressors.

Table 1–7. Cultural influences on transference and countertransference

	Interethnic effects	Intraethnic effects
Transference	Overcompliance Denial of ethnocultural factors Mistrust Hostility Ambivalence	Omniscient-omnipotent therapist The traitor Autoracism Ambivalence
Countertransference	Denial of ethnocultural factors Clinical anthropologist syndrome Guilt or pity Aggression Ambivalence	Overidentification Distancing Cultural myopia Ambivalence Anger Survivor's guilt

Source. Adapted from Comas-Diaz and Jacobsen 1991.

who have clarity about their own cultural identity and their own role in mental health treatment are in a better position to anticipate these cultural dynamics and subsequently diminish the negative outcomes and enhance the positive outcomes of the clinical exchange. Part of this process involves maintaining an awareness of the clinician's own biases, attitudes, and stereotypes. It also is important to consider the cultural influences on transference and countertransference in the clinical exchange (Table 1–7). Comas-Diaz and Jacobsen (1991) discuss these potential influences.

Interethnic transference involves the patient's response to an ethnoculturally different clinician. *Overcompliance,* for example, may occur when there is a sociocultural power differential between patient and clinician, resulting in superficial agreement on treatment in the clinical setting but nonadherence to treatment at home. *Denial of culture and ethnicity* is shown when the patient avoids discussing issues related to ethnicity and culture with the culturally different clinician, making cultural assessment more difficult. *Mistrust and hostility* may also occur in the context of the sociopolitical history between the patient's and clinician's respective cultural groups. Unacknowledged cultural differences may exacerbate the suspicion. *Ambivalence* describes the patient's struggle with negative feelings about the culturally different clinician while he or she is also developing attachment to the clinician. Likewise, ethnoculturally different clinicians may respond in a nontherapeutic manner, what Comas-Diaz and Jacobsen refer to as *interethnic* countertransference. Examples of this include a *denial* of ethnocultural differences in which the clinician maintains that the clinical encounter is not influenced by the cultural and social factors. Conversely, the *clinical anthropologist syndrome* occurs when the therapeutic process is derailed by an inordinate devotion to inquiring about the patient's cultural background to the exclusion of other interventions. The clinician may also have unresolved *guilt* about his or her cultural or social privilege in society, or pity the patient's position in society. This may manifest in either *pity* or *aggression* toward the patient.

Although ethnocultural matching between patient and clinician can have significant therapeutic benefits (Takeuchi et al. 1995), there is also potential for destructive transference and countertransference. Comas-Diaz and Jacobsen describe the potential negative transferences associated with this dyad. One such involves the *omniscient-omnipotent therapist* phenomenon, in which the patient overidealizes the clinician because of their shared cultural background. Alternatively, the patient may perceive the clinician as a traitor because he or she has sold out to their shared culture. *Autoracism* can occur in transference as well, manifesting as the patient's belief that he or she is getting inferior treatment because the clinician is of the same ethnic group. The patient may also have ambivalent feelings about the therapist, at once appreciating the shared cultural background and being apprehensive about too much psychological closeness.

The clinician must also be aware of his or her negative countertransferences when treating patients from a similar ethnocultural background. Without this awareness, the clinician risks *overidentifying* with the patient by choosing an activist approach when other approaches would be more beneficial. The clinician may also become judgmental of the patient. "If I've been able to overcome these cultural barriers, my patient should do the same." This "us versus them" mentality is an extreme form of overidentification. In contrast, *distancing* can occur when the clinician has fears of overidentifying with the patient. *Cultural myopia* occurs when the clinician frames the therapy in cultural terms to the exclusion of other clinical perspectives. Further, the patient's experiences, shared from an ethnocultural perspective, may bring up painful memories for the clinician, which may result in *anger* or *guilt* toward the patient. Finally, the clinician's own experience with unresolved cultural conflicts may emerge as *ambivalence* when addressing similar experiences of the patient.

The case of X.W. illustrates some of the potential cultural conflicts that can arise between patients and clinicians from differing backgrounds, as well as the therapeutic potential of further cultural inquiry.

X.W.'s treating clinicians were troubled by her husband's seemingly paternalistic attitude. On further inquiry, this was found to be consistent with the traditional role of the husband in Chinese culture as the protector of and spokesman for his family. As the treatment team became more accepting of the husband's traditional role, he became more interested in understanding more about the patient's emotional state and in learning about possible follow-up. This process was facilitated by one of the clinicians, who was Chinese American and Mandarin-speaking.

The Mental Status Examination and Psychological Assessment

The cognitive and descriptive aspects of the mental status examination were developed in Western European, British, and American settings to describe the various cognitive, linguistic, perceptual, and affective domains of brain function. The result is that the exam is culturally biased. Accordingly, mental status measures must be elicited, described, and integrated in ways sensitive to the patient's cultural identity and milieu. Patients' responses are shaped by their culture of origin, educational level, and level of acculturation. For example, asking patients to state today's date checks for the patient's level of orientation. The patient may use a different calendar, such as the lunar calendar, and may not feel that dates are important information to recall. Some cultures do not use clocks, and seasons vary around the world, depending on latitude (Westermeyer 1993). For some societies with strong oral history traditions, the patient's date of birth is irrelevant information. The interpretation of tests of abstraction, commonly tested by proverb interpretation, is difficult to assess because the meaning and wording of proverbs varies widely among different societies and language groups. Using serial 7s to assess patients from illiterate cultures may be meaningless if their education has been limited to arithmetic with single digits. Differences in educational background may further limit the general usefulness of questions that assess fund of information. It is often an incorrect assumption that most people know much geography (Escobar et al. 1986). The patient's ability to name objects or remember items in short-term memory tests is affected by his or her familiarity with the items chosen. Similarly, three-step commands should be adapted to be very simple (Hughes 1993). Escobar and others (1986) concluded that the Mini-Mental State Examination (MMSE) was influenced by age, educational level, ethnicity, and the language of the interview and recommended that it be revised to remove educational, social, and cultural artifacts if it is to be used in a Hispanic population.

Marsella and Kameoka (1989) observed that many of the tests and self-assessment questionnaires used in research have been developed on Western subjects and are not appropriate for use among ethnic minority patients because they lack cultural equivalence. Merely translating the items was stated to be insufficient and to result in linguistic inequivalence, because meanings and connotations changed and idioms of expression differed between languages. Rating scales for symptoms can be used if the scales are translated, back-translated, and validated (Marin and Marin 1991). Excellent examples of culturally appropriate tests include the Hopkins Symptom Checklist-25 translated into Vietnamese, Laotian, and Cambodian (Mollica et al. 1987) and the Harvard Trauma Questionnaire translated into the same three languages (Mollica et al. 1992). Finally, the interpretation of the results can be affected by using improper norms. Often, translated tests are not standardized for the testing group and must be properly normed on a representative patient group for meaningful results. Other sources of error have included biased analysis, inaccurate assumptions and translation, and inappropriate instruments (Rogler 1989). The use of translated editions of existing rating scales must be viewed with extreme caution unless these concerns are addressed.

Language Barrier and Use of Interpreters

Effective communication is essential for a successful therapeutic interaction. In a mental health setting, communication has both verbal and nonverbal components and is highly influenced by cultural nuances. For patients with English as a second language, mental health encounters are even more difficult than standard medical interviews, since communicating emotional and social distress essential to a psychiatric interview requires more than Basic English proficiency. Hence, interpretation is critical for providing adequate care to patients who are monolingual or have only Basic English proficiency. The *therapeutic triad* incorporates the interpreter as an essential team member (Lee 1997b).

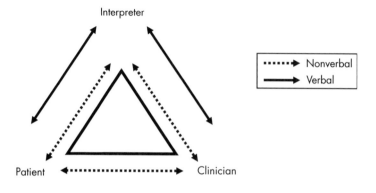

Figure 1–2. The therapeutic triad model.

Source. Adapted from Lee 1997.

Figure 1–2 illustrates the importance of the positioning of individuals in the clinical triad. Each individual should have a clear view of the others in order to effectively communicate and receive *nonverbal* communication. The interpreter provides the critical verbal communication link between clinician and patients, in addition to helping to contextualize nonverbal communication when appropriate (see section below on cultural informants).

Interpreters should be trained in a set of competencies (Table 1–8) that clearly extend beyond simply speaking the patient's language. There are significant problems in using an untrained interpreter, such as a family member, a stranger in the vicinity, or an untrained staff member, because they likely lack the necessary technical vocabulary or dual fluency. Problems may arise with confidentiality as well. Accuracy may also be affected if the ad hoc translator avoids communicating potentially embarrassing information. This can be particularly problematic when using family members, such as young children or spouses.

In addition to including an appropriately trained and matched interpreter, the clinician should be aware of the three phases of the interpreted interview: preinterview, interview, and postinterview (Lee 1997b). Prior to the clinical interview, the clinician should take time to prepare the interpreter by discussing issues such as the objectives of the interview, topics to be covered, the patient's background and current difficulties, interpreter's cultural knowl-

Table 1–8. Competency criteria for interpreters

Technical
- Good command of spoken and written English and language of the patient, including dialectical nuances
- Ability to translate fine shades of meaning and nonverbal communication
- Familiarity with psychiatric terminology and procedures

Cultural
- Intimate knowledge of his or her ethnic community, including illness models, social/power structures, cultural values
- Familiarity with culture of mainstream society and mental health service
- Ability to act as a cultural broker

Interpersonal
- Ability to get along with peers/staff and deal with conflicts arising from unrealistic expectations from clinician or patient
- Understanding of own communication style and awareness of personal values, attitudes, and bias
- Ability to assess areas of incompatibility with clinician or patient and react accordingly

Ethical
- Ability to maintain a code of ethics that includes confidentiality, impartiality, and professional conduct

Other
- Ability to effectively advocate for patient
- Fine attention to detail and good memory
- Flexibility in handling diverse situations

Source. Adapted from Lee 1997b.

edge about these issues, and the desired length of the interview. This pre-interview phase allows for rapport building in addition to helping the participants use the interview time more effectively. During the actual interview, as noted above, it may be helpful for the clinician, interpreter, and patient to sit in a triangular formation so that each can have face-to-face contact with the others. The clinician-interpreter team can use a number of translating formats depending on the situation (Lee 1997b).

Verbatim translation involves minimal participation by the translator and can be useful when attempting to translate factual or technical information.

This can be done softly while the patient is speaking (which saves time but increases the chance of miscommunication) or after the patient speaks (which can potentially double the interview time).

Summary interpretations emphasize the main points that the patient is attempting to communicate. This method can save time, but it increases the margin of error. This method is particularly helpful when the patient requires a length of uninterrupted time to speak, as during an emotionally charged topic.

Cultural interpretation involves conveying the patient's statements as well as his or her cultural contexts so as to more accurately reflect the patient's experience. After the interview is finished (during the postinterview phase), the clinician and the interpreter should review the interview to clarify potential areas of confusion. Clinician and interpreter should also discuss their experience of working with each other in order to help build rapport and lay groundwork for future sessions utilizing the interpreter. After the interview, or during key moments in the interview, the interpreter may be able to act as a *cultural informant* to help the clinician gain a better sense of the norms and values of the patient's ethnic or cultural group.

Pitfalls in the Use of Interpreters

The common practice of relying on young members of the family, who are more likely to be proficient in English, as interpreters for the older members tends to create confusing roles and responsibilities within the family system's dynamics. Obviously, in situations in which an interpreter is not available on staff, the disadvantages of using a family member may be outweighed by the benefits of ensuring effective communication.

Another common practice in clinical settings is using bilingual staff members who are not professional interpreters and who are temporarily used in this role as needed because of their bilingual skills. This practice also presents several limitations, such as the inability to check for accuracy of translation, as well as ethical concerns about using employees to provide services for which they are not being adequately compensated.

There are numerous challenges even in the use of professional interpreters. Particularly relevant to mental health, concerns about confidentiality may inhibit some of the personal information that a patient may provide with a third party present. It is not uncommon, especially in some neighborhood health clinics, that patients and interpreters are members of the same community, which may present serious confidentiality issues. Further, despite the assumed neutrality of the interpreter, he or she creates a triad that challenges some of the basic elements and assumptions of the more conventional therapeutic dyad. For example, differences and similarities between the interpreter and the patient in terms of nationality and socioeconomic, educational, or geographic (urban versus rural) background may create particular interpersonal dynamics that become part of the clinical encounter. Such dynamics need to be adequately identified and analyzed because they may influence the information provided by the patient, as well as his or her behavior.

Cultural Informants

Cultural informants, also referred to as cultural brokers or cultural consultants, are not limited to interpreters. They can be members of a cultural group with various other roles, including religious or community leaders, primary care or mental health providers, or peers. Their function is to provide information and clarification about attitudes and perspectives of the patient's cultural group(s). Their expertise is derived from their level of participation within the cultural group. Cultural informants may not necessarily have specific knowledge of or training in mental health. Hence, clinical questions about the broker's assessment of the patient's mental illness may be inappropriate. However, inquiries about the cultural group's general attitudes toward mental illness, explanatory models, and treatment pathways can be invaluable in helping the clinician understand and contextualize the cultural information that is obtained during an evaluation.

E. Overall Cultural Assessment for Diagnosis and Care

The overall assessment should highlight the key issues illustrated in the previous sections of the cultural formulation. Treatment planning should provide options that address these key issues without further exacerbating cultural conflicts or creating new ones. The treatment plan may involve culturally specific treatment pathways (such as traditional healers or religious interventions); appropriate application of ethnopharmacological principles, as discussed in Chapter 6; the use of cultural consultants; and the use of culturally appropriate services. Often, interventions that are focused on a family or social level can be very helpful for patients as well. The formulation of overall assessment and treatment plans is illustrated below with reference to the case example.

X.W. struggles with balancing three important roles in her life: worker, mother, and wife. She demonstrates an all-or-nothing strategy to cope with this struggle, which ultimately proves to be maladaptive for her, leading to further social isolation and distancing from her daughter. After her injuries, Ms. W. is under significant stress because she is now unable to work and remains far from her daughter. She will likely continue to experience alienation from the mainstream society. To some degree, she remains "a stranger in a strange land." Because of this, she is at significant risk for worsening depression. However, her husband has become more available to her with her physical injuries, and presently he is her most important source of support. A cultural assessment reveals several areas in which interventions will likely be helpful:

1. Although Ms. W. reports feeling disappointed in her relationship with her husband, she would benefit from the treatment team's efforts to bolster what is currently working in their relationship rather than to destabilize the relationship in this time of crisis. Such efforts will involve validating and encouraging the husband's role in her care as a protector and a caregiver. It is important for both the patient and the husband to have a positive and validating experience with the mental health system. If the husband feels alienated or "to blame" for the patient's injuries and distress, he may disengage from the treatment, resulting in destabilization of the family system and ultimately in a failure to follow through with mental health services. At a later point, when the family system is more stable and the patient has other sources of support, they would benefit from marital therapy.

2. The patient might benefit from exploring how she defines being a mother, a wife, and a worker, since she is presently experiencing role conflict. Eventually she might be encouraged to redefine her expectations of herself to facilitate a more balanced integration, hence mitigating the cultural conflicts arising from these different identities.

3. The patient should be reunited with her family. They will become an even more important source of validation now that she will be unable to work for some time. Consideration should be given to helping facilitate her return to Hong Kong. The patient has experienced significant migration stress in her transition to the United States and will likely continue to experience this stress if she remains here.

Conclusion

Culture has an influence at every level of the mental health system. Its effects mediate access, service delivery, evaluation, treatment, and follow-up. Moreover, mental illness affects an individual's role in his or her cultural system. In the best-case scenario, the cultural system can respond with a bolstering of sociocultural supports, but too often, the individual risks becoming stigmatized by his or her community. By understanding the individual's culture, the clinician will gain insight into the complex interplay between culture and mental illness, which will ultimately improve his or her ability to care for the individual. Although the ongoing pursuit of learning about the major cultural groups to which one's patients belong is important, that knowledge is often incomplete. The DSM-IV-TR Outline for Cultural Formulation discussed in this chapter provides a framework that helps guide and organize the clinician's exploration of an individual's multifaceted culture. The case example of X.W. illustrates the practical application of the Outline for Cultural Formulation, and the sections on working with interpreters and cultural informants are intended to help clinicians make optimal use of the available resources. These tools and guidelines, when used with an attitude of openness to learn from the patient and his or her community, will significantly improve the clinician's ability to assess and treat the increasingly heterogeneous and multicultural patient community.

References

Adebimpe VR: Overview: white norms and psychiatric diagnosis of black patients. Am J Psychiatry 138:279–285, 1981

Alarcon RD, Westermeyer J, Foulks EF, et al: Clinical relevance of contemporary cultural psychiatry. J Nerv Ment Dis 187:465–471, 1999

American Psychiatric Association: Diagnostic and Statistical Manual of Mental Disorders, 4th Edition. Washington, DC, American Psychiatric Association, 1994

American Psychiatric Association: Appendix I: Outline for cultural formulation and glossary of culture-bound syndromes, in Diagnostic and Statistical Manual of Mental Disorders, 4th Edition, Text Revision. Washington, DC, American Psychiatric Association, 2000, pp 897–903

Berry JW: Immigration, acculturation, and adaptation. Applied Psychology: An International Review 46:5–68, 1997

Cheung FM: Conceptualization of psychiatric illness, and help-seeking behavior among Chinese. Cult Med Psychiatry 11:97–106, 1987

Comas-Diaz L, Jacobsen FM: Ethnocultural transference and countertransference in the therapeutic dyad. Am J Orthopsychiatry 61:392–402, 1991

Du N, Lu F: Assessment and treatment of posttraumatic stress disorder among Asian Americans, in Working With Asian Americans: A Guide for Clinicians. Edited by Lee E. New York, Guilford, 1997, pp 275–294

Eisenberg DM, Kessler RC, Foster C, et al: Unconventional medicine in the United States: prevalence, costs, and patterns of use. N Engl J Med 328:246–252, 1993

Escobar JI, Vega WA: Mental health and immigration's "AAA's": where are we and where do we go from here? J Nerv Ment Dis 188:736–740, 2000

Escobar JI, Burnam A, Karno M, et al: Use of the Mini-Mental State Examination (MMSE) in a community population of mixed ethnicity. J Nerv Ment Dis 174:607–614, 1986

Fabrega H: Culture and history in psychiatric diagnosis and practice. Psychiatr Clin North Am 24:391–405, 2001

Gaw AC: Concise Guide to Cross-Cultural Psychiatry. Washington, DC, American Psychiatric Publishing, 2001

Group for the Advancement of Psychiatry Committee on Cultural Psychiatry: Cultural Assessment in Clinical Psychiatry. Washington, DC, American Psychiatric Publishing, 2002

Hsu FL: Rugged Individualism Reconsidered: Essays in Psychological Anthropology. Knoxville, University of Tennessee Press, 1983

Hughes CC: Culture in clinical psychiatry, in Culture, Ethnicity, and Mental Illness. Edited by Gaw AC. Washington, DC, American Psychiatric Press, 1993, pp 3–41

Kinzie JD: The historical relationship between psychiatry and the major religions, in Psychiatry and Religion: The Convergence of Mind and Spirit. Edited by Boehnlein JK. Washington, DC, American Psychiatric Press, 2000, pp 3–26

Kirmayer LJ: Cultural variations in the clinical presentation of depression and anxiety: implications for diagnosis and treatment. J Clin Psychiatry 62 (suppl 13):22–28, 2001

Kleinman A: Rethinking Psychiatry: From Cultural Category to Personal Experience. New York, Free Press, 1988

Kulhara P, Chakrabarti S: Culture and schizophrenia and other psychotic disorders. Psychiatr Clin North Am 24:449–464, 2001

Lee E: Assessment and treatment of Chinese-American immigrant families, in Minorities and Family Therapy. Edited by Saba GW, Karrer BM, Hardy KV. New York, Haworth, 1990, pp 191–202

Lee E: Chinese-American families, in Working With Asian Americans: A Guide for Clinicians. Edited by Lee E. New York, Guilford, 1997a, pp 46–78

Lee E: Cross-cultural communication: therapeutic use of interpreters, in Working With Asian Americans: A Guide for Clinicians. Edited by Lee E, New York, Guilford, 1997b, pp 477–489

Lu FG, Lim RF, Mezzich JE: Issues in the assessment and diagnosis of culturally diverse individuals, in American Psychiatric Press Review of Psychiatry, Vol 14. Edited by Oldham JM, Riba MB, Washington, DC, American Psychiatric Press, 1995, pp 477–510

Lukoff D, Lu FG, Turner R: Cultural considerations in the assessment and treatment of religious and spiritual problems. Psychiatr Clin North Am 18:467–485, 1995

Marin G, Marin B: Research With Hispanic Populations. Newbury Park, CA, Sage, 1991

Marsella AJ, Kameoka VA: Ethnocultural issues in the assessment of psychopathology, in Measuring Mental Illness: Psychometric Assessment for Clinicians. Edited by Wetzler S. Washington, DC, American Psychiatric Press, 1989, pp 229–256

Matsumoto D: Culture and Psychology. San Francisco, CA, Brooks/Cole, 1996

Mezzich JE, Otero AA, Lee S: International psychiatric diagnosis, in Comprehensive Textbook of Psychiatry, 7th Edition. Edited by Kaplan HI, Sadock BJ. Baltimore, MD, Williams & Wilkins, 2000, pp 839–853

Mezzich JE, Berganza CE, Ruiperez MA: Culture in DSM-IV, ICD-10, and evolving diagnostic systems. Psychiatr Clin North Am 24:407–419, 2001

Mollica RG, Wyshak G, De Marneffe D, et al: Indochinese versions of Hopkins Symptom Checklist-25: screening instrument for psychiatric care of refugees. Am J Psychiatry 144:497–500, 1987

Mollica RG, Caspi-Yavin Y, Bollini P, et al: The Harvard Trauma Questionnaire: validating a cross-cultural instrument for measuring torture, trauma, and posttraumatic stress disorder in Indochinese refugees. J Nerv Ment Dis 180:111–116, 1992

Muskin PR: Complementary and Alternative Medicine and Psychiatry (Review of Psychiatry Series, Vol 19; Oldham JM and Riba MB, series eds). Washington, DC, American Psychiatric Press, 2000

Phinney JS: Ethnic identity and self-esteem: a review and integration, in Hispanic Psychology: Critical Issues in Theory and Research. Edited by Padilla AM. Thousand Oaks, CA, Sage, 1995, pp 57–70

Rogler LH: The meaning of culturally sensitive research in mental health. Am J Psychiatry 146:496–303, 1989

Rogler LH: Culture in psychiatric diagnosis: an issue of scientific accuracy. Psychiatry 56:324–327, 1993

Takeuchi DT, Sue S, Yeh M: Return rates and outcomes from ethnicity-specific mental health programs in Los Angeles. Am J Public Health 85:638–643, 1995

Ton H: Health and cultural change: perspectives of a Vietnamese and Vietnamese-American extended family. Master's thesis, Division of Health and Medical Sciences, University of California, Berkeley, School of Public Health, 1996

U.S. Census Bureau: Census 2000 Summary File 1. Washington, DC, U.S. Census Bureau, 2000. Available at: http://factfinder.census.gov/servlet/DatasetMainPageServlet?_ds_name=DEC_2000_SF1_Uand_program=DECand_lang=en. Accessed February 14, 2005.

U.S. Census Bureau: Table 1a. Projected Population of the United States, by Race and Hispanic Origin: 2000 to 2050. Washington, DC, U.S. Census Bureau, 2004. Available at: http://www.census.gov/ipc/www/usinterimproj/natprojtab01a.pdf. Accessed February 14, 2005.

U.S. Department of Health and Human Services: Executive summary, in Mental Health: Culture, Race, and Ethnicity. A Supplement to Mental Health: A Report of the Surgeon General. Rockville, MD, U.S. Department of Health and Human Services, Public Health Service, Office of the Surgeon General, 2001. Available at: http://www.surgeongeneral.gov/library/mentalhealth/cre

Westermeyer JJ: Psychiatric Care of Migrants: A Clinical Guide. Washington, DC, American Psychiatric Press, 1989

Westermeyer JJ: Cross-cultural psychiatric assessment, in Culture, Ethnicity, and Mental Illness. Edited by Gaw AC. Washington, DC, American Psychiatric Press, 1993, pp 125–144

PART II

Cultural Issues in Assessment and Treatment

2

African American Patients

Annelle B. Primm, M.D., M.P.H.

African Americans are a heterogeneous group who trace their ancestry to Africa. With the dispersal of African people around the world, U.S. residents with African ancestors include both those born in the United States of slave ancestry and others who are relatively recent immigrants from other nations. In this chapter, the term *African American* will be used to encompass the wide range of people of African descent who live in the United States. The overwhelming majority of African Americans are U.S.-born descendants of slaves, primarily of West African origin. Adding diversity to this group are individuals from Caribbean nations and Central and South America, who may also consider themselves Hispanic, as well as those from South and East Africa, who tend to be more recent immigrants. Collectively, they represent multiple variations in national origin, religious beliefs, and customs.

Despite the diversity within the African American population, global racism and the history of people whose ancestors were from Africa inform the African American experience to a large extent. People are judged socially by how they appear phenotypically. This has a major impact on all aspects of the lives of African Americans, especially their mental health.

Approximately 34 million people (12% of the population in the United States) identify themselves as African American, a figure that probably is underestimated—especially among younger and middle-aged males—because of the high number of homeless and incarcerated as well as those who are unwilling to participate in the census. According to the 2000 census, 53% of all African Americans live in the South, 19% in the Midwest, 18% in the Northeast, and 10% in the West. Fifteen percent reside in rural areas, compared with 23% of whites and 25% of all Americans (U.S. Department of Health and Human Services 2001b).

African American physicians are five times more likely than white physicians to treat African American patients. However, only 2% of psychiatrists, 2% of psychologists, and 4% of social workers reported being African American, implying that many African Americans in need of mental health treatment do not have access to services (U.S. Department of Health and Human Services 2001b).

Historical Context

The majority of today's African American population traces its ancestry to the slave trade from Africa. The Fourteenth Amendment to the U.S. Constitution extended citizenship to African Americans and forbade states to take away civil rights. The Fifteenth Amendment prohibited disenfranchisement on the basis of race. However, the "Jim Crow" laws (or "black codes") that were enacted in many southern states prevented African Americans from bettering themselves.

As late as 1910, 89% of all blacks lived in legalized subservience and deep poverty in the rural South. Migration to the northeastern and midwestern states began with World War I, and after World War II, blacks moved to selected urban areas in the West, mostly in California (U.S. Department of Health and Human Services 2001b).

In 1954, the U.S. Supreme Court declared racially segregated education unconstitutional, and the Civil Rights Act of 1964 prohibited both segregation in public accommodations and discrimination in education and employment. The use of voter qualification tests was suspended in 1965 with passage of the Voting Rights Act.

The legacy of slavery and discrimination continues to influence the social and economic standing of African Americans in the United States, and their mental health status can be appreciated only within this historical context. It is important to note that classic psychiatric care did not exist for African Americans until the desegregation of state mental hospitals. Community mental health centers played an important role in expanding access.

Many African Americans have been able to overcome adversity and to maintain a high level of mental health because of their resilience and their ability to forge social ties. They have shown extraordinary individual and collective strengths that have enabled many to survive and to do well, often in the face of enormous odds. Through mutual affiliation, loyalty, and resourcefulness they have developed adaptive beliefs, traditions, and practices. For example, nearly 85% have described themselves as "fairly religious" or "very religious" and have identified prayer as among their most common coping responses. Other preferred coping responses include confronting problems rather than shrinking from them and turning to family, friends, neighbors, and community institutions and associations for aid—a strategy that evolved from the experience of having to rely on one another often for their very survival (U.S. Department of Health and Human Services 2001b).

African Americans have developed a capacity to downplay stereotypical negative judgments about their behavior and to rely on the beliefs and behavior of other African Americans as a frame of reference. They have a collective identity and perceive themselves as having a significant sphere of collectively defined interests. Such psychological and social frameworks have enabled many African Americans to overcome adversity and sustain a higher degree of mental health.

Myths and Stereotypes

Despite the development of positive coping responses among African Americans, the clinician should be aware that myths and stereotypes still exist that can affect assessment and treatment.

The Evil Black Woman

In this description, *evil* describes someone who is mean, irritable, "ugly acting," and cranky. Although the connotation of evil in the occult sense does not apply here, someone who is evil is considered to be a bad person, someone to be avoided. The term *evil* often is used to describe women, particularly those who are difficult to get along with either acutely or chronically; in the latter case, this can be a label that sticks. In the author's experience this label is most often applied to describe dark-skinned women, as if to suggest that blackness and possessing African facial features and hair texture makes one more prone to being evil. This association of evilness with more African-appearing individuals may be a manifestation of internalized racism wherein dark-skinned, African traits are regarded as bad and undesirable while individuals with lighter skin complexion and more European facial features are regarded as good and desirable.

The Angry Black Male

Stereotypical descriptions of African Americans who receive mental health services have included angry, lazy, limited in intelligence, and lacking the capacity to be introspective. In particular, the angry black male is often misunderstood. The clinical presentation of African American men with depression may include anger, which represents a depressive equivalent. Being sad or weak, more often associated with the diagnosis of depression, is the last way in which a black man in America wants to appear. Rather, maintaining a perpetual mask of invincibility and strength is the preferred mode of presenting and expressing oneself. Unfortunately, angry black men in the United States are feared and are more likely to be seen as bad people who need to be sent to the criminal justice system rather than as depressed individuals who need treatment in the mental health system.

"Flash of the Spirit"

A book entitled *Flash of the Spirit* (Thompson 1989) captures the essence of black culture. It describes the African American tendency to be expressive, vocal instead of quiet, decorative instead of minimalist, colorful instead of plain, creative instead of rote or routine. This tendency, apparent in black cultural expression in music, art, fashion, and personal communication style, may underlie the influences of black music and fashion trends on national style.

A case example of how the "flash of the spirit" may be misunderstood is an incident that I experienced personally. One of my patients came to see me for a session, "dressed to the nines" in numerous colors with dramatic flair. A colleague of mine saw this individual and remarked to me that the person must be manic. That was not the person's diagnosis at all. The stereotype that dressing in colorful clothing was pathognomonic for mania surprised me and led me to realize that I had seen the patient through a different lens, a culturally normed lens that saw her dressed in a fancy way, but not one that would signify pathology. My colleague needed to understand this aspect of the "flash" of spirit in African and African American culture that glorifies and takes delight in embellishment and adornment.

The Myth of the African American Superwoman

A syndrome common among African American women and particularly problematic for those with depression is the *superwoman complex*. In this syndrome, women feel that they have to do everything for everyone, not for only members of their nuclear family but also for an extended family network of relatives, friends, neighbors, and coworkers. They typically feel guilty if they say no when asked, and they may even volunteer to help. In many ways, this syndrome is an exaggerated caricature of what black women are supposed to be within the cultural frame, "the mammy" taking care of their own children as well as the Master's children. This is a syndrome of selflessness and martyrdom that is a cultural norm in a sense. However, it can be destructive because it may lead the individual down a path of exhaustion, accompanied by inappropriate denial of one's needs, postponement of one's pleasures, and outright self-neglect, leading indirectly to self-destruction. Women who want to break out of this syndrome have to be reminded to set limits, to have a clear understanding of what their responsibilities are, and not to enable helplessness in people who are capable of taking care of themselves. Taking this approach can help preserve the person's energies and strength to take care of her own needs and those of her dependents without going overboard and risking her physical and mental health.

Current Context

Family Structure

In the year 2000, there were approximately 9 million African American families in the United States, and 65% of these families had 3 or more members.

Nonetheless, only 38% of African American children lived in two-parent families, compared with 69% of all children in the United States. African American children who lived with only one parent were most likely to live with their mothers; hence the myth of the matriarchal family. African Americans participate extensively in family foster care—although this practice is eroding because of the burden of problems brought on by urban poverty and the relative youth of many grandmothers, who continue to work outside the home (U.S. Department of Health and Human Services 2001b).

Socioeconomic Status

Census data from the year 2000 show that 79% of African Americans age 25 or over had earned at least a high school diploma, and 17% had received bachelors' or graduate degrees (U.S. Census Bureau 2000). Nearly 25% of all African Americans had incomes over $50,000 in 1997, and the median income of African Americans living in married-couple households was 87% of that of comparable white households. Nearly 32% of African Americans lived in the suburbs. At the other extreme, in 1999, approximately 22% of African American families had incomes below the poverty line. African Americans are more likely to move in and out of poverty because they have relatively few assets to protect them when they are unemployed, and many become homeless.

Many African Americans still live in segregated neighborhoods, and poor African Americans tend to live among other African Americans who are poor. Poor neighborhoods tend to have few resources, a disadvantage reflected in high unemployment rates, homelessness, crime, and substance abuse. Children and youth in these neighborhoods often are exposed to violence. They are more likely to suffer the loss of a loved one, to be victimized, to attend substandard schools, to experience abuse and neglect, and to encounter too few opportunities for safe, organized recreation and other constructive outlets. Personal vulnerabilities are exacerbated by problems at the community level that are beyond the sphere of individual control.

On the other hand, stronger African American communities, both rich and poor, possess cohesion and informal mechanisms of social control, sometimes called *collective efficacy.* Evidence indicates that collective efficacy can counteract the effects of disabling social and economic conditions and form the foundation for community-building efforts.

Physical Health Status

In general, the health status of African Americans is worse than that of whites, and African Americans are more likely to have comorbid conditions such as diabetes, heart disease, HIV/AIDS, prostate cancer, and breast cancer. Their mortality rates from these diseases are higher than those of other Americans. To compound this situation, they are less likely to have a regular source of medical care and more likely to obtain their health care from hospital outpatient departments and emergency departments (U.S. Department of Health and Human Services 2001b).

Mental Health Status

Historical and Sociocultural Factors

Poor mental health is more common among the impoverished than among the more affluent. African Americans are more likely than whites to become homeless or incarcerated or to have children who come to the attention of child welfare authorities and are placed in foster care. Factors associated with increased risk for mental disorders in African Americans include 1) racism, discrimination, and prejudice; 2) lower socioeconomic status, with resultant environmental stressors such as chronic exposure to violence and increased likelihood of having witnessed or been a victim of violence; 3) more comorbid medical problems, as well as feelings of isolation, loneliness, and alienation for elderly African Americans who live alone; and 4) biases, stereotypes, and misperceptions held by some health care professionals and some patients about African Americans and mental illness. An additional problem is over-representation of African Americans in the rural South, especially in impoverished areas where safety-net services are limited if they exist at all.

Epidemiology

Schizophrenia, unipolar depression, anxiety disorders, bipolar disorder, multi-infarct dementia, Alzheimer's disease, trauma-related disorders, and substance abuse are the more common problems seen in African Americans. Two major epidemiological surveys, the Epidemiologic Catchment Area Study (ECA; Robins and Regier 1991) and the National Comorbidity Survey (NCS; Kessler et al. 1994) have shed some light on the distribution of mental disorders among African Americans. Both surveys found that African Americans had rates of major depression similar to those of whites (U.S. Department of Health and Human Services 2001b).

The ECA found that African Americans had higher 6-month prevalence rates of cognitive impairment, drug abuse, panic attacks, and phobia. Rates of major depression and schizophrenia across all age groups were lower than those for non-Hispanic whites but higher than those for Hispanics (Griffith and Baker 1993). The higher prevalence of cognitive impairment in African Americans has been hypothesized to be caused primarily by alcoholic dementia, multi-infarct dementia, and impairment in attention and registration resulting from anxiety, phobias, and panic attacks, and by medical problems such as obesity, diabetes, and hypertension. The role of accidents involving head trauma also must be considered (Griffith and Baker 1993).

Psychotic disorders have been documented as being higher in prevalence and incidence among African Caribbeans than among Europeans (Shaw et al. 1999). However, less attention has been given to the more common mental disorders. In general, Shaw and colleagues (1999) found similar prevalence of mood disorders between groups, although in African Caribbeans, anxiety disorders were less common and depression was more common than in white Europeans.

African Americans have reported more severe phobic avoidance, higher rates of comorbid posttraumatic stress disorder (PTSD), more intense levels of numbing and tingling, greater fears of dying and of going crazy, increased rates of isolated sleep paralysis, and decreased response to standard treatments (Scott et al. 2002).

In the aggregate, these studies appear to indicate that there is no overall difference in the prevalence rate of mental illness between African Americans and whites. However, this finding can be called into question given the overrepresentation of African Americans in high-need populations such as those in psychiatric hospitals, prisons, and poor urban and rural areas, who are not readily accessible to survey researchers.

Disparities in Mental Health Care

Use of mental health services by African Americans is a reflection of their adverse social and economic circumstances and the social disability associated with having a mental illness, being African American, and living in poverty. Compared with whites, African Americans are four times more likely to be confined in prison and two times more likely to be inpatients in mental hospitals. They are more likely to be counted in institutional surveys and left out of community surveys, thereby skewing estimates of service use. Without adjustment for sociodemographic differences, African Americans are found to have a mixed pattern of use of mental health services. However, when sociodemographic variables are controlled for, community-residing African Americans are less likely to seek mental health services than whites. When incarcerated individuals are added to the analysis of service, the disparity in specialty mental health services usage is diminished (Snowden 1999).

Blacks are less likely than whites to see a health care provider, and they are significantly less likely to receive appropriate care (Young et al. 2001). The NCS found that only 16% of African Americans with a diagnosable mood disorder saw a mental health specialist, and fewer than one-third consulted a health care provider of any kind. A number of studies reinforce this latter point. Although 83% of individuals with probable depressive or anxiety disorders saw a health care provider, most visited primary care providers only. Of that group, only 19% received appropriate care, compared with 90% of individuals who visited mental health professionals. Appropriate treatment was less likely for men and for individuals who were black, less well educated, younger than age 30, or older than age 59 (Young et al. 2001).

Compared with white populations, people of African descent enter mental health treatment at a later stage in the course of their illness, are more often misdiagnosed by mental health practitioners, use fewer treatment sessions for their mental health problems, receive most of their care through emergency visits, overutilize inpatient psychiatric care in state hospitals, underutilize community mental health services of all kinds, and are more often diagnosed with severe mental illness (U.S. Department of Health and Human Services 2001a). The African American patient is likely to seek care later in the course of illness and to have some constraints with regard to available resources (Griffith and Baker 1993). Patients' fears of addiction to antidepressant medications and of mental illness–associated stigma, their reliance on spiritual beliefs to cope with depression, and their concerns about trust and other aspects of relationships with health care providers are potentially important personal barriers to treatment of depression in African Americans (Primm et al. 2002).

African Americans receive accurate diagnoses less frequently than white Americans when they are experiencing depression and are seen in primary care (Borowsky et al. 2000) or are seen for psychiatric evaluation in an emergency department (Strakowski et al. 1997). African Americans with mental health problems are more likely to consult their primary care providers than mental health professionals. When they are hospitalized, African Americans are more likely than whites to be committed involuntarily. After eliminating the impact of sociodemographic differences and differences in need, the proportion of African Americans receiving treatment from any source was only about one-half that of whites.

Compared to whites with similar symptoms, blacks are more likely to receive a diagnosis of a severe mental disorder such as schizophrenia; to be diagnosed with substance abuse, even though the rates are the same for both groups; to be diagnosed with anxiety disorder; to be misdiagnosed, hospitalized, hospitalized involuntarily, receive seclusion and restraints, and receive inadequate treatment for the severity of their diagnosis; to be discharged earlier, without follow-up care; to be overmedicated with psychotropic medications; to terminate treatment earlier; and to underutilize specialized mental health facilities. They are also less likely to seek help for their children. (Chung 1995; Diala et al. 2002; Lawson 1999; Schneider et al. 2002; Strakowski et al. 2003; U.S. Department of Health and Human Services 2001b.)

These phenomena may be possibly or partially explained by a difference in physician referral patterns, a tendency for African Americans to delay seeking help, use of more informal supports, preference to seek help from non–mental health sources, and stigma and social embarrassment about seeking psychological help (Primm et al. 2002).

In a study of black patients and white patients consecutively admitted to an inpatient psychiatric facility, Chung and coworkers (1995) found that nonpsychotic African American patients had shorter lengths of stay than white patients with similar disorders. White patients were more likely to be placed on one-to-one observational status, and clinicians were more likely to order urine drug screens for African American patients with high socioeconomic status than for comparable white patients. African American patients with schizophrenic disorders received higher doses of neuroleptic medications than white patients with similar diagnoses. However, the authors found racial differences related to the detection, phenomenology, treatment, and course of psychotic disorders and to the diagnosis and management of alcohol and drug use disorders and personality disorders. Schneider and colleagues (2002) found that blacks were less likely than whites to receive follow-up after hospitalization for mental illness.

Applying the DSM-IV-TR Outline for Cultural Formulation

A. Cultural Identity of the Individual

Understanding identity and self as products of culture and race are essential for improving the quality of mental health services. Racial identity and cultural identity are both necessary descriptors for use in formulations to increase reliability of the DSM-IV-TR diagnoses and conceptualizations (Dana 2002). The following case illustrates how racial and cultural identities emerge as an important aspect of mental health as described in the first part of the DSM-IV-TR Outline for Cultural Formulation (American Psychiatric Association 2000).

> Ms. T is a dark-skinned African American woman in her forties who grew up in a large family in an urban setting. The skin color of people in her family is like a rainbow, ranging from people who are very fair and light-skinned, who could pass for white, to those with "caramel complexions" and those described as "dark as a skillet." Ms. T is on the darker end of the spectrum. As a child, her family members and schoolmates ridiculed her because of her dark skin color. Her short, tightly curled hair was often compared with that of her siblings, which was long and wavy. "Why couldn't you have 'good' hair, like so-and-so?" was a frequent question. She also couldn't help but notice the favoritism with which her lighter-skinned siblings were treated. This was a source of hurt and gave her the sense of being alienated from her own flesh and blood. Although she embraced her racial identity as an African American, much of the time she felt that her skin color was some sort of dark prison that put her at others' mercy. It felt like a badge of shame. Her skin color "preceded" her in public. When shopping, she would be watched like a hawk, as if the salespeople thought she would steal something. She longed to have a romantic relationship with a man but felt passed over by men who preferred women with more Caucasian features. She read somewhere that as a black woman of her age, she is more likely to be murdered than to find a marriage partner. In this regard, she felt her skin pigmentation placed her at an extreme disadvantage. At times, she wished she were white, or at least light-skinned. It seemed that that would make her life so much easier. When she thought that way she felt very guilty, especially when she thought about the sacrifices her ancestors made during slavery, as well as those of freedom fighters in the civil rights movement. This mix of feelings—of not belonging, of not melting in the so-called melting pot, rejection by her family and society, and guilt

about wishing she were of another race—left her in a no-man's land. These feelings generated a chronic, smoldering depression that eventually drove her to seek help from a psychiatrist.

Racial identity is focused on racial consciousness, a collective interpretation of group experience that includes grievances concerning disadvantaged status and continuing power differentials. Racial consciousness is considered to be essential for health because it externalizes stress. The spectrum of racial consciousness typically ranges from the militancy encompassing the psychological and sociopolitical dimensions invoked by the terms *Afrocentrism* to the acquiescence to or acceptance of a European American construction of reality by African Americans. Although racial consciousness can be marginalizing, in its healthiest manifestation it can enrich, empower, and endow individuals with meaning, dignity, history and group integrity contained in a sense of self (Dana 2002).

Race supersedes all other experiences for people of color in the United States and has become the designation of choice and pride for many, as an insistence on acknowledgment of a history of oppression as well as a call for justice and equity. Many African Americans prefer the term *racial identity* because racial *status* has been the index of acceptance in white America (Dana 2002).

African Americans struggle with issues of self-identity and self-determination. When working with persons who appear "black," it is important to establish the special heritage within the patient's family of origin. Having patients describe their heritage and cultural background, and that of their parents and grandparents, is important in order to have a context for understanding their behavior, defenses, expectations, vulnerabilities, and anger (Baker 1988).

Culture is embodied in the individual cultural self as a consequence of transformations due to acculturation or development of racial identity. Therefore, it is important to explore the level of acculturation/assimilation. An Afrocentric worldview embodies psychobehavioral modalities of groupness, sameness, and commonality; includes values and customs relevant to cooperation, collective responsibility, and interdependence; and includes an ethos of tribal survival and oneness with nature.

Bicultural African Americans know the "rules" for good functioning in both African American and white social contexts, although they may be more comfortable in one milieu or the other—or in neither. *Assimilated* African

Americans refers to those who are more comfortable in the Anglo-American world (Dana 2002).

It is important to explore whether the patient prefers to be referred to as black or African American. The latter term is less stigmatizing to some because it includes reference to cultural heritage and formalizes the African connection (Paniagua 1998).

Communication and language are important aspects of identity. African American patients prefer personalized interactions that include a greeting, an introduction of the provider to the patient, and a handshake. They may prefer to be greeted by their surnames, and in the South as *sir* or *ma'am* (Kaiser Permanente 1999).

African Americans may use street talk, Black English, or Ebonics, which are variations of nonstandard English that may be difficult to comprehend. If the therapist cannot understand the patient, it is important to ask directly about whatever specifically is not understood. It is important that the patient understand that the therapist is not questioning the correctness of his or her use of language but rather is trying to facilitate communication between the two so that the patient's main concerns can be understood (Paniagua 1998).

Nonverbal communication refers to gesture, posture, eye contact, and interpersonal distance. It is not uncommon for African Americans to use subverbal utterances, like *"umnh, umnh, umnh"* or grunts and other nonverbal sounds to indicate, without talking, that they are listening or to convey an emotional response to something that has been said. African Americans tend to prefer a narrower space between conversants, in contrast to a preferred wider distance among whites (Primm et al. 1996). The potential risk in cross-cultural situations is a mismatch in preferred distance, giving the African American patient a sense of being rejected by the therapist and the therapist a sense of being crowded. Such a situation could result in difficulties in establishing a therapeutic alliance, in misdiagnosis, or in early termination by the patient.

Eye contact is another manifestation of nonverbal communication to which mental health professionals pay close attention. African Americans, like other nonwhite racial groups, consider sustained, direct eye contact rude and disrespectful to authority. Touching between patient and therapist is usually considered taboo in the mental health encounter. However, among African Americans, a touch or embrace is an acceptable and desirable way to convey warmth, acceptance, and consolation (Primm et al. 1996).

The concerns of Ms. T are not uncommon among African Americans. Racial consciousness and pride can be challenged by the way in which society, including African American society, views African Americans. The self-hatred that underlies the rejection Ms. T experienced from her own family is a vestige of the higher social status afforded to racially mixed African Americans, dating back to slavery. The adoption of European standards of beauty by some African Americans also fuels the ridicule that she experienced. The challenge for the therapist is to help the patient to preserve and expand on her sense of racial identity and pride, to build her self-esteem, and to develop a support system that validates her as a valuable human being.

B. Cultural Explanations of the Individual's Illness

In the second part of the DSM-IV-TR Outline for Cultural Formulation, it is vital to understand the patient's and the patient's family's understanding of the patient's illness.

Mr. B is a 26-year-old man who was born and raised in Jamaica and migrated to the United States as an adult. He and his family are extremely religious, and his mother, with whom he lives, is studying to be a minister. He earns his living as a truck driver and prides himself on a new rig he just bought. Things were going well with him until he began to have trouble sleeping, racing thoughts, auditory hallucinations, and feelings of suspiciousness toward others around him, including his family. These experiences were out of keeping for him, and his family noticed the change in his behavior. He began drinking excessively and at one point was charged with driving while intoxicated. Mr. B was devastated when he lost his license to drive, which forced him to stop working as a truck driver. His mother helped him make ends meet once he no longer had a source of income. However, she blamed his predicament on his not attending church, losing his faith, and not praying hard enough. She believed strongly that his strange behavior and his misfortune were a result of his "not living right" in God's eyes. According to his mother, he would achieve reversal of his circumstances if he would start praying and return to church. Mr. B, on the other hand, had a different explanation for his troubles and a different method for curing them. He believed that someone from Jamaica who didn't like him had placed a curse on him. When he heard voices, he felt that ghosts, or "duppies," were visiting him. He wanted to find an *obeah* woman, to help him remove the curse. When he discovered that none were available in the area where he lived, he despaired. After he had been out of work for a while, his mother couldn't stand his acting strangely and cleaning

Table 2–1. Help-seeking pathways for African Americans

- The spiritualist, who is the most commonly consulted.
- The "old lady," who generally deals with common ailments, provides advice, and gives herbs. Young mothers most frequently consult her.
- The voodoo priest or "hougan," who has more formal training in the selection of plants for healing purposes, prescribes the ingestion of organs or parts of certain animals to treat a particular problem, and has the skills to deal with individual or family problems.
- The minister. Alternatively, individuals may attend prayer meetings or Bible study groups.

the house all day and decided to bring him to a mental health center for evaluation. Initially he was reluctant to accept mental health services, but he later relented when he realized that he wouldn't be able to visit a healer. On the basis of the evaluating psychiatrist's pathological interpretation of his beliefs in ghosts, Mr. B was diagnosed with schizophrenia and his symptoms of bipolar disorder and mania were ignored.

Religion is important in explanatory belief models as well as in treatment. Some African Americans believe that illness results from discordant relations between a person and his or her natural or social world, or that mental problems are caused by religious or spiritual factors. When they seek help for problems, they may consult any of the following: a spiritualist, an "old lady," a voodoo priest, or a minister (see Table 2–1) (Paniagua 1998).

There is less reporting of culture-bound syndromes in African Americans than in other groups. Five relevant syndromes are included in DSM-IV-TR in the Glossary of Culture-Bound Syndromes (American Psychiatric Association 2000). One of these is *falling out*, defined as lapsing into a state of semiconsciousness, which is thought to represent an extreme method of denial and escape from an unbearable environment (Gaw 2001). Another culture-bound syndrome is *brain fag*, found primarily in Nigeria and other African cultures. It is a cluster of symptoms including poor concentration, memory, and thinking that results in "fatigue" in the brain and difficulty with reading, comprehending, and overall intellectual functioning. Some people with brain fag report feeling as if worms were crawling in their heads. Most symptoms center on the head and neck region and may include pressure, tension, pain, blurred vision, and a burning sensation. *Spell*, a culturally specific syndrome seen in African American populations, particularly in the South, involves a state of trance and communication with deceased relatives or spirits. *Boufée delirante* is a syndrome found in West Africa and Haiti that is composed of a sudden onset of agitation and aggression, severe disorganized behavior, and psychomotor changes that may be accompanied by paranoid ideas or hallucinations in the auditory and visual spheres. These attacks are similar to brief psychosis. *Rootwork* is a culture-bound syndrome involving symptoms of mental illness believed to be caused by a hex.

African Americans have a prevalence of isolated sleep paralysis of approximately 41%, and those with this condition are more likely to suffer from panic disorder (Baker and Bell 1999). The high proportion of African Americans with isolated sleep paralysis may represent a form of a culture-bound syndrome.

The African American tradition of folk medicine reflects knowledge of plants and herbs that African ancestors applied to the indigenous plants of the American continent. Use of herbal medicine is still referred to as "doctoring." "Working of roots" involves the use of plant roots to prepare potions that are employed to bring about either good or evil.

African Americans see the maintenance of good mental health as depending on a person's ability to stay in harmony with the magico-religious world. The biopsychosocial perspective is particularly pertinent for elders. The Task Force on Black and Minority Health pointed out that ethnic elders and their families do not define mental disorders as "illnesses" to be treated by Western medicine with diagnostic tests and medications but rather as conditions that bring shame on the family (Baker and Lightfoot 1993). People with psychiatric illnesses are managed within the family until it is no longer possible to contain their symptoms (Griffith and Baker 1993). Accepting the patient's beliefs about causation and treatment, rather than trying to counter them, can enhance assessment and treatment.

The case of Mr. B illustrates how culturally based explanatory models can have an impact on conception of mental illness as well as on help-seeking patterns and mental health service use. Religion and spirituality play a central role in the lives of people of African descent. Many believe that worship and prayer are central to maintaining health and balance and that not engaging in religious activity is a recipe for ill health. Often, African Americans with mental illness rely on faith-based solutions to their mental health problems, to the exclusion of professional sources of help. Mr. B's beliefs in sorcery and magico-spiritual practices are found among many cultures of people from the African diaspora. These beliefs in supernatural powers and healing practices have many similarities and range from "duppies" (a Caribbean form of ghosts), *obeah* (traditional healing), voodoo (practiced by people of Haitian descent), and hoodoo or rootwork (practiced by African Americans primarily in the South), to *santería* (a Cuban syncretism of ritual sacrifice of animals and worship of multiple African deities) and *espiritismo* (practiced by people from Puerto Rico).

Given that belief in duppies and *obeah* are accepted among some people from Jamaican culture, they should not be regarded as evidence of psychosis but rather should be understood as a way in which illness is explained within a cultural context.

C. Cultural Factors Related to Psychosocial Environment and Levels of Functioning

In the third part of the DSM-IV-TR Outline for Cultural Formulation, the clinician assesses how the patient relates to his or her environment and delineates stressors and supports.

> Ms. J is a 60-year-old woman who is loving and kind to everyone. She has always taken her maternal role seriously, and she openhandedly nurtures all those with whom she comes in contact. She feels obligated to do everything for everybody and often overcommits herself to a variety of tasks and favors for family, coworkers, friends, sorority sisters, and fellow church members. She doesn't feel she has the right to say no, and when she does say no to people, she is plagued with guilt. Her problems arose because her giving to others, while benevolent, had a negative impact on her mental health. She was tired all the time and frequently worked herself into a state of exhaustion. She made no time to pamper herself or to exercise and became extremely overweight. When she felt anxious and frustrated, she ate large amounts of food. After being diagnosed with diabetes, she was unable to deal with the demands on her to maintain a special diet, exercise, take her medication, watch her blood sugar counts, or even keep up with her doctor visits. She ignored her diabetes after a while and kept on with her extensive activities and good-doing, even while remaining depressed and anxious. She developed a sore on her foot that didn't heal for a long time no matter what she put on it. Despite urging from her family to get it checked out by her physician, she let it go, stating, "I'll put it in the Lord's hands." She prayed about it, but the sore developed into a severe infection, and when she finally went to her physician, she was told that her foot would have to be amputated.

Psychosocial stressors experienced by African Americans are related to socioeconomic status, residence in high-crime areas, perceived racial discrimination, and perceived limitations on attainments (Baker and Bell 1999). These stressors can be exacerbated in certain phases of the life cycle, especially youth and old age.

African American children comprise about 45% of the children in public foster care and more than half of all children waiting to be adopted. Garland and colleagues (1998) reported that approximately 42% of children and youth in child welfare programs met DSM-IV criteria for a mental disorder.

Perhaps because of a lack of health insurance, few African American children are in psychiatric inpatient care, but there are many in residential treatment centers for emotionally disturbed youth. In many cases, it is not parents but child welfare authorities that initiate treatment for African American children.

Little is known about the mental health problems of older African Americans. The ECA study found that they had a higher prevalence of severe cognitive impairment. Cognitive impairment is strongly related to education. Therefore, simple measures may fail to fully assess the long-term impact of excluding African Americans from good schools because of segregation. For the most part, ethnic minority elders have survived great difficulties (U.S. Department of Health and Human Services 2001b).

Among African Americans, both the nuclear family and the extended family are important. The extended family often includes nonbiological members such as friends, clergy, and godparents. It is important for the therapist to formulate a genogram that emphasizes the extended family rather than a simple biological family tree. Role flexibility is important in the African American family, and the father may not be the head; role flexibility is often extended to include the parental role assumed by the grandfather, grandmother, aunts, and cousins.

The church often is a very important part of the family, and it is important to explore whether the patient includes the church in his or her extended family. The majority of African Americans belong to the Baptist or the African Methodist Episcopal denomination (Paniagua 1998).

A study of daily stress and experience of discrimination found that African Americans perceive greater distress triggered by racism than do European Americans. These findings add support to the notion that discrimination presents a unique stressor in the lives of African Americans. Three basic assumptions underlie research on racism and the mental health of African Americans. They are that 1) striving for upward social mobility is a widely shared cultural value in the United States, 2) racial discrimination prevents many African Americans from achieving their mobility goals, and 3) African Americans suffer psychological damage because of unsuccessful attempts at upward mobility (Neighbors et al. 1996).

Ms. J is a classic version of the African American "superwoman" who goes out of her way to help others and fulfills a stereotype of the black mother figure, all-knowing and all-giving. She is over-responsible for others' problems and is the ultimate, benevolent enabler whose helping of others defines her existence. Her depression and anxiety are overlooked, most likely, because she is so functional. If her depression had been recognized and treated early, she might have enjoyed a better quality of life and learned to maintain appropriate boundaries and set reasonable limits on people's demands of her. The loss of her foot is tragic because it was a treatable condition. Her religious beliefs led her to pray for her foot infection to heal. The delay in addressing this issue aggressively may have resulted from a lack of treatment for her depression (Neighbors et al. 1996).

D. Cultural Elements of the Relationship Between the Individual and the Clinician

Part D of the DSM-IV-TR Outline for Cultural Formulation has enormous impact on the treatment of African Americans, both by non–African American clinicians and by African American clinicians.

> Mr. S is a 50-year-old divorced African American man who lives in a northern city with a very small African American population. He went to a mental health center after losing his job following an altercation with his boss, a white female. The patient maintains that he was falsely accused of stealing and (based on his previous experience) that being the only African American male in his workplace placed him at risk of being blamed whenever something went awry. Ever since he was fired, Mr. S has been depressed and consumed with anger. His heart disease has flared up and he frequently experiences chest pain. Mr. S constantly worries about how he will make ends meet and how he will be able to afford health insurance now that he is without a job. He has been having trouble sleeping, and because nothing he could obtain over the counter was working, he decided to drink alcohol to help him sleep.

Mr. S has been very concerned about drinking again because he has had a problem with alcohol in the past. He also notices that his cigarette smoking has increased as his drinking has increased. Initially, he was ambivalent about seeking mental health care. He felt he should be able to just continue working out to relieve his stress. But when exercise proved to be insufficient in quelling his anxiety and anger, he felt he had no choice. On meeting his therapist, Ms. A, he was very disappointed. Here was another white female in a position of authority over him, and he was uncertain how she could help him and what his outcome would be. He had to admit, though, that she was nice enough in their initial meeting, and he didn't mind looking at her.

As they began to work together, he made it a point to talk about his life almost exclusively in a racial context. He frequently talked about slavery and all the global permutations of racism that he could think of. He saw himself as a black man in white-dominated society who is a victim of racism and a member of an endangered species. His experience in the workplace only served to galvanize that belief. The therapist found the patient's anger to be remarkable. Whenever he would elaborate his insights on global racism, she would feel her skin tingle uncomfortably and she knew her face was flushed and red. She couldn't help it. Several years ago, while working on a psychiatric inpatient unit, she was hit in the face by a psychotic African American male patient, and she only recently had felt comfortable enough to work with patients again. It was an effort to resist the urge to run out of the room or hit the emergency call bell when Mr. S would become loud about how he felt he had been wronged. She turned to her own religion and spirituality to help her get through each session. The therapist even encouraged the patient to pray and consider going to church again. The patient was resistant to this idea and resentful that the therapist would suggest it. At one point, she gave him a poem about African American racial identity, which he found offensive and utterly useless. Surprisingly, he kept his appointments, accepted antidepressant medication from her psychiatrist supervisor, and over several weeks appeared to have an improvement in mood.

A black patient entering treatment expects the therapist to have some knowledge of the effects of racism and their implications for African Americans in American society. If a black patient feels rejected or devalued by the therapist, he or she is likely to discontinue treatment. The therapist must be empathic, sensitive, and inquiring in his or her concern. Black patients' adherence to treatment is influenced by the quality of the interaction between the therapist and the patient. Ease of psycholinguistic communication, mutual understanding of cultural references, and avoidance of confounding the transference-countertransference issues with ethnocentrism (racial stereotyping) will facilitate the formation of a therapeutic alliance (Baker 1988).

Prior to accepting services, an increasing number of African Americans seek affirmation of a clinician's humanity, cultural knowledge, and relative freedom from prejudice and stereotype. Clinicians should communicate an understanding of the pervasive effects of racism and discrimination in the daily lives of their patients as further evidence of credibility. Psychiatrists treating black male patients reported the following factors as most important in successful treatment of black males: empathy, patience, supportiveness, tolerance, and the ability to listen and indicate directions without leading. These therapists also noted that racial issues must be put in perspective, that the therapist must be knowledgeable, and that he or she must gain the patient's trust. Given that elderly patients have special needs, clinicians need to elicit their histories carefully in order to form a contextual background and increase the ability to form a therapeutic alliance (Dana 2002).

When assessing a patient, it also is important to *listen* rather than immediately trying to understand the patient; to define the roles of those who accompany the patient to the sessions; to emphasize strengths rather than deficits; to be present-time focused; and to suggest a brief, focused intervention to deal with the presenting problem quickly. African Americans tend to believe that emotional problems are caused by environmental factors. They tend to prefer *concrete suggestions* regarding solutions rather than causal explanations. Recommended modalities of therapy are problem-solving and social skills training and family therapy. It is important to emphasize empowerment to help the patient gain the skills needed to make important decisions in his or her own life and the lives of other family members. Assisting with the development of skills that could help the patient take back control of his or her family is crucial (Paniagua 1998).

It is extremely important to handle family secrets with care and to wait for them to be revealed. Listen carefully, pay attention to the amount of silence when the patient is queried about issues that appear to be sensitive, and don't ask questions that may imply the revelation of family secrets—especially if others are present.

Given the important role of religion and spirituality in the lives of many African Americans, it is important to consider these factors in evaluation and treatment. African Americans may present with psychiatric symptoms that they attribute to lack of faith or reduced participation in religious activities. Patients may also rely on their church community for support for and endorsement of their acceptance of psychiatric treatment, specifically medication. When religious factors impede progress in clinical care, it is important to obtain consultation from religious leaders or cultural brokers, or to make accommodations to treatment within acceptable ethical boundaries. Accommodation may take the form of incorporating prayer into treatment, but only *at the patient's request.*

It can also be helpful to assess whether the patient is a member of a particular church and whether the church can provide emotional and financial support. Inviting the patient to bring church members to subsequent sessions can help with assessment and treatment. If the patient has no church, the clinician can help him or her find one and can then obtain help from the minister in keeping the patient in treatment. It is important to obtain the patient's consent before doing this.

After the initial evaluation, it is important for the therapist to review the findings in understandable language and to discuss the prescribed treatment and its length. With the patient's consent, it is essential to take the time to explain the treatment process to the extended family and essential others of the African American family and to encourage their involvement in the treatment process. Both patients and their family members or caregivers should be included in educational programs about the patient's illness and the effects of medication.

The impact of racism must always be considered in the assessment of African Americans, regardless of whether or not it is a presenting problem or a contributing factor to psychopathology. African Americans may present as highly suspicious of others with different ethnicity and values. This is known as the "healthy paranoia effect" and results from adaptation to the effects of slavery and racism. If patient and therapist are not of the same race, it is important that the therapist acknowledge the difference during the first session and encourage the patient to talk about his or her feelings concerning the issue (Dana 2002).

An example of institutional racism can be found in the old diagnosis of *drapetomania.* This term was used to describe a disease that caused black slaves to run away from their masters. The construct was based on the theory that because blacks are by nature subservient, those who try to escape from slavery are behaving contrary to their natural tendencies and must be ill. This "diagnosis" and others were based on racist notions of black inferiority that undergirded the warnings that treating black slaves as equals to whites could induce diseases such as drapetomania.

Black patients can be defensive, hostile, and nonverbal in an initial meeting in a new setting, thereby adapting to powerlessness. They often experience fear and distrust of white therapists. If black patients believe the goal of therapy is to maintain the status quo and their place in society, they may be suspicious of the motives of white as well as black psychiatrists.

When treating an African American patient, an African American therapist also needs to establish him- or herself as a credible therapist. This should be done by presenting a set of verbal and nonverbal behaviors that establish the therapist as a peer rather than assuming the patient will consider him or her a peer simply because he or she is an African American. Another suggestion is to avoid sitting behind a desk, a practice that tends to create distance and a power differential between therapist and patient. It is important to distinguish between discussion of racial issues to facilitate assessment and treatment and the therapist's explicit or implicit role as a "protector of the race." Mixing discussion of these two sets of issues should be avoided.

Rosenheck and colleagues (1995) found race to be an important factor in the treatment of PTSD in outpatient settings. In a study of veterans with war-related PTSD, black veterans who were paired with white clinicians received fewer services and had significantly higher rates of termination. This example of problems related to racial pairing is likely indicative of fears of white clinicians with respect to black veterans and the suspiciousness and lack of trust that black veterans have toward white clinicians. The finding that black veterans had lower attendance and less participation and involvement in their care than whites, *regardless* of the race of their therapist, suggests a cultural adaptation to play one's cards close to the vest, maintaining personal business and secrets at all costs in order to avoid "playing" oneself into a position of greater vulnerability (Rosenheck et al. 1995).

Stereotypes and prejudice are part and parcel of the training that mental health professionals receive. Stereotypes of African Americans as violent people are abundant, resulting in misinterpretations of ambiguous behavior (Whaley 1998). Because violence is a major factor driving decision making in mental health settings, this misinterpretation results in higher risk of African

Americans receiving severe diagnoses and restrictive interventions. This phenomenon is reflected in high rates of the misdiagnosis of schizophrenia and in the patterns of utilization of mental health services and institutionalization among African Americans—namely, overrepresentation in the criminal justice system (where there are high rates of comorbid mental illness and substance abuse), disproportionately high rates of involuntary hospitalization, and low rates of tenure in outpatient care (Whaley 1998).

Other manifestations of misperceptions about African Americans are the delivery of less professional treatment, greater use of pharmacological agents with greater risk of irreversible adverse effects (such as tardive dyskinesia associated with antipsychotic medications), and higher hospital recidivism rates. In addition, there are stereotypes that African Americans are lacking in physical attractiveness and in suitability for psychotherapy, leading to the discomfort of therapists working with patients of African descent. It is important to minimize stereotyping and bias in decision making in clinical care. The training of mental health professionals must address the impact of societal racism on patients and clinicians.

The case of the patient Mr. S and the clinician Ms. A offers an opportunity to explore transference and countertransference with a racial theme. In many ways, the patient's relationship with Ms. A was a mirror image of his relationship with his previous boss, given that she, too, was a white female with some control over him. It is surprising that Mr. S did not specifically request an African American therapist so as to avoid reminders of his unpleasant experience in the workplace. But as in many areas of the country with small black populations, African American therapists are in short supply. Mr. S interpreted all his conflicts through the lens of racism. He also exhibited anger and feelings of victimization, at times directed toward Ms. A, which were transferential in nature. While acknowledging the impact of racism on Mr. S's life and allowing him to ventilate, Ms. A could have done a better job of helping him explore other important themes in his life. Her own countertransference, based on her fear of Mr. A when he talked loudly about racism, was provoked by her memories of being assaulted by a black male patient. Although her response was psychological and physiological, Ms. A maintained her professionalism rather than fleeing. Ms. A assumed that Mr. S was a religious person, based on the stereotype that all African Americans are religious. It is more appropriate to explore the role of religion and spirituality in a patient's life before making the assumption that the person has a religious orientation. Her effort to engage him with the poem on African American identity was a well-meaning gesture, but to Mr. S it seemed like an effort to control the terms of even his identity. He was justified in rebuffing this offering.

The cross-racial therapeutic relationship is a laboratory of interplay between that which is seen and that which is not seen. It is the therapist's responsibility to maintain appropriate boundaries between self and patient, past and present, and impulse and reason. Also, in developing healthy empathy, the therapist must find a way to appreciate what the patient is going through and try to see the world through his or her eyes. Once that is accomplished, the therapist can gain the patient's trust and begin to guide the patient toward the accomplishment of his or her goals, one hopes in a realistic context. When the therapist experiences a countertransference reaction that is difficult to contain, it is important that he or she work this through in supervision. If this cannot be achieved, arrangements should be made to transfer the patient.

E. Overall Cultural Assessment for Diagnosis and Care

Part E of the DSM-IV-TR Outline for Cultural Formulation addresses the question of how cultural factors affect our diagnosis and treatment of African American patients.

> Mr. W is a 30-year-old man of large stature who has a history of heroin and cocaine abuse and incarceration. He had experienced multiple losses and traumas in his life: his father was physically and emotionally abusive during his childhood; he spent several years in foster care; his marriage ended in divorce; and his son and niece were murdered. He made one suicide attempt with an overdose of heroin when he was in his late teens. He was treated in an emergency room but was let go without psychiatric evaluation or mental health follow-up. While attending a substance abuse treatment program after his release from prison, he stayed in an affiliated shelter for homeless men and began having frequent disagreements with the residents there. He was on the verge of being thrown out of the shelter for bad behavior when an astute substance abuse counselor became concerned that he might have mental health needs and referred him to a psychiatrist for evaluation. In order to reduce the stigma, the psychiatrist agreed to see the patient in the primary care suite of the substance abuse program, where he was being treated for hypertension and diabetes.

The psychiatrist found the patient to be extremely angry, presenting himself with a very hard, "macho" veneer and a stoic reserve. He complained of poor sleep, poor appetite and weight loss, backaches, and headaches; however, he was quite guarded. As the psychiatrist kept pushing to obtain more details of the history, the patient became tearful. This was a breakthrough for the psychiatrist because prior to that, he had come to the conclusion that the patient was just a typical substance abuser with a bad attitude and antisocial personality traits. The psychiatrist began to formulate the patient as having major depression and started him on an antidepressant. Given his large size, the psychiatrist estimated that he would need a high dose of antidepressant medication at the initiation of therapy.

Mr. W was started on the medicine and returned a week later even more angry and threatening never to return. He complained that the medication made him sick and couldn't understand why the psychiatrist put him on medication that made him feel worse. The psychiatrist expressed empathic concern about the patient's bad experience and reduced the dose after convincing him not to give up on the medication and psychiatric treatment altogether. He reassured Mr. W that thereafter they would increase the dose in small increments in an effort to minimize uncomfortable side effects. The patient agreed to try again at a lower dose. As his dose was titrated upward slowly and he began individual psychotherapy with a social worker, the depressive symptoms began to remit.

The therapist arranged for case management services to assist the patient in obtaining independent housing, entitlements, and benefits. Eventually, Mr. W revealed to the social worker that he had great difficulty reading, which was a major source of anxiety and humiliation for him. The therapist identified a program to help him work on his literacy skills and prepare him for a general equivalency diploma (GED).

At one point, the patient became frustrated with his mental health services when his therapist moved to another city and he was reassigned. Mr. W also began seeing a new psychiatrist who felt that his guardedness and concreteness were evidence of a psychotic disorder. The new psychiatrist reformulated the patient as having schizoaffective disorder and added an antipsychotic medication to his antidepressant regime. The patient began having additional side effects, including extreme sedation, which interfered with his performance in his GED class. Mr. W began noticing that the therapist would arrange for him to see the psychiatrist at a certain time but would keep him waiting without letting him know what was happening or how long a wait to expect. This made the patient feel as if the therapist were disrespecting his time. On several occasions, out of frustration, he left without being seen by the psychiatrist. The patient confronted the new therapist about this and threatened to leave treatment with her altogether if this was not addressed.

African Americans are more likely to be diagnosed with schizophrenia than with major depressive disorder. It therefore is important to screen carefully for depression in order to reduce misdiagnosis and labeling of psychotic disorders. Alcoholic hallucinosis or alcohol withdrawal states may mimic the hallucinations and agitation of an acute psychotic episode. Withdrawal delirium and paranoid psychosis may be seen among patients who abuse alcohol. Other substances of abuse and dependence may confound evaluation and diagnosis. Cocaine-induced mood disorder with intense dysphoria and suicidal ideation is a frequent complaint of cocaine-dependent persons evaluated in emergency medical settings. Paranoid psychosis with a clear sensorium may be seen among users of crystal methamphetamine (Baker and Bell 1999).

It is crucial to pay close attention to the differences in response to psychopharmacological treatment in African Americans, given that they have been found to be poor metabolizers of psychotropics based on genetic polymorphism of liver enzymes involved in drug metabolism. This observation dictates that psychiatrists use lower starting doses (paying attention to adverse effects and poor adherence), slower upward titration, and plasma level monitoring. The higher sensitivity to these medications is manifested in a faster and higher rate of response and more severe side effects, including delirium, when black patients are treated with doses commonly used for whites. Nonetheless, clinicians in psychiatric emergency services and inpatient services prescribe more and higher doses of oral and injectable antipsychotic medications to African Americans than to whites.

Additional consideration should be given to the effects on medications of nutrition, diet, tobacco use, and alcohol and illicit drug consumption. Alternative and complementary therapies also can have significant effects on the metabolism of psychotropic medications (Strickland et al. 1997).

Many elders in populations of color have multiple health problems and require comprehensive diagnostic assessments to rule out underlying medical problems. They should also receive thorough medication reviews. It is important for the evaluating psychiatrist to be aware that African American elders may also be seeing traditional healers. What the healers prescribe may increase the potential for drug-drug interactions, and therefore it is important to have the patient bring in all the medications that he or she is taking (Baker and Lightfoot 1993).

In a nationwide telephone and mail survey, African Americans were found to be less likely than white Americans to receive appropriate care for depression and anxiety (Young et al. 2001). African Americans were less likely to receive an antidepressant when their depression was first diagnosed (27% vs. 44%). Of those who did receive antidepressants, African Americans were less likely than whites to receive selective serotonin reuptake inhibitors. In a large longitudinal study of older community residents, whites were nearly twice as likely as African Americans at the beginning and four times as likely at the end to use antidepressants (Blazer et al. 2000).

The case of Mr. W embodies many important themes that may arise in the psychiatric diagnosis and treatment of African American patients. Black patients with substance use disorders frequently have underlying mood disorders and anxiety disorders that are overlooked. Mr. W was almost expelled from the shelter where he was living because of "bad behavior." It did not occur to anyone that being argumentative was uncharacteristic for Mr. W, who was usually an easygoing person. Anger has been termed an idiom of distress among African Americans and can be seen as a presenting symptom of mood disorder, as opposed to the more familiar presenting symptom of sadness. Typically, the last thing a black man wants to do is present himself as sad because of the association of sadness with weakness and vulnerability. Mr. W's psychiatrist almost accepted the stereotypes of black substance abusers being bad people as opposed to people who may have mental health needs. Certainly, the bravado style that Mr. W uses is similar to the "cool pose" described by Majors and Billson (1992) in their book of the same name. *Cool pose* describes the tendency for African American males to present themselves in a cool, confident way at all times to maintain a tough, impermeable image. This image can obscure underlying dysfunction and despair or can masquerade as evidence of psychopathy. Misinterpretation of *cool pose* could account for the high percentage of African American males in the criminal justice system and high rates of involuntary treatment.

The psychiatrist was not familiar with racial and ethnic differences in metabolism mediated by the cytochrome P450 enzyme system (discussed in further detail in Chapter 6) and thus was unaware of the need to be cautious and gingerly in initial dosing with African Americans, even when using medications like selective serotonin reuptake inhibitors that are known to have a relatively tolerable side-effect profile. African Americans are more likely than whites and Asians to be poor metabolizers; poor metabolizing can result in high plasma levels and potentially more side effects and higher toxicity. This applies to antidepressants and antipsychotic medications alike. Given the mistrust that many African Americans feel toward mental health providers and their ambivalence about mental health services, practitioners cannot afford to be too aggressive in dosing strategies and risk losing the patient altogether. Therapists must be proactive in linking patients who have a low income or limited resources to needed services and resources. Mr. W's concerns about his ability to read and the therapist's response are critical to the accomplishment of any vocational goals he may have in the future. For an African American male just being released from the criminal justice system, the need for linkage with community resources is even more critical.

The patient's diagnosis was reformulated as schizoaffective illness with a thin rationale. Certainly, guarded affect alone does not indicate psychosis. His concreteness could have been related to inadequate education and may not have been an aspect of a psychotic disorder. Practitioners should always be wary of making the diagnosis of schizophrenia or purely psychotic disorders in African American patients, given the long history of misdiagnosis and over-diagnosis of this group. As for the long waiting times and the patient's leaving without being seen, it is important not to assume that an African American patient will be late or will tolerate being kept waiting without receiving appropriate courtesies. The patient's interpretation of the way he was being treated was that his time was not regarded as valuable. The best quality of care involves, first and foremost, treating individuals with respect and valuing them and their time.

The stigma of mental illness is high among African Americans, who see the individual with mental health problems as "going off," "having trouble," or "not being right in the head." Clinicians should be prepared to explore antipsychiatry feelings with their African American patients in an effort to counteract the negative effects of antipsychiatry propaganda that they may have heard.

Suicide among African American male adolescents is on the rise (U.S. Department of Health and Human Services 2001b). Suicide rates have always been lower among African Americans than other racial groups, and many African Americans were unaware that suicide occurred in the black community at all. However, rates of suicide among black male adolescents, while lower than those of white males of the same age group, rose steeply from 1986 to the end of the twentieth century, when they began to plateau. The rise in suicide among black adolescents was a wakeup call to pay greater attention to the mental health of black youth and to design suicide prevention programs for the black community. The National Organization for People of Color Against Suicide (NOPCAS) has taken the lead in increasing awareness about this issue.

African Americans' attitudes toward mental illness are a major barrier to accessing care. Mental illness retains considerable stigma, and seeking treatment is not always encouraged. Sussman and colleagues (1987) found that the proportion of African Americans who feared mental health treatment was 2.5 times greater than the proportion of whites who feared such treatment. A study of parents of children meeting criteria for attention-deficit/hyperactivity disorder discovered that African American parents were less likely than white parents to use specific medical labels to describe their child's difficulties and were more likely to expect a shorter-term course of treatment (Bussing et al. 1998). Zylstra and Steitz (1999) found that older African Americans were less knowledgeable about depression than elderly whites.

African Americans in the general community, as well as those who were diagnosed with depression, had more positive views about seeking mental health care than did their white counterparts. This seems somewhat paradoxical given that African Americans were less likely to use mental health services (Diala et al. 2002). Further, compared with whites, African Americans who had used mental health services were more likely to have negative attitudes and were less likely to continue with treatment. African Americans were also less likely than whites to have positive attitudes about friends having knowledge of their mental health help-seeking, and, overall, African Americans had lower likelihood of using mental health services.

African Americans are affected especially by the amount of time spent with their providers, by a sense of trust, and by whether the provider is an African American (Keith 2000). African American focus group participants reported being more likely than whites to describe stigma and spirituality as affecting their willingness to seek help (Cooper-Patrick et al. 1997).

Stigma can be overcome only by education about and exposure to African American patients for psychiatrists and other mental health clinicians, along with widespread education of patients, their families, and the general public about mental illness in African Americans, the reasons for seeking treatment early, and why they should not feel ashamed. Provider education can take the form of case presentations and discussion, as well as the use of popular books and films that focus on racial issues and mental health. Radio, television, newspapers, and popular magazines can be used for public education. For those of low literacy, videotapes such as *Black and Blue* can be quite useful (Primm et al. 2002).

Conclusion

This chapter has provided a framework and context for understanding African Americans and their knowledge, attitudes, beliefs, and behaviors about mental health and mental illness. Some epidemiological and clinical material also has been provided. Readers are encouraged to learn more, and we hope that some will contribute to the growing body of literature about the mental health issues of people of African descent.

References

American Psychiatric Association: Appendix I: Outline for cultural formulation and glossary of culture-bound syndromes, in Diagnostic and Statistical Manual of Mental Disorders, 4th Edition, Text Revision. Washington, DC, American Psychiatric Association, 2000, pp 897–903

Baker FM: Afro Americans, in Clinical Guidelines in Cross-Cultural Mental Health. Edited by Comas-Diaz L, Griffith EHE. New York, Wiley, 1988, pp 151–181

Baker FM, Bell CC: Issues in the psychiatric treatment of African Americans. Psychiatr Serv 50:362–368, 1999

Baker FM, Lightfoot OB: Psychiatric care of ethnic elders, in Culture, Ethnicity, and Mental Illness. Edited by Gaw AC. Washington, DC, American Psychiatric Press, 1993, pp 517–552

Blazer DG, Hypes CF, Simonsick EM, et al: Marked differences in antidepressant use by race in elderly community sample. 1986–1996. Am J Psychiatry 157:1089–1094, 2000

Borowsky SJ, Rubenstein LV, Meredith LS, et al: Who is at risk of no detection of mental health problems in primary care? J Gen Intern Med 15:381–388, 2000

Bussing R, Schoenberg N, Rogers KM, et al: Explanatory models of ADHD: do they differ by ethnicity, child gender or treatment status? Journal of Emotional and Behavioral Disorders 6:233–242, 1998

Chung H, Mahler JC, Kakuma T: Racial differences in treatment of psychiatric inpatients. Psychiatr Serv 46:586–591, 1995

Cooper-Patrick L, Powe NR, Jencke MW, et al: Identification of patient attitudes and preferences regarding treatment for depression. J Gen Intern Med 12:431–438, 1997

Dana R: Mental health services for African Americans: a cultural/racial perspective. Cultur Divers Ethnic Minor Psychol 8:3–18, 2002

Diala C, Muntaner C, Walrath C, et al: Racial differences in attitudes toward professional mental health care and the use of services, in Race, Ethnicity and Health. Edited by LaVeist TL. San Francisco, CA, Jossey-Bass, 2002, pp 591–560

Garland AF, Ellis-MacLeod E, Landsverk JA, et al: Minority populations in the child welfare system: the visibility hypothesis reexamined. Am J Orthopsychiatry 68:142–146, 1998

Gaw AC: Culture-bound syndromes, in Concise Guide to Cross-Cultural Psychiatry. Washington, DC, American Psychiatric Publishing, 2001, pp 73–97

Griffith EHH, Baker FM: Psychiatric care of African Americans, in Culture, Ethnicity, and Mental Illness. Edited by Gaw A. Washington, DC, American Psychiatric Press, 1993, pp 147–174

Kaiser Permanente: A Provider's Handbook on Culturally Competent Care: African American Population. Kaiser Permanente, 1999. For copies, phone (510) 271-6663.

Keith V: A profile of African Americans' health care, in Minority Health in America. Edited by Hogue C, Hargraves MA, Collins KS. Baltimore, MD, Johns Hopkins University Press, 2000, pp 47–76

Kessler RC, McGonagle KA, Zhao S, et al: Lifetime and 12-month prevalence of DSM-III-R psychiatric disorders in the United States: results from the National Comorbidity Survey. Arch Gen Psychiatry 51:8–19, 1994

Lawson WB: Psychiatric diagnosis of African Americans, in Cross Cultural Psychiatry. Edited by Herrera JM, Lawson WB, Sramek JJ. New York, Wiley, 1999, pp 99–104

Majors R, Billson JM: Cool Pose: The Dilemmas of Black Manhood in America. New York, Lexington Books, 1992

Neighbors HW, Jackson JS, Broman C, et al: Racism and the mental health of African Americans: the role of self and system blame. Ethn Dis 6:167–182, 1996

Paniagua F: Guidelines for the assessment and treatment of African-American clients, in Assessing and Treating Culturally Diverse Clients. Thousand Oaks, CA, Sage, 1998, pp 20–37

Primm AB, Lima BR, Rowe CR: Cultural and ethnic sensitivity, in Integrated Mental Health Services: Modern Community Psychiatry. Edited by Breakey W. New York, Oxford University Press, 1996, pp 146–159

Primm AB, Cabot D, Pettis J, et al: The acceptability of a culturally tailored depression education videotape to African Americans. J Natl Med Assoc 94:1007–1016, 2002

Robins LN, Regier DA: Psychiatric Disorders in America. New York, Free Press, 1991

Rosenheck R, Fontana A, Cottrol C: Effect of clinician-veteran racial pairing in the treatment of posttraumatic stress disorder. Am J Psychiatry 152:555–563, 1995

Schneider EC, Zaskavsky AM, Epstein AM: Racial disparities in the quality of care for enrollees in Medicaid managed care. JAMA 287:1288–1294, 2002

Scott EL, Eng W, Heimberg R: Ethnic differences in worry in a nonclinical population. Depress Anxiety 15:79–82, 2002

Shaw CM, Creed F, Tomenson B, et al: Prevalence of anxiety and depressive illness and help seeking behaviour in African Caribbeans and white Europeans: two phase general population survey. BMJ 318:302–305, 1999

Snowden LR: African American service use for mental health problems. J Community Psychol 27:303–313, 1999

Strakowski SM, Hawkins JM, Keck PE, et al: The effects of race and information variance on disagreement between psychiatric emergency service and research diagnoses in first episode psychosis. J Clin Psychiatry 58:457–463, 1997

Strakowski SM, Keck PE, Arnold LM, et al: Ethnicity and diagnosis in patients with affective disorders. J Clin Psychiatry 64:747–754, 2003

Strickland TL, Stein R, Lin K, et al: The pharmacologic treatment of anxiety and depression in African Americans. Arch Fam Med 6:371–375, 1997

Sussman L, Robins L, Earls F: Treatment seeking for depression by black and white Americans. Soc Sci Med 24:187–196, 1987

Thompson RF: Flash of the Spirit: African and Afro-American Art and Philosophy. New York, Vintage, 1984

U.S. Census Bureau: Census 2000 Summary File 1. Washington, DC, U.S. Census Bureau, 2000. Available at: http://factfinder.census.gov/servlet/DatasetMainPageServlet?_ds_name=DEC_2000_SF1_U and_program=DECand_lang=en

U.S. Department of Health and Human Services: Cultural Competence Standards in Managed Mental Health Care: Four Underserved/Underrepresented Racial/Ethnic Groups (DHHS Publ No SMA00–3457). Rockville, MD, Center for Mental Health Services, Substance Abuse and Mental Health Services Administration, 2001a. Available at: http://www.mentalhealth.samhsa.gov/publications/allpubs/SMA00-3457/default.asp

U.S. Department of Health and Human Services: Mental Health: Culture, Race and Ethnicity. A Supplement to Mental Health: A Report of the Surgeon General. Rockville, MD, U.S. Department of Health and Human Services, Public Health Service, Office of the Surgeon General, 2001b. Available at: http://www.surgeon-general.gov/library/mentalhealth/cre

Whaley AR: Racism in the provision of mental health services: a social cognitive analysis. Am J Orthopsychiatry 68:47–57, 1998

Young AS, Klap R, Sherbourne CD, et al: The quality of care for depression and anxiety disorders in the United States. Arch Gen Psychiatry 58:55–61, 2001

Zylstra RG, Steitz JA: Public knowledge of late life depression and aging. J Appl Gerontol 18: 63–76, 1999

3

Asian American Patients

Nang Du, M.D.

Asian Americans are the third largest and the fastest-growing minority group in the United States, with a population of 10.2 to 11.9 million according to Census 2000 (U.S. Census Bureau 2002, 2004). The category of Asian American includes at least 43 ethnic subgroups (S.M. Lee 1998) with many different languages and dialects, religious beliefs, immigration patterns, socioeconomic statuses, and traditional patterns of seeking healthcare. These cultural and social variables affect psychiatric disorders in Asian Americans' manifestation of psychiatric symptoms, help-seeking behaviors, treatment strategies, compliance, and outcomes. This chapter will provide an overview of the historical backgrounds of the various groups and some culturally appropriate practical assessment techniques and therapeutic approaches organized around the DSM-IV-TR Outline for Cultural Formulation (American Psychiatric Association 2000).

Table 3–1.   Major Asian groups and their population and percentage of Asians in the United States, 2000

Group	Population (millions)	U.S. population (%)	Asian population (%)	Mixed race (%)
All Asian	11.9	4.2	100	10.3
Chinese	2.9	1.0	23.8	15.4
Filipino	2.4	0.8	18.3	21.8
Asian Indian	1.9	0.7	16.2	11.6
Vietnamese	1.2	0.4	10.9	8.3
Korean	1.2	0.4	10.5	12.3
Japanese	1.15	0.4	7.8	30.7

Source.   US. Census Bureau 2002, 2004.

Overview of the Asian American Population: Immigration Patterns

In 1970, the Asian American population was reported to be 1.5 million; in 1980, this number had exploded to 3.5 million, and by 1990, that number more than doubled to 7.2 million. Census 2000 reported 10.2 million Asians alone and an additional 1.7 million who identified themselves as Asian alone or in combination with another race. Most Asian Americans live in California, New York, Hawaii, Texas, New Jersey, Illinois, Washington, Florida, Virginia, and Massachusetts. They are concentrated in metropolitan areas. New York City and Los Angeles are the U.S. cities with the largest Asian American populations (U.S. Census Bureau 2002). See Table 3–1 for data on specific groups within the Asian American population.

Immigration Patterns

Asian Americans came to the United States at different periods, by different routes, and under different circumstances. Some came for economic reasons, others seeking safe haven and freedom from persecution. Many Asian Americans who have survived flights from their home countries have suffered traumatic experiences caused by famine, war, political imprisonment, and persecution. American domestic and foreign policy, along with global political and economic events, have strongly influenced Asian American immigration and population growth in the United States. Understanding the historical context of an Asian patient's immigration to the United States is crucial to understanding his or her experiences. The following section contains a brief historical introduction to the major Asian American groups.

Chinese Americans

The Chinese were the first Asian group to come to the United States. The political unrest and depressed economy in China, combined with the need for cheap labor in the United States, led large numbers of Chinese to immigrate to the West Coast during the Gold Rush period (1848–1882) (Takaki 1998). The Chinese, mostly men, worked as hand laborers in the mining, farming, and railroad industries. They contributed significantly to agricultural success in California and to the construction of the Union Pacific Transcontinental Railroad.

The flow of Chinese immigration ceased in the latter half of the 1800s, a period of economic recession in the United States when cheap Chinese labor was considered a threat to American workers. This threat led to the passage of several discriminatory laws to limit Chinese civil rights and the flow of immigration. The Chinese Exclusion Act of 1882 and several other immigration and naturalization acts that were enacted and enforced over the next 60 years prohibited Chinese from bringing their families to the United States, owning land, and becoming American citizens (Gaw 1993; Takaki 1998).

Despite harsh treatment from the government, thousands of Chinese, along with other Asian groups, mainly Filipino Americans and Japanese Americans, joined the U.S. army during World War II to prove their loyalty to the United States. Asian Americans' participation in the war campaign against Germany and Japan led to a more favorable attitude toward Asians in America. The U.S. Congress eventually repealed all 15 Chinese Exclusion Acts in 1943. The subsequent enactment of the War Bride Acts in 1945 allowed many Chinese and Japanese wives of Asian American and American servicemen to come to the United States. During the Chinese civil war between the Kuomintang and Communists in China in 1949, large numbers of highly educated Chinese students, visitors, and seamen were granted permanent residence in the United States. The political uncertainty and upheaval in China during and after the Cold War continued to feed the flow of Chinese immigrants to America, most notably after the massacre in Tiananmen Square in June 1989. The subsequent crackdown on the democratic movement in China after 1989 also led many Chinese scholars and students to seek political asylum in the United States. Recently, many Hong Kong immigrants chose to come to the United States because of fears of living under the Chinese Communist regime when the British government returned Hong Kong to China in 1997.

Filipino Americans

Filipino immigration began in the early 1900s with small numbers of seamen and laborers (Arameta 1993; Takaki 1998). More Filipino immigrants came during the second wave, 1906–1934, to fill in as cheap laborers in the farms and canning industries after the Gentlemen's Agreement between the United States and Japan limited the immigration of Japanese laborers. The third wave, comprising Filipinos who served alongside U.S. servicemen who fought against the Japanese in the South Pacific, arrived in the United States after World War II. The fourth wave arrived after 1965, when the immigration quota was lifted; unlike previous waves, this group of Filipino immigrants consisted of highly educated professionals such as doctors, engineers, and nurses who fled the depressed economy and the political repression of the Marcos regime. They came with the dual purpose of enhancing their professional skills and filling the employment gap in the United States during the economic boom of the 1960s and 1970s.

South Asian Americans

Asian Indians immigrated to the United States in small numbers during the 1800s (Juthani 1992; Prathikanti 1997). A larger influx of Asian Indians, mostly young professionals, occurred during the late 1960s and early 1970s. From 1980 to the present, many Asian Indians who immigrated were computer science engineers and workers who contributed significantly to the boom in the high-technology industry during the 1990s. A large proportion of the new immigrants during this time were family members and relatives of the Asian Indian professionals who immigrated during the 1960s. These family-sponsored immigrants were less well educated than the earlier immigrants and were unfamiliar with Western culture.

Southeast Asian Americans

The Southeast Asian Americans came to the United States not as immigrants but as war and political refugees. At the end of the Vietnam War in 1975, hundreds of thousands of Vietnamese fled the country to escape the Communist regime (Cima 1989; Ross 1990; Savada 1995). This first wave of refugees comprised mostly well-educated, high-ranking government and military officers and their immediate families. The second wave arrived from 1978 to 1982 and consisted of Vietnamese, Vietnamese Chinese, Cambodian, and Laotians, who were less well educated and were unfamiliar with Western culture. They were "boat people" who risked their lives on rough seas to escape the political, religious, and racial discrimination and persecution of the Communist regimes in Vietnam, Cambodia, and Laos. The third wave of Southeast Asian refugees, mostly Amerasian children of American servicemen and Vietnamese women, concentration reeducation camp survivors, political refugees, and families of refugees from the previous waves, came after 1985. Southeast Asian refugees, especially those from the second wave, experienced untold traumas related to their uprooting from the war-torn countries and during their escape journey. The ones who made it to the United States faced tremendous stress in adjusting and adapting to American life (E. Hsu et al. 2004).

Korean Americans

The first significant wave of Korean immigrants came to the United States between 1903 and 1905 (L.I.C. Kim 1993). They were mostly uneducated men employed by sugar plantations in Hawaii. These laborers contributed significantly to the movements to liberate Korea from the Japanese colonial occupation. The second wave of Korean immigrants arrived between 1951 and 1964, after the Korean War, as wives of American servicemen, orphans, and students. The third wave consisted of Koreans who came to the United States after 1965, when the immigration quota imposed on Asians was lifted.

Japanese Americans

The Japanese immigrated to the United States in large numbers between 1880 and 1920 (O'Brien and Fugita 1991; Takaki 1998). Many Japanese sought a better life away from the depressed economy during the Meiji era when Japan rapidly transformed from a feudal, agrarian society to a democratic, industrialized one. They worked as hand laborers in sugar plantations, farms, mines, canning factories, and the railroad industry. Unlike the Chinese immigrants, who were mostly men, Japanese immigrants sent for wives from their own country. Many of these women came as "picture brides" who had not previously met their husbands. Japanese immigrants experienced harsh treatment similar to that faced by other Asian immigrants in the United States. They were ineligible for citizenship and were prohibited from owning land or marrying whites. Many were prevented from obtaining jobs commensurate with their skills. The most traumatic discriminative act occurred during World War II, with the implementation of Executive Order 9066 in 1942 that forced more than 100,000 Japanese Americans into internment camps. The internment camp experience had dramatic and lasting effects on that generation and on subsequent generations of Japanese Americans (Nagata 1991). Today, most Japanese Americans are well assimilated, with more than half married to non-Japanese Americans.

Pacific Islanders

Pacific Islander Americans are neither refugees nor immigrants. They are the descendants of indigenous peoples on Pacific islands that were conquered by European explorers, missionaries, and colonists. In the late 1760s and 1770, Captain James Cook discovered Hawaii and Tonga. He and his crew brought previously unknown diseases to the natives on these islands, decimating their populations. Subsequent to these discoveries, missionaries and traders followed to colonize the islands and to impose new religions, cultures, and laws on the islanders. They occupied and took away the islanders' land ownership (U.S. Department of Health and Human Services 2001).

Pacific Islanders are diverse in languages and cultures. They consist of three large groups: Polynesians, Micronesians, and Melanesians (U.S. Census Bureau 2001). The Polynesians are most numerous and include Hawaiians, Samoans, Tongans, and Tahitians. The Micronesians, the second largest group, consist of Guamians (or Chamorros), Marianas Islanders, Marshall Islanders, Palauans, and other smaller groups. The third group is Melanesian, mainly from the Fijian population. Hawaii has been a state of the United States since 1959. The other islands remain as free associated states affiliated with the United States. Their people elect their own legislatures and governors, and the U.S. Department of the Interior has administrative responsibility for coordinating federal policy.

Because of the wide variety of experiences among Asian Americans, knowledge of Asian American background and pre-immigration experience is essential in understanding possible traumatic experiences during the immigration process and journey, as well as post-immigration acculturation and assimilation stress.

Applying the DSM-IV-TR Outline for Cultural Formulation

The DSM-IV-TR Outline for Cultural Formulation and the biopsychosocial model are particularly useful to clarify Asian American patients' dynamics, diagnosis, and treatment plans. Culture, religion, and philosophy of life intertwine to shape Asian American health beliefs and health care–seeking behaviors. The DSM-IV-TR Outline for Cultural Formulation is an excellent tool for cultural assessment. It aids the clinician in evaluating a patient's ethnic identity, cultural explanations of the illness, cultural factors related to psychosocial environment and levels of functioning, and cultural elements of the relationship between the individual and the therapist (Group for the Advancement of Psychiatry Committee on Cultural Psychiatry 2002; Lu et al. 1995). A thorough psychiatric interview to obtain information for a DSM-IV-TR diagnosis and cultural formulation is necessary to understand the Asian American dynamic, to formulate the case, and to strategize the treatment course.

A. Cultural Identity of the Individual

The cultural identity of the individual is shaped by several cultural variables distinctive to that person's ethnicity, age, gender, sexual orientation, socioeconomic status, educational achievement, and philosophical, religious, and spiritual beliefs.

Cultural/Ethnic Identity

Ethnic identity is defined as a person's sense of belonging with other members of the ethnic group and the extent to which that person embraces and practices his or her ethnic cultural tradition (Marsella 1993). Asian American ethnic identity depends on each person's degree of assimilation or acculturation to American culture. In general, new, recent, and elderly immigrants are very traditional with reference to their original culture. Immigrants who are from urban areas and well educated in Western culture and younger immigrants who were raised in the United States can embrace both traditional and American cultures and become bicultural.

Preferred Terms

Most traditional Asian Americans prefer to be referred to as people from their home countries, for example, Chinese American, Japanese American, Filipino

American, and Korean American. There are also subgroups. For example, Chinese Americans differentiate among themselves based on their origins in China or their speaking dialects. The most prominent Chinese groups in the United States are the Cantonese, Toisanese, Fukienese, Amoy, Taiwanese, Shanghainese, Hakka, and Szechuanese. In addition to their regionally specific dialects, many Chinese also speak Mandarin, which is the official national language (Gaw 1993).

Southeast Asians (Indochinese) include Vietnamese Americans, Cambodian Americans, and Laotian Americans. The Cambodians like to be called "Khmer" because that more closely represents the authentic and original name of people in the country called Kampuchea (the Khmer Empire in the past). The French changed the name *Kampuchea* to *Cambodia* during the colonial period. The term *Cambodian* continues to be used more commonly in the West. The Laotians in the United States consist of lowlander Laotian, highlander Hmong, middle-lander Mien, and Khmu (Cima 1989; Ross 1990; Savada 1995).

Asian Americans who have been in the United States for several generations and are well acculturated prefer to be referred to as Americans.

Culture, Spirituality, and Religion

Two distinct civilizations, the Chinese and the Indian, influence the majority of Asian Americans. The Chinese Confucian, Buddhist, and Taoist philosophies exert a strong influence on social, family, and individual values as well as on art, literature, and languages among Japanese, Korean, Vietnamese, Mien, and Hmong societies. The Japanese, Korean, and old Vietnamese (*chu nom*) scripts were derived from Chinese ideographs. The current Vietnamese romanized written language was not developed until the seventeenth century when French and Portuguese missionaries introduced it for use in evangelism (Cima 1989). The Mien and Hmong have no indigenous written script. They rely on oral history and tradition to transmit their culture from one generation to another. The Hmong use story quilts to keep their history. Their shamans keep their intellectual and cultural records in written Chinese characters (Ross 1990). Mien language has been romanized to written language since 1982, but the use of the romanized Mien language remains unpopular among the Mien Americans (Moore and Boehnlein 1991). The Cambodian and Laotian cultures are deeply rooted in Asian Indian civilization. The Cambodian written language is derived from Sanskrit script, and the Laotian use Pali script (Ross 1990; Savada 1995).

With regard to religion, most Chinese, Japanese, Korean, and Vietnamese worship their ancestors, follow Confucian teachings, and believe in Mahayana Buddhism. Many Japanese Americans follow Shintoism and Zen Buddhism. Most Filipino Americans are Catholic. More than 70% of Koreans in the United States are Protestant Christians (L.I.C. Kim 1993). Most Hmong and Mien believe in animistic and supernatural causes. The Cambodians and Laotians are followers of Brahmanism of the Hindus and Theravada Buddhism (Ross 1990; Savada 1995). Among Asian Indians, Hinduism is the major religion (Juthani 1992; Prathikanti 1997). The Pakistanis are mostly followers of Islam.

Hierarchy

Traditional Asian Americans strongly respect hierarchical order in family and society. It is crucial for the therapist to identify and show respect to the person who is head of the hierarchy in order to conduct family or group therapy. Most of the time the elder, grandfather, father, or oldest son is the one who makes decisions for the group. In the United States, family members develop different levels of acculturation. The younger member who is bilingual and bicultural or is the breadwinner may have more influence in family decision-making matters. Culturally, younger Asian Americans assert their influence behind the scenes to show their respect to elders. The wife will persuade her husband when they are alone. The son will discuss matters with the father separately, not in front of the family. Clinically, the patient may show respect to the therapist by not voicing objections to certain things but then may not carry out fully what has been discussed and agreed on in the session. The therapist should always ask the patient about adherence to treatment recommendations in a supportive and nonconfrontational manner with which the patient feels comfortable.

Asian Virtues (Modesty, Humility, Politeness)

Asian cultures are vastly diverse, yet they have in common the teaching that a person should be modest, humble, and polite. Individuals should put the needs of family and community first and live in harmony with others and nature. One should not speak first in the group, out of respect for hierarchy and the virtues of modesty and politeness. Traditional Asian American patients may look shy, passive, and anxious in therapy. They wait for the therapist to speak and provide guidance. Depending on their level of acculturation, Asian Americans need encouragement to participate in discussions. They express their own opinions when they feel safe and permitted to speak. The degree to which the Asian American patient spontaneously engages in conversation can be used to measure progress in therapy.

B. Cultural Explanations of the Individual's Illness

Asian Americans' health explanatory systems for illnesses and psychiatric disorders originate from their religious and spiritual beliefs. These beliefs are associated with their expressions of illness and health-seeking behaviors.

Traditional Healing Methods, Spiritual Healing, and Herbal Treatment

Substantial numbers of Asian Americans seek traditional treatment before coming to see Western doctors (U.S. Department of Health and Human Services 2001). The therapist should respect and ask about past and current traditional treatment. This is an opportunity to understand different methods of treatment from different cultures. The therapist's sincere effort to learn a different point of view will make the patient feel that the therapist is empathetic with his or her struggle to get well. A consultation with the spiritual healer, if necessary, can help in providing holistic spiritual, psychological, and biological care for the patient.

A large percentage of Asian Americans may use herbal medicine concurrently with Western medicine. The interactions between herbs and Western medicine have not been fully studied. Some of the herbs with atropine-like anticholinergic effects can cause anticholinergic psychosis, particularly when used simultaneously with tricyclic antidepressants or low-potency typical neuroleptics. Some of the herbs also interfere with the metabolism of psychotropic medications (K.M. Lin et al. 1997) (see Tables 6–9 and 6–10 in Chapter 6, "Ethnopsychopharmacology," in this volume). The therapist should obtain an herbal medication history and explain the possible adverse effects to the patient. If there is no issue of danger to self or others, it is prudent to give the patient an opportunity to choose to pursue one kind of treatment at a time to see which one works for him or her.

Idioms of Distress and Culture-Bound Syndromes

Idioms of Distress–Somatization. Asian cultures consider emotional expression as personal weakness and highly stigmatize mental illness (U.S. Department of Health and Human Services 2001). With the concept of unity of mind, body, and soul, Asian Americans express their psychological distress mostly through somatic complaints (Conrad and Pacquiao 2005; E.H.B. Lin et al. 1985; Mak and Zane 2004; Nguyen 1982). Exploring and clarifying somatic complaints helps the therapist understand the dynamics of emotional disturbance and stress. These somatic complaints should be examined and worked up thoroughly to rule out possible medical illness before proceeding with psychiatric treatment and therapy. Even if the results of the somatic workup are negative, the attention to somatic complaints will show the patient that the therapist can provide a total care treatment plan that includes mind and body. This will reinforce the therapeutic alliance and the patient's trust in the therapist.

For example, traditional Asian Americans may show their depression by complaining of severe, constant headaches, muscle aches, joint pains, backache, fatigue, low energy, dizziness, tired eyes, blurred vision, or confused and overwhelmed thoughts. Anxiety can also cause an increased frequency of urination, constipation, or diarrhea. Frustration, anger, or feelings of disgust can lead to repeated vomiting or complaints of a "hot stomach." It is not uncommon to hear the patient express anger or frustration as "my frustrated 'qi' is up to my chest"; these symptoms can cause shortness of breath and breathing difficulty even when a workup for chest pain reveals no organic cause. Somatic symptoms tend to be exacerbated at night, when the patient may have difficulty sleeping and has more time to think about the troubling issues.

Somatic manifestation can be interpreted according to the belief of integration of mind and body. As one patient said: "depression or distress penetrates painfully to all my muscles, joints, and deep to my bones. The stresses are so much that I feel overwhelmed, unable to think or to hear and to see clearly. The distresses are so heavy that I am exhausted of all my physical energy. I feel so weak, barely able to move my limbs."

Culture-Bound Syndromes. Asian Americans can also exhibit a variety of psychiatric syndromes that are strange to Western culture but are appropriate to their beliefs. These culture-bound syndromes will not be discussed in detail

Table 3–2. Culture-bound syndromes

Name	Country where seen	Characteristics
Amok	Southeast Asia	Acute display of rage or sudden outburst of aggressive and violent behaviors
Dhat	South Asia	Severe anxiety and hypochondriasis reaction, often leading to a discharge of semen, whitish coloration of urine, and feelings of weakness and exhaustion
Hwa-byung	Korea	Insomnia, indigestion, dyspnea, anxiety or panic attacks, feelings of impending death, feelings of a mass in the abdomen, somatic pain or aching
Koro	China and Southeast Asia	Fear that sexual organs and appendage are shrinking into their body, resulting from secondary symptoms of insomnia, restlessness, anxiety or panic attacks, paranoia, or a hallucinative state
Latah	Malaysia, Indonesia, Philippines, Thailand, Southeast Asia, Japan, and Mongolia	Hypersensitivity to being startled; reaction with echolalia, echopraxis, coprolalia, command obedience, and dissociative or trance-like behaviors
Qi-gong-induced psychosis	China	Improperly practiced qi-gong can cause severe headache, chest pain, abdominal pain, nocturnal emission, respiratory difficulty, anxiety, hallucination-like symptoms, mood disturbance, memory impairment, and thought disorder as well as autonomic, primitive, reflective movements, and emotional outbursts such as crying, laughing, shouting, or dancing.

Table 3–2. Culture-bound syndromes *(continued)*

Name	Country where seen	Characteristics
Shenjing shuairuo (neurasthenia)	China	Feelings of general weakness or fatigue accompanied by a variety of physical and mental symptoms, such as dizziness, gastrointestinal problems, sexual dysfunction, sleep disturbances, diffuse aches and pains, irritability, poor concentration, and memory loss
Taijin kyofusho	Japan	A variant of social phobia; the patient is self-conscious about his or her own manner, displays unreasonable fear of offending or displeasing other people, and is afraid of direct eye contact, blushing, giving off odor, or having an unpleasant facial expression or a poorly shaped physical feature.

Source. Akhtar 1988; Bernstein and Gaw 1990; Caiyun et al. 1988; Chang et al. 2005; Huaihai et al. 1988; Hughes et al. 1996; Kleinman 1986; K.M. Lin 1983; K.M. Lin et al. 1992; T.Y. Lin 1992; Ng 1999; Russell 1989; Tseng 2001a, 2001b; Tseng et al. 1988; Westermeyer 1973; Yamamoto 1992.

in this chapter. More information can be found in Table 3–2 and in Appendix I of DSM-IV-TR. (The Glossary of Culture-Bound Syndromes from Appendix I is reproduced in Appendix C of this volume.) The principle of evaluation and treatment in medicine and psychiatry is to do no harm and to prevent misdiagnosis and the use of inappropriate medication. Hence, culture-bound syndromes should be thoroughly evaluated and managed in the context of Asian American health beliefs.

Religion and Philosophy

Religion and spiritual philosophies have a strong influence on an Asian American's health beliefs and practices. A brief review of the relationship of health issues to religion and of Asian cultures is necessary to understand Asian American help-seeking behaviors. A brief summary can be found in Table 3–3.

Confucianism. Confucianism originated from the philosopher Confucius (Master K'ung, full name Ch'iu K'ung; 551–479 B.C.), in China. Confucian teaching developed a standard of a civil code of conduct that has deeply in-

Table 3–3. Religious philosophies

Religion	Beliefs	Clinical consequences
Confucianism	Reciprocity, benevolence, and filial piety, respect for authority, self-development, scholarship	Elder brother, parents may discourage patient from taking medications.
Buddhism	Human life is full of sorrows caused by family's deeds, one's own karma and expectations, or one's desires.	Patient accepts mental illness in a fatalistic manner and passively does nothing.
Taoism or the Way	Yin is the female energy, representing softness, darkness, and coldness. Yang is the male energy, representing strength, lightness, and heat. The balance is achieved by moving the vital energy qi (or chi).	Patient may seek alternative healing methods to balance qi.

fluenced the Chinese and the people of Korea, Japan, and Vietnam. Confucianism emphasizes reciprocity, benevolence, and filial piety, respect for authority, self-development, and scholarship. It advocates maintaining peace and harmony in society by practicing and respecting a hierarchical order. In the family, a woman should listen to her father until she marries, then to her husband after marriage, and to her son after her husband's death. At the national level, the people should respect the authority of the political leader, the teachings of the teacher, and the orders of the father. The community and familial needs are placed higher in priority than the individual's (D.D. Huang and Charter 1996). Traditional Asian Americans who follow Confucian teachings consider the therapist an authority figure and a teacher who will give them guidance to relieve their suffering or to help resolve their conflicts. At the same time, traditional Asian American families and patients deny or hide their mental illness because the bizarre, disorganized, impolite, and disruptive behaviors of the patient or family member in public will bring shame to the whole family.

Buddhism. Buddhism is one of the ancient religions. Founded in India about 2,500 years ago by Siddhartha Gautama, it has spread through China, Korea, Japan, and Southeast Asian countries. Buddhism holds that human life is full of sorrows and proceeds through stages of birth, age, sickness, and death. Suffering does not arise independently but comes through chains of causation due to the family's deeds, one's own karma and expectations, or one's desires. To free the self from life's cycle of suffering, one needs to follow Buddha's Four Noble Truths, to do good deeds and to give up desires, greed, ambitions, and high expectations (Canda and Phaobtong 1992). Asian Americans who practice Buddhism consider mental illness to be a suffering caused by one's own misdeeds in the past, by too much desire, or by the deeds and wills of dead ancestors. Buddhist beliefs can affect patients in several ways:

1. The mentally ill patient and his or her family feel shame and guilt that inhibits them from revealing the illness, because it could be perceived as indirect proof of wrongdoings in the past. Mental illness thus becomes a stigma of bad karma. The family and the patient will try to hide or to deny the illness.

2. The patient accepts mental illness as a punishment of past karma. The patient follows Buddha's teachings to cultivate good deeds and to lower or extinguish unrealistic desires or high ambitions.

3. The patient accepts mental illness in a fatalistic manner and passively does nothing.

Taoism or the Way. Taoism is a spiritual philosophy practiced and taught by Lao Tzu and his followers in China. It has strong influence in China, Korea, Japan, and Vietnam. Taoism is the way to achieve a peaceful, contented, everlasting life in harmony with nature. According to Taoism, the body is a microcosm of the universe that is governed by the balance of two principal forces: *yin,* the female energy, representing softness, darkness, and coldness; and *yang,* the male energy, representing strength, lightness, and heat. The balance is achieved by moving the vital energy *qi* (or *chi*) from one vital organ or site to another through a complex network of channels (*luo*), meridians (*jing*), and capillaries (*mai*) interlacing the entire body (D. Reid 1994). The imbalance of yin and yang or the blockage of qi causes illnesses.

The yin-yang theory is the foundation of traditional Chinese medicine, which advocates meditation, tai chi breathing and body movement exercises, and qi-gong breathing exercise that directs the qi to the appropriate paths to preserve good spiritual, mental, and physical health. Traditional Chinese treatment uses herbal medicine, food ingredients, or acupuncture to preserve, improve, or restore the balance of yin and yang in the body.

Hinduism and Ayurveda.   More than 80% of South Asians follow Hinduism, which is one of the most ancient religions, predating 3000 B.C. The Hindus believe in one god, Brahman, who is the origin of all existence, and follow the teachings of the Vedic scriptures (Vedas). They view physical and mental illnesses as caused by God's punishment, violation of religious doctrines, bad karma, or suffering of the spirit (Conrad and Pacquiao 2005). Suffering from the illness affects the whole triad of body, mind, and soul. Somatization in mental illness is considered as the body manifestation of the distress of the mind and soul.

Ayurveda (*ayur:* longevity; *veda:* knowledge) is a medical system that originated from Hinduism. The central concept of Ayurveda is that there are three vital humors in the body representing the three cosmic elements in the universe: breath for air or wind, bile for fire, and phlegm for water. Good health is the balance of this triad of vital humors and the harmony of mind, soul, and body with the natural environment and community. Ayurveda is still very popular among South Asians (Juthani 1992; Prathikanti 1997). Traditional therapies aim at keeping or correcting the delicate balance inside the body in harmony with outside forces of nature and conflicts in the community. Proper diet, breathing exercises, meditation, and yoga practices are the traditional methods to enrich the body humors' homeostasis and restore vital energy. Ayurveda's goals are to prevent illness, treat sickness, and rejuvenate the body for longevity.

Health Beliefs and Practices

Table 3–4 provides a brief summary of health beliefs and practices.

Naturalistic Beliefs.   Naturalistic theory is a common health belief among Chinese, Southeast Asians, and Filipinos. Health is considered the balance and harmony between the human body and natural forces. Changes in the weather or in the physical condition of the environment can cause physical and mental illnesses. The theory of "hot and cold" balance energy in the body and among vital organs is very similar to the yin and yang principles in Taoism. Eating excessive foods that have too much "hot" or "cold" energy will upset the balance in certain organs and cause illness. Frequent exposure to "bad, cold" wind or "damp, wet" environment will result in bad cold, fever, chills, or rheumatism. The naturalistic theory speculates that "bad wind" can penetrate into the body openings such as the mouth, ears, nose, and anal and gen-

Table 3–4.   Alternative beliefs and healing strategies

Belief system	Beliefs	Healing strategies
Naturalistic	Health is considered the balance and harmony between the human body and natural forces. Causes of illness can be changes in the weather, eating excessive foods that have too much "hot" or "cold" energy, frequent exposure to "bad, cold" wind or "damp, wet" environment, surgery, giving birth, or exhaustion due to overwork or stress. Therapy seeks to remove the "bad wind."	*Coining:* using a coin to scratch superficially on a certain area on the body until the skin turns deep red *Pinching:* traditional care provider uses fingers to pinch the skin in sensitive areas until a contusion occurs *Cupping:* applying heated cups on the back, forehead, or abdomen *Moxibustion:* using burning incense or combustible herbs to cause superficial small burns on the torso, head, and neck
Animism	Illness is attributed to the punishment of the gods, ancestor spirits, evil spirits, or the loss of one's soul.	A shaman will perform specific ceremonies to ask for forgiveness from the gods and/or ancestors and to chase the evil spirits away or call one's soul back to the body.
Ayurveda	Three vital humors in the body represent the three cosmic elements in the universe: breath for air or wind, bile for fire, and phlegm for water.	Proper diet, breathing exercises, meditation, and yoga practices are the traditional methods to enrich the body humors' homeostasis and restore vital energy.

ital orifices. The body becomes more vulnerable to "bad wind" after surgery, giving birth, or exhaustion due to overwork or stress.

Several traditional methods of treatment using naturalistic theory common among Asian Americans include coining, pinching, cupping, and moxibustion.

- *Coining* is the practice of using a coin or similar dull-edged object (e.g., a silver coin or ceramic soup spoon) to scratch superficially on a certain area on the body until the skin turns deep red (i.e., develops petechiae) to get the "bad wind" out of the body. The deeper the redness on the skin, the more "bad wind" has been released from the body. Coining is applied mostly on the back, along the intercostal spaces on both sides of the spine, or at the back of the neck.
- *Pinching* is similar to coining. The traditional care provider uses fingers to pinch the skin in sensitive areas until a contusion occurs, indicating that the "bad wind" has been removed or released.
- *Cupping* is a method of applying heated cups on the back, forehead, or abdomen to suck out the "bad wind."
- *Moxibustion* is a method of treatment that uses burning incense or combustible herbs to cause superficial small burns on the torso, head, and neck to remove the "bad wind."

Animism.   Animism is popular among rural Laotians, Hmong, Cambodians, and Vietnamese (Aronson 1987; Westermeyer 1988). Animists believe that human beings, animals, and inanimate objects all possess souls and spirits. Illness is attributed to the punishment of the gods, ancestor spirits, evil spirits, or the loss of one's soul. Traditional treatment will involve calling on the assistance of a shaman, who is knowledgeable in how to discover the causes of the illness, and then performing specific ceremonies to ask for forgiveness from the gods and/or ancestors and to chase the evil spirits away or call one's soul back to the body.

Pacific Islanders' View of Health and Illness.   Native Hawaiians believe that the psyche and the body are inseparable, and they believe that good health is the harmonic integration of the person with the natural and spiritual worlds. The disturbance of these balances causes physical or mental illnesses.

Samoans believe in germ theory for certain diseases. They also think that overwork, lack of sleep, exposure to bad weather, or "bad blood" is the cause of physical illness. Samoans value close relationships in their family and responsibility in their community. They attribute serious illnesses to interpersonal conflicts in the family or among friends or to violation of social laws or God's laws (Cook 1983).

C. Cultural Factors Related to Psychosocial Environment and Levels of Functioning

Despite the vast diversity in origins, immigration history, degree of acculturation, socioeconomic status, and level of education of different Asian American subgroups, these groups' family structures and developmental processes share traditional values that are rooted in agricultural and feudal cultures and in Eastern religions and philosophies.

Family Structure

Asian American families appear to occupy a high place in the socioeconomic structure of the United States. Taken as a whole, they have higher median household income ($52,626) than all other U.S. ethnic groups ($42,409), due to a combination of higher educational achievement and having more household members in the labor force. As individuals, however, Asian Americans have an average per capita income that is similar to the national average (U.S. Census Bureau 2003). These statistics show that even in the United States, Asian Americans continue to remain in extended-family households where several generations live together under the same roof.

In a traditional extended Asian family, the hierarchy of authority is very important and is established according to age, sex, and order of birth. A male elder, usually a grandfather, father, or oldest son, assumes responsibility as a breadwinner and protector of the family; he makes most of the important family decisions. The older children are expected to assume more responsibility in helping their parents and in caring for younger siblings. Family members are interdependent and supportive of each other until an individual becomes self-sufficient. The family structure mirrors the teaching of filial piety, which expects children to obey and respect their parents and elders and to provide care for their parents in their old age (E. Lee 1996). It is common to see the adult Asian American settling down near his or her extended family to maintain family ties and to provide support to siblings and parents. The degrees of acculturation and education of family members affect how the traditional family evolves to adopt different values in Western culture.

Intergenerational Conflicts

Clinically, examples of intergenerational conflicts are evident when parents enforce strict traditional values while children adapt to American values of individualism, autonomy, assertiveness, and open communication. Such conflicts are seen most often with adolescents, as discussed later in this chapter. Intergenerational conflicts are much less pronounced in families where parents have been well acculturated or assimilated to American culture and in Asian American families that have been in the United States for several generations. Recently, there has been an increase in the number of successful Asian American interracial families. Family problems can arise if there are conflicts about racial and cultural values, communication styles, and child-rearing issues (Crohn 1997; E. Lee 1996).

Developmental Issues

Asian American Children.　Although traditional Asian American families prefer male children because they can carry on the surname of the family, highly acculturated and bicultural Asian American families value male and female children equally. In addition to the parents, other extended family members play a prominent role in providing love and care for the child. In return, children are taught to respect and listen to the elders in the family and to keep the tradition of filial piety. Children learn to honor the family's name by showing good behavior in the family and community. Values such as high achievement, hard work, responsibility, obedience, respect, and filial obligation are encouraged and praised. Problematic behaviors such as aggression, antisocial behaviors, disobedience, irresponsibility, and poor performance in school bring shame to the family. Modesty is encouraged, to the point that even though Asian American parents are proud of their children's academic achievement, they rarely praise them directly. Thus, children are taught to be humble instead of arrogant; the rationale is that the less the praise, the harder the children will strive for higher achievements. Such traditional expectations by parents living in the United States put tremendous stress on Asian American children. Fear of failure, starting with academic failure at an early age, leads to guilt, shame, self-blame, and low self-esteem (Chung 1997).

Asian American Adolescents.　During adolescence, Asian Americans often face the double stresses of living up to family traditional expectations at home and having to adapt to Western cultural values at school. These diverging cultural expectations can cause identity crises for youths. Examples of possible reactions to these dual stresses include 1) marginalization and alienation from both Asian and American cultures, as seen in some gang members, 2) withdrawal into Asian culture and rejection of the American culture, and 3) acculturation to American culture and rejection of Asian traditional values. Adolescents who are able to overcome these stresses and integrate well in both cultures will eventually become the liaison for the family with the outside society. Parents depend on these children to provide interpretation and assistance to obtain health care, welfare, and social supports. This role reversal not only gives the children who are bilingual/bicultural more participation in family decision-making processes, it also puts more burdens on the youth, in addition to the stresses of growing up and schooling. Often, conflicts and stresses from attempting to adapt to both cultures can result in poor academic performance, dropping out of school, using drugs, joining a gang, or running away from home (L.N. Huang 1997).

Special attention should be given to Southeast Asian children who have experienced the trauma of forced labor, starvation, uprooting, separation, and loss of family. These Southeast Asian children and adolescents show a high prevalence of depression and posttraumatic stress disorder (PTSD) symptoms, making the acculturation process particularly challenging for them and their families (E. Hsu et al. 2004; Kinzie et al. 1986, 1989; Sack and Clarke 1996).

Asian American Young Adults.   Asian American young adults face the stress of compromising personal independence and family obligation. Besides having high academic achievement expectations, they have to make a career choice, build a social life, choose their friends and partnerships, and find a marriage partner. In addition, they face stress caused by racism and discrimination in school and at work (Wong and Mock 1997).

Asian American Elderly.   Traditionally in Asian society, the elderly are respected for their lifelong contributions to the family and the community, as well as revered for their life experiences. The family and community take their words of advice very seriously. Whereas in America old age is associated with conservatism, noncreativity, nonproductivity, and dependency, it is regarded as a sign of distinction, deserving of respect, in Asian culture; hence Asian American adults continue to seek the advice of the elderly, even those far advanced in age.

Attention should be paid to Asian Americans who came to the United States in the 1920s to work as railroad and mining laborers, who faced the greatest amount of brazen racism and discrimination. They tended to live in ethnic Chinese enclaves well into their old age without adequate health care and welfare support (Chen 1976; Kao and Lam 1997). Unlike these men, the Asian Americans who came to the United States in the latter decades of the twentieth century brought along their children. As the children grew into adulthood, they became more acculturated and served as intermediaries in helping their elderly parents adjust to Western culture; issues of intergenerational gap are less prominent among this group. In contrast, Asian American elders who were sponsored to come to America by their immigrant children often find the intergenerational gap too wide to bridge, and traditional expectations clash with Western values on a regular basis, leading to stress on both adult children and elderly parents (Kao and Lam 1997; Leong and Lau 2001).

Gender Issues

Asian American Women.   In most Asian societies, women have a lower status than men. Asian women often assume responsibilities for domestic affairs, providing love and caring for the whole family. They are expected to be modest, supportive, and protective. Women sacrifice their personal needs for the success of their husbands and children. Asian American immigrant women face a host of cultural challenges that can lead to stress. In addition to the stress of learning a new language and culture, many women work outside the home to support the family financially. Exposure to Western values of independence and individual rights, along with their discovery of self-worth, can lead them to be more confident and outspoken in the home. These values often clash with Asian traditional values, particularly in cases where women are the main breadwinners for the family, essentially reversing roles with the men. The role reversal may cause a shift of domestic power and a strain in the marital relationship that can lead to domestic violence (Homma-True 1997; Masaki and Wong 1997).

Immigrant women from Southeast Asia, who have experienced uprooting from their countries, death of family members, separation, abuse, and other kinds of war trauma, face tremendous adjustment problems. Severe chronic PTSD and depression are particularly pronounced among this group (E. Hsu et al. 2004; Rozee and Van Boemel 1989). U.S.-born Asian American women do not have to deal with the stress of cultural adjustment; nevertheless, they still have to struggle with racism, sexism, and discrimination on a daily basis.

They have to overcome dual negative stereotypes: the submissive, passive, helpless, and obedient woman and the stereotypical "dragon lady" who is evil and untrustworthy. Cultural differences and stereotypes lead to many problems for Asian American women who have interracial marriages, particularly in issues related to communication, childrearing, and coping with in-laws (Homma-True 1997).

Asian American Gays and Lesbians. Homosexuality has been documented in Chinese, Japanese, Filipino, and Asian Indian literatures, but the concept of same-sex relationship has been discouraged in all Asian cultures (Nakajima et al. 1996). Homosexuality is considered to go against several Asian religions and philosophies. A same-sex relationship does not fit into Confucian family hierarchical order and traditional gender roles in society. A traditional Asian woman is supposed to get married and to bear children. Traditional expectations for an Asian man, especially an eldest son, are to get married and have children, especially sons, to carry on the family name. Asian American gays and lesbians face tremendous parental pressure to fulfill their traditional roles (Aoki 1997). A homosexual relationship is considered to be sexual lust in Buddhism, a breach of the harmonious balance of yin and yang in Taoism, and a sin in Christianity. Traditional Asian parents often make gay and lesbian children feel guilty about their sexual orientation. They disapprove of homosexual life styles and consider a same-sex relationship a shame to the family's name. Asian American gays and lesbians face tremendous obstacles in overcoming family bias and traditional societal discrimination to "come out" (Nakajima et al. 1996).

D. Cultural Elements of the Relationship Between the Individual and the Clinician

Stereotypes, cultural health beliefs, and culture-based role expectations can influence the interaction between the patient and the therapist, regardless of cultural similarity. The use of the biopsychosocial model as a standard therapy model needs to be tailored appropriately to patients from Asian cultures to provide effective treatment.

Expectations of Mental Health Practitioners

Assimilated Asian Americans tend to seek mental help at earlier signs of distress than do traditional Asian Americans. Most traditional Asian Americans and their families seek advice from elders in the family or in the community or from friends or relatives and look for traditional treatment first. They seek Western health care as a last resort, when the patient shows inappropriate or dangerous behavioral problems or the family is unable to care for him or her. Often they hesitate to get help sooner because of the stigma of mental illness as well as the fear that Western medications are too strong and not as "natural" as herbal medicine (Barry and Mizrahi 2005; Conrad and Pacquiao 2005; Tracy et al. 1986; Westermeyer et al. 1983; Ying and Miller 1992).

Most traditional Asian American patients who have made the decision to come to the clinic or hospital expect to get treatment with medication. However, therapists must consider several cultural issues in the psychopharmacological treatment of Asian American patients, especially recent immigrants and those who remain closely tied to traditional health practices. Traditionally oriented Asian patients expect medication to relieve their symptoms in a short period of time. Psychotropic medications will not be considered as "good" medication unless there are immediate therapeutic effects. Thus, it is important to explain at the beginning of treatment that psychotropic medications take several weeks to build up and to exert their maximal effect. The psychiatrist should also tell the patient which target symptoms can be expected to improve. Involving the patient in understanding the treatment and monitoring the target symptoms will increase the patient's feeling of control and participation and assist in the patient's adherence with the treatment.

Traditional Asian American patients believe that Western medicines are synthetic chemical substances or pure essences of herbs that are too strong for their smaller bodies and can cause severe side effects. Several studies have shown that Asian Americans require lower doses of antipsychotics and antidepressants to achieve therapeutic effects (K.M. Lin and Finder 1983; K.M. Lin and Shen 1991; K.M. Lin et al. 1989, 1993). The average textbook dosages can be too large, and they can cause severe side effects. Patients or family members will often reduce the dose or stop the medication if the patient experiences uncomfortable side effects. To avoid unnecessary side effects, the dose should initially be as low as possible, then be slowly and gradually increased until therapeutic effects are obtained. To ensure adherence with treatment, the most common side effects of the medication should be explained clearly at the patient's level of understanding. Incorporation of cultural beliefs, such as "hot" and "cold" theory, in the explanation will greatly increase the patient's trust and compliance.

Table 3–5. Common beliefs about medications and strategies

Traditional belief	Strategy to approach belief
They are too strong	Prescribe small doses
They should act immediately	Inform about duration of effect
They are not needed after the symptoms are gone	Inform of chronic nature of illness
They are not "hot" or "cold"	Explain by using terms "hot" and "cold"

Traditionally oriented Asian American patients think of psychiatric pharmacotherapy as similar to medical pharmacological treatment. They expect immediate alleviation of psychiatric symptoms and eventually a cure of their illnesses. They will stop taking the medication once their psychiatric symptoms have improved. It is important to explain to patients the chronic nature of mental illnesses and the need for long-term treatment and follow-up. The clinician should discuss in an open manner the limitation of current psychopharmacotherapy in the treatment of mental illnesses and encourage participation in other psychosocial treatment modalities that can provide additional improvement of symptoms. See Table 3–5 for a summary of medication beliefs that could lead to nonadherence and strategies to address them.

Psychosocial approaches are quite strange to traditional Asian Americans, who rarely hear of "talk therapy." Because of the cultural differences, traditional Asian American patients find it difficult to believe that their symptoms will be improved by talking out their problems. They see their therapists as having different expectations than typical Western psychotherapy goals, which are to listen and guide patients to their own solution—contrary to these patients' expectations that the therapist will tell them what they should do (the authoritarian model).

- They respect the therapist as an authority figure, a knowledgeable expert who can understand their physical and emotional disturbances based on an examination, laboratory tests, and verbal and nonverbal expressions, without much detailed questioning.
- They expect the therapist to make an accurate diagnosis of their problems and then suggest a clear, reasonable course of treatment for them and their family to follow. They will doubt the therapist's capability if the therapist,

out of respect for individualism and freedom of choice, keeps asking them, "What do you want to do?" Their thought process is, "I have sought help from you as a last resort, and if I knew what to do I would not come to therapy to seek help."

- They expect the therapist to act as an authority figure who has power to judge and to solve their interpersonal conflicts or family problems.
- They expect the therapist to provide information and to advocate for their social welfare entitlements.

Knowledge of Asian Americans' health beliefs and expectations can lead to a more culturally appropriate approach that will increase the likelihood of patients' involvement and the maintenance of their treatment.

Clinical Methods

Initial Contact.   Most traditional Asian Americans present themselves as polite, anxious, and shy in the first contact. To show respect for the authority of the therapist, they will wait quietly and patiently for the therapist to initiate the session. They will rarely ask questions because they expect to be under the care of a capable expert who can understand their problems and provide suitable treatment. A limited, self-revealing introduction of the therapist's credentials, experience, and familiarity with the patient's life experiences, situation, or problems can help to gain the patient's trust in therapy. In the initial session, the therapist should educate the patient about the medication treatment course and the therapy process, and encourage the patient's participation. A calm, gentle, and supportive approach will put patients at ease and build up the therapeutic alliance for successful later sessions.

Expectations about personal appearance: Traditional Asian Americans place very high value on the therapist as an authority figure. They expect the therapist to appear clean, confident, and organized. Patients are unlikely to show their trust and bring up their problems if the therapist looks untidy or acts improperly (Marsella 1993).

Styles of Communication.   Asian Americans' styles of communication are very diverse. Well-acculturated Asian Americans can be more direct, whereas traditional Asian Americans tend to use more metaphors and more nonverbal communication.

Verbal communication: Verbal communication is crucial in counseling and psychotherapy. Asian Americans' verbal communication styles are strongly influenced by their cultural practice of hierarchy, modesty, and harmony in life. Communication style is correlated to their level of assimilation and acculturation.

- Listening. Asian cultures do not encourage individuals' overt expression of thoughts and feelings. For traditional Asians, showing feelings could be interpreted as weakness or a loss of self-control. Traditional Asian Americans listen to their elders in the family and to authority figures in their community. They are modest in voicing their opinions when being asked by others, particularly those more senior or having higher status. In therapy, traditional Asian American patients revere the authority of the therapist and consider the therapist an expert with profound wisdom and high education. They tend to respond passively to questions rather than to actively express their feelings or complain about their discomforts. They expect the therapist to ask the proper questions and to address their problems, instead of directly telling the therapist their problems immediately. They show their respect by using a low voice to answer the therapist's questions. Hence, the therapist's gentle and empathetic speaking tone and nonconfrontational approach will help patients to feel at ease and secure in therapy.

- Silence. Asian tradition teaches individuals to live in harmony with nature, with family, with community, and in interpersonal relationships. Confrontation is discouraged, especially with authority figures and in public places. Disagreement or embarrassment should be expressed discreetly, or in some cases through a mediator. Contrary to Western communication, where no objection means agreement, the traditional Asian American patient's silence can be a nonconfrontational way of expressing disagreement. The therapist should be gentle and patient in exploring the patient's stance on the issues on which patient and therapist disagree, as indicated by the patient's silence.

- Metaphors. While the use of metaphors exists in both the West and the East, Asians place a particularly strong emphasis on the use of literary metaphors, fables, fairy tales, religious stories, and ethical scenarios to teach people culturally appropriate conduct and ways of life. These metaphors are further enforced by a history of strong oral tradition that passes these stories from one generation to another. To apply these Asian stories as an analogy to clarify the patient's conflicts and to suggest guidance is an effective method to communicate with Asian patients in an indirect and nonconfrontational way.

Nonverbal communication: To traditional Asian Americans, nonverbal communication is as important as verbal communication. Nonverbal behaviors are used to express emotions, feelings, and thoughts discreetly and politely without showing weakness or confrontation. Following are some examples of common nonverbal communication among Asians.

- Eye contact. Direct eye contact is considered disrespectful to another person who is of equal status or of higher status and authority because it conveys a message of challenge. Asian parents use a stare or a stern glance to express their disapproval or disappointment to their children in public instead of verbally scolding them. In therapy, traditional Asian Americans will avoid eye contact to show respect to the therapist. They will glance occasionally toward the therapist to indicate interest and attention to the conversation. Intensely staring at an Asian American patient can cause feelings of anxiety, fear, and discomfort.
- Physical contact. To show their respect for hierarchy and authority, Asian American patients keep some distance from the therapist. A gentle gesture of the therapist to invite the patient to take a seat is enough to make him or her feel at ease. A young patient will politely wait for the therapist to sit first. The therapist should show respect to elder patients by insisting that they be seated first. Shaking hands, as a Western gesture of greeting, sometimes makes traditional Asian Americans feel uncomfortable; it is more acceptable to male than to most female Asian American patients.

Biological Treatment Approach.   Traditional Asian Americans who take herbal medicine consider Western biological treatment methods unnatural and too potent. To ensure a culturally appropriate biological approach, the therapist should acknowledge the patient's concerns about the strong effects of the Western medication. The therapist should explain to the Asian American patient how the medication will improve and change the chief complaints or target symptoms, but that results will not be immediate and may take weeks. The medication should be started at the lowest dosage and gradually increased to a therapeutic dosage to avoid overdosing and unwanted side effects. Information concerning side effects should be given to the patient and discussed at his or her level of understanding. The therapist should suggest measures that help patients to cope with these uncomfortable side effects. Incorporating the patient's health beliefs, such as "hot" and "cold" theory, in explanation of the medication and side effects will increase the patient's trust of and adherence to treatment recommendations. The therapist must pay attention to somatic pain complaints and provide an appropriate workup and symptomatic treatment to relieve the symptom temporarily while waiting for the psychotropic medications to take effect. When the patient has improved, the therapist should remind the patient to continue with medication because of the chronic nature of mental illness.

Mr. K.N. is a 51-year-old Vietnamese American man who has had diagnoses of major depression and posttraumatic stress disorder. He had been seen by several clinics and doctors but did not stay in treatment for long with anyone. He described several years' history of depressed mood, insomnia, muscle aches, joint pain, backaches, general weakness, feeling cold, poor concentration, and low energy. He had been unemployed for 12 years since he and his family settled in America. His wife reported that he would wake up at night because of vivid nightmares of a scene of the atrocities in concentration camps or combat. He would hear the sounds of guns, airplanes, voices of Communists shouting and of dead soldiers and friends; yet he had told no one because he was afraid that they would think of him as "crazy." The patient believed that "cold wind" had infiltrated his body because while in the army he frequently slept on the damp, wet ground, and while in the concentration camps he had to do hard labor and did not have enough clothing to keep him warm. After evaluation, the therapist explained his findings and treatment as follows:
"Mr. K.N., I agree with your belief that your symptoms are probably caused by severe 'bad cold wind or energy' that has been penetrating into your body for so long. The symptoms that you are suffering are what we call posttraumatic stress disorder and major depressive disorder. It is very fortunate that you survived your battles in the war and the Communist concentration camps. However, these horrible experiences in the war and the concentration camps can have a forceful impact and cause traumatic shocks to your brain and mind. You must have been very strong to survive for all these years to bring your family to America. Now you and I have to fight these symptoms

together. I am going to prescribe to you a low dose of risperidone to reduce the voices and noises and gradually make them go away. I will give you paroxetine to make you feel less depressed, have more energy, and be able to concentrate better. I will also give you trazodone to help you sleep better at night. When you have a headache, muscle ache, or backache you can take acetaminophen for pain. The medications that I give you have 'hot energy' qualities [most anticholinergic effects are considered as 'hot energy' qualities]; they may cause dry mouth, constipation, dizziness, and palpitations. You will need to drink a lot of water to counteract these effects and to help the 'hot energy' spread throughout the body. The 'hot energy' medications are good for you because they will balance the 'bad, cold energy' that caused your illness. I can assure you that you are not 'crazy.' Your illness can be treated but it requires patience and perseverance. I wish I had the 'magic pills' that work immediately, but our science has its limitations. The medication that I give you will work, but slowly. It takes 4 to 6 weeks or longer to see its maximal effects. You will see the effects of the medication to help you sleep better in 3 to 4 days, but your mood and other symptoms will take a longer time to improve. Please be patient with yourself, and with me. We will work together to monitor your symptoms closely and to adjust your medication dosage carefully to prevent unnecessary side effects. I will see you again in 2 weeks; please call me if you have any concerns about your medication or illness."

Mr. K.N. told his wife that he thought the "doctor of the head" had been able to understand his illness. He was glad to know that he was not "crazy" because that thought has bothered him for so long. He took his medication daily and kept his return appointment 2 weeks later.

Psychological Approach.   Western psychodynamic concepts have been found to be foreign to traditional Asian concepts of medicine, where mind, body, and soul are inseparable. Western psychology, based on Western culture, emphasizes individualism, freedom of choice, and mastery of nature. Asian culture emphasizes the values of the extended family group, acceptance of one's own fate due to one's karma, and living in harmony with nature (Kinzie 1978; Kinzie and Fleck 1987). Furthermore, traditional Asian virtues of self-control, humility, and loss of face (loss of reputation) to self and family make it difficult for Asian Americans to talk about their mental problems. Because of these differences, traditional Asian Americans find it hard to reveal their conflicts and difficult to believe that "talk" therapy will relieve their symptoms or help to solve their problems.

Several methods of therapy have been proposed to work with Asian Americans. J. Hsu and Tseng (1972) suggested a problem-solving approach, while

S.C. Kim (1983) advocated for an Eriksonian hypnotic framework for Asian Americans, and Tang (1997) advised psychoanalytic psychotherapy. Asian Americans can benefit from a combination of different approaches if therapists are able to flexibly apply traditional Asian health beliefs and philosophies of life in therapy. At the early stages of therapy when the patient finds it difficult to open up to a stranger, it is appropriate to use supportive, problem-oriented therapy where the therapist is actively engaged in identifying the problems and providing support and guidance in solving conflicts. This approach matches the Asian American patient's expectation that the therapist will be an authority, expert, and teacher. The therapist should work to build trust and a therapeutic alliance to allow deeper exploration of interpersonal or family conflicts. Then the therapist will have the flexibility to take a directive approach to provide psychoeducation and to teach the patient certain cognitive-behavioral techniques for correction of maladaptive behaviors. Employment of Asian cultural relaxation techniques that advocate integration of body and mind are familiar to and readily accepted by Asian Americans.

Culturally accepted methods such as sitting-meditation or walking-meditation, yoga, qi-gong, and tai chi exercises are very helpful to reduce stress, anxiety, and depression. Gentle inquiries to clarify the conflicts in a nonjudgmental and nonconfrontational manner will help stimulate the patient to gain insights without feeling embarrassment or shame. The therapist can employ an indirect approach using metaphors, fables, Buddhist or Zen religious stories, proverbs, or sayings from Confucius and ancient sages to stimulate thinking or to unearth the unconscious conflicts. The technique and art of teaching by using metaphors, stories to "wake up" the students' unconscious thoughts and help them reach enlightenment, have been widespread in Asian religious, literature, and philosophical training.

Here are two Zen stories that are used to show different patients that their thoughts affect their mood and actions. The message in the first is that if the patient can free his thoughts, he can achieve peaceful emotion.

C.L. is a 49-year-old Chinese American with a diagnosis of bipolar affective disorder who has been stabilized on lithium for several years. However, he quickly feels irritable and angry at home and at work whenever someone does or says things that he dislikes. He takes trivial matters personally and feels miserable, angry, and upset for a long time. His therapist offers him the following Zen story to help him let go of his unpleasant emotions:

"One morning after the spring rain, two Zen monks took a walk out of the temple to enjoy the fresh air and beautiful scenery. On their way, they saw a pretty young girl, lovely in a new light pink kimono. She looked anxious and hesitant beside the street that had become muddy after the rain. One monk asked her what was wrong and whether he could help. She replied that she would like to cross the street but was afraid that she would ruin her new kimono. He offered to carry her to the other side of the street. With her consent, he lifted her up and held her in his arms to walk across the street. The girl thanked him and happily hurried on her way. Both monks went on to enjoy the spring scenes and sounds.

"After more than an hour, the other monk seemed very annoyed and could not hold his disturbing thoughts any longer, he asked: 'Brother, I have been thinking about what happened. We are not supposed to touch women. How could you hold her in your arms?' His friend turned to him and said: 'Oh, brother! While I think you have been enjoying the smell of fresh air, sounds of birds, scenes of flowers, green grass, and beautiful butterflies on our walk, you have been preoccupied with unpleasant thoughts. I did a good deed to help a little girl. My mind is clean and happy. You see, I put her down in one minute after we crossed the street, but you have carried her in you for more than an hour!'"

The therapist's interpretation could be stated as: "I hope you will think about this story whenever you think that someone or something has made you angry for a long time, because it isn't them but rather your prolonged preoccupation that has disturbed and bothered you."

L.P. is a 25-year-old Chinese American male student who was referred to therapy for his drug abuse problems. The therapist told him this story to imply indirectly that the patient needed to be responsible for his treatment:

"Once, there was a young man who accidentally fell into an abandoned well. He yelled loudly for help. The villagers ran over and formed a human chain to rescue him. They were short just an arm's length of reaching him. They called him to extend his arm to grasp the hand so they could pull him up. If he reached out to them, he would live, but if he waited until they could reach him, he probably would have to wait forever and would be dead."

For this story, the therapist's interpretation could be stated as: "Do you see that your family, relatives, and friends, all wanted to help you? Now it is up to you whether to grasp their hands or not."

Asian Americans, especially Southeast Asians, who suffer from posttraumatic stress disorder cannot tolerate confrontational insight-oriented therapy, which can increase anxiety and exacerbate their symptoms. Research from the Indochinese Refugee Clinic in Oregon (Kinzie et al. 1980), the Indochinese Psychiatric Clinic in Boston (Mollica and Lavelle 1988), and New South Wales Service for the Treatment and Rehabilitation of Torture and Trauma Survivors (STARTTS) (J. Reid et al. 1990) showed that Asian PTSD patients will benefit from a multimodal, supportive, activity-oriented combination of individual and group therapy. Asian American patients with PTSD will feel safe and less anxious in supportive, cultural activity-oriented groups where they can relate to others who encountered the same traumatic experiences and have suffered similar PTSD symptoms. Working together on small projects where they can feel worthy, contribute to the group, and be productive will help their self-esteem. The safe and empathetic environment of the activity-oriented groups will facilitate verbal communication among group members, who can safely recall their trauma and express their sufferings under the supervision and guidance of group therapists.

Social Approach. In Asian cultures, the individual is closely tied to family and community. Thus, the involvement of family and use of supportive community resources are critical in therapy.

Family involvement: In a family meeting, the therapist should identify the authority figure or the decision maker in the family, who will most likely be an elder, father, oldest son. Gaining trust from the decision maker is crucial in asserting the therapist's authority appropriately in conducting the meeting. E. Lee (1997b) proposed a structured, time-limited, problem-solving psychoeducational approach to solve family conflicts, to help the family understand the patient's symptoms and needs, and to provide information to the family about community resources.

Community supports: Social support in the community is very important for the Asian American patient and family. The Chinese have created several support systems based on the same language dialect (e.g., Fukienese Association, Hakka Association) or the same surname (e.g., Lee Association, Wu Association, Yee Association). The Vietnamese have organized mutual associations of people who came from the same province or school alumni association. The Laotians and Cambodians have developed their support systems around their Buddhist temples (Canda and Phaobtong 1992). Protestant Koreans and Catholic Vietnamese have relied on their churches for support. Therapists should encourage patients to go to temples or churches, to participate in cultural activities, traditional holidays, and ceremonies. These activities are helpful to give patients a sense of belonging, to help them regain social functioning, and to increase the meaningfulness of their life.

Therapy Issues.   Working with Asian Americans requires an understanding and respect of their ethnocultural and health beliefs. Several therapy issues and several stereotypes need to be considered in therapy.

Ethnic psychopharmacology: Recent pharmacokinetic and pharmacogenetic studies on the enzyme system of cytochrome P450 (CYP) polymorphism show that some Asian Americans are slow metabolizers of psychotropic medication because they have low amounts or a deficiency of enzyme activities, mostly of isoenzymes CYP2D6 and CYP2C19. This leads to a high serum concentration of psychotropics in some Asian Americans and can cause severe side effects. This issue is discussed in detail in Chapter 6.

Taboo issues: Asian Americans do not want to reveal problems of the group members to outsiders. They practice tolerance and nonconfrontation to live in harmony with others. The therapist needs to be aware of several types of unmentionable issues that the patient will not bring up spontaneously:

- Family conflicts. Family members suppress family conflicts to save the face and name of the whole family. It is more difficult to bring up conflicts if they involve elders—for example, those between wife and mother-in-law, children and parents, or wife and husband.
- Intergenerational differences. Asian Americans acculturate at a variety of different rates depending on age, age at arrival, how long they have lived in the United States, socioeconomic status, family structure, and level of education. In general, the younger children learn a foreign language more easily and acculturate faster. The wife may need to go out to work to support the family while her husband still struggles to find a job. Elders who come to the United States to reunite with their children's family may still keep all the traditions of the old countries, which are quite different from the children's and grandchildren's experiences in America. Highly educated individuals may have more advantages that help them to acculturate faster. Different levels of acculturation can create role reversal of the hierarchy. The grandfather or father might depend on the grandchildren or

children for support and connection to outside communities and resources where the family can obtain social, economic, and legal assistance. Husbands might depend on wives who have now become principal breadwinners for the family.

- Domestic violence. Domestic violence is common and tolerated in several Asian cultures. A generation gap, the stress of adaptation, and role reversal can easily break the husband's tolerance. The wife and children can become scapegoats and hence the objects of domestic violence. Domestic violence can be carried out psychologically by verbal abuse, threats to harm, intimidation, and degradation, or physically by hitting, beating, and keeping family members hostage in the house. In some cases the husband's entire family abuses the wife and treats her as a domestic slave. The family or the husband holds the children as hostages and keeps the wife's identification and passport to prevent her from leaving. Families have kept domestic violence a family secret for fear of shame, losing face in the community, and repercussions (Masaki and Wong 1997).

- Homosexuality. As discussed earlier in the gender issues section, it is very difficult for the Asian American patient and family to bring up homosexuality issues in therapy. Asian American gays, lesbians, and their families need tremendous support to come to terms with same-sex relationships and lifestyles (Nakajima et al. 1996).

- Youth delinquency. Asian Americans value their children and place great value on their education. Teaching children is the responsibility of the entire extended family. Youth delinquency goes against the family teaching and hierarchy and causes pain and shame to the extended family. The family might consult elders to enforce discipline and mobilize relatives to "reform" the delinquent. Having the adolescent go to counseling or therapy is the last resort. Asian youth usually join an Asian gang in search of a substitute for the traditional hierarchical structure that somehow has become dysfunctional because of the acculturation stress (Landre et al. 1997; Le 2002).

- Substance abuse. Substance abuse is another secret to keep in the Asian American family. The family tends to minimize the abuse and discreetly ask for help from trusted elders and relatives to talk to and reform the substance abuser. Drug abuse therapy is the last consideration and is turned to only after the family cannot care for the substance abuser or if the person becomes violent or suicidal (Ja and Aoki 1993; Nemoto et al. 1999).

Alcohol consumption has a long history in Asian cultures. Confucian teachings and Taoism accept moderate use of alcohol at home and in ceremonies. In Japan and Korea, heavy or social alcohol consumption is considered the norm. Alcohol drinking and abuse are tolerated in Asian communities. Asian Americans seldom think of seeking help for problem drinking.

- Gambling. Gambling is a problem to many Asian American families. Whether it is pathological gambling, which causes big financial losses, or impulsive gambling, a gambling problem is considered shameful but is tolerated in the family. The family rarely mentions it or asks for help, probably because gambling involves mostly Asian American males and heads of the family. Gambling behavior and financial loss causes stress to the family members that can lead to a disruption of familial hierarchy, separation, or divorce (Petry et al. 2003).

Stereotypes: Interaction in therapy between the Asian American patient and the therapist who have different cultures and philosophies has the potential to stir up stereotypes on both sides that manifest as transference and countertransference in therapy.

- Transference. The traditional Asian American patient considers the therapist to be an expert, teacher, and guru who provides teaching and guidance to find the solutions for the problems. The therapist is expected to mediate family discord, to judge, and to solve family conflicts. On the totem pole of traditional Confucian hierarchical order in society (king, teacher, father), the therapist as a teacher is respected just below the king. Asian American youth and well-acculturated Asian Americans may develop transference to consider the therapist as an elder in family. Most Asian Americans expect to see the therapist keep a warm, supportive, empathic, but authoritarian attitude to ensure their respect and trust (Juthani 1992; Marsella 1993). Asian American refugees and PTSD patients whose lives have been traumatized by war, imprisonment, or flight experiences may bring into therapy feelings of mistrust, suspicion, and hostility. Their needs for therapy go beyond help for their psychiatric problems. In some cases, they may also look at the therapist as a benevolent teacher who will help them get support and assistance to stabilize their living situation (Du and Lu 1997; Kinzie and Fleck 1987)

• <u>Countertransference</u>. Facing the complicated and unfamiliar Asian cultural and health beliefs, the therapist may develop a defensive response of denial, wherein the therapist thinks that all patients are the same and ignores cultural factors in therapy. The therapist may also develop the opposite attitude, becoming overly curious about the Asian cultures and spending substantial time to explore the culture instead of focusing on the patient's conflicts. American therapists who work with Southeast Asian refugees may develop feelings of guilt, pity, shame, or anger, depending on their political point of view about the Vietnam War. A therapist may become emotionally numbed and not know how to respond while hearing extraordinarily horrible war and escape stories from refugees; or the therapist may become fascinated with the traumatic stories and explore for more when the patient is not ready to reveal much. Asian American therapists who share a similar ethnic background with the patient may overly identify with the patient's struggles and conflicts and thus can stir up feelings of anger, guilt, or overprotection. In other cases, Asian American therapists may try to distance themselves from the patient to avoid overidentification, thus causing feelings of guilt and denial (Comas-Diaz and Jacobsen 1991). The Asian American therapist may also have blind spots, not asking particular questions because they think they know the answers or they assume that the subject is taboo.

Therapist Authority. Therapist authority is very important in working with traditional Asian American patients. The "blank slate" approach in therapy may work for Asian American youth and well-acculturated Asian Americans but does not work well with traditional Asian Americans, who may feel confused, anxious, and awkward if treated as an equal to the therapist. They will doubt the therapist's credentials and ability to understand and handle their problems (Marsella 1993). The therapist should maintain a warm, gentle, and supportive but authoritative attitude in therapy to build the therapeutic alliance, trust, and adherence. See Table 3–6 for a summary of tips for psychotherapy with Asian Americans.

Language and the Use of Interpreters. The use of interpreters in evaluation and treatment is inevitable because Asian Americans speak many languages and dialects. E. Lee (1997a) recommended the *therapeutic triad,* or the

Table 3–6.   Ten tips for psychotherapy with Asian Americans

1. Patients will normally be quiet and make poor eye contact.
2. Therapists should self-reveal their credentials.
3. A calm, gentle and supportive manner helps to build a therapeutic alliance.
4. A specific treatment plan should be outlined.
5. The individual should be treated as a part of a family and community system.
6. Problem-solving approaches may be helpful.
7. Directive or cognitive-behavioral techniques can be used later in therapy.
8. Use Asian metaphors.
9. Group therapy may be helpful in patients with posttraumatic stress disorder.
10. Consider the exploration of "taboo" subjects.

"triangle model," where the clinician, patient, and interpreter are seated in an equilateral triangle, as discussed in Chapter 1.

The following clinical case demonstrates countertransference and inappropriateness in an interpreter.

> K.L. is a 21-year-old single Korean male who was admitted to the hospital for a suicide attempt in which he overdosed with over-the-counter sleeping pills. A Korean interpreter was called to help in the evaluation. The assessment showed that the patient was the oldest son in the family who felt extremely guilty and stressed at home because his family disapproved of his homosexuality. His family had pressured him to marry a girl in Korea "to cure the problem." After interpreting the reason for the stress and the patient's suicide attempt, the interpreter began a lengthy conversation with the patient, then turned to the treatment team and said, "He will be fine. If you need to talk to his family, I am available for help." A Korean American medical student in the team told us that the interpreter is a pastor's wife. She gave the patient a moral lecture on homosexuality and told him that if he would like to get out of the hospital, he should not tell the doctor that he was suicidal.

E. Overall Cultural Assessment for Diagnosis and Care

Working with Asian Americans and understanding their vastly diverse cultures and health beliefs is fascinating and challenging. Before the therapist can provide culturally appropriate treatment, he or she faces challenges to make an accurate evaluation, to overcome stigma, and to ensure compliance.

Misdiagnosis

Asian Americans seek treatment at the late stages of mental illness, when all other resources for help and alternative treatments have been exhausted. Evidence of traditional treatments using coining, pinching, or cupping that leave contusions, bruises, and petechial marks on the skin can be mistaken for signs of battering or abuse (Gellis and Feingold 1976; Yeatman et al. 1976). Similarly, moxibustion can leave small, light burns on the skin that also may be mistaken for abuse. To avoid misdiagnosis, the therapist needs to investigate the use of traditional cures and herbal medicines that can cause severe psychotic symptoms (K.M. Lin and Cheung 1999). Culture-bound syndromes that manifest differently from Western psychiatric disorders may be considered bizarre and psychotic, thus leading to misdiagnosis and an inappropriate treatment approach. Culturally appropriate beliefs such as feeling the presence of dead family members or seeing or hearing from the dead during the time of an anniversary of their deaths may be mistaken for psychosis (T.Y. Lin and Lin 1980). The therapist should approach Asian American patients with an open mind and listen with empathy to their cultural health beliefs to avoid misunderstanding and misdiagnosis.

The following is a case of "qi-gong deviation syndrome":

G.L. is a 42-year-old married Asian American woman who was brought to the hospital by her family because she developed bizarre symptoms of uncontrollable and nonpurposed hand and arm gestures, episodes of fainting in the middle of her work, and sudden trance-like spells during conversation. According to her family, over the last 6 months she had experienced increased moodiness, irritability with labile affect, crying spells, and poor memory and concentration. The patient reported that she felt uncomfortable because of pressure on the top of her head, dysphoric mood, and low energy. She indicated that she could not control her irritability or crying spells. She did not recall much about her episodes of fainting and trances but said that the uncontrollable gestures in her hand and arms happened soon after she started practicing qi-gong breathing by herself 8 or 9 months ago. She said that she did not have these movements when she learned qi-gong in China. She had stopped practicing qi-gong for more than 5 years after she immigrated to the United States and resumed the practice of qi-gong as a method to calm herself at work and relieve her anxiety about having slightly high cholesterol and high blood pressure. Results of a physical examination, including neurological and cardiac examinations, were within normal limits except for mildly high blood pressure of 140/88. The patient was noticed to have bizarre danc-ing-like gestures of both hand and arm. She had episodes of falling suddenly into a trance during interviews and occupational therapy groups and com-plained of loss of appetite, insomnia, palpitation, anxiety, weakness, and tremor in every limb. She was scared about what was happening to her. She reported hearing noises, but not voices. She denied visual hallucinations and suicidal or homicidal thoughts. She was alert and oriented to name, time, and place. Her treatment in the hospital included lorazepam to calm her anxiety and help her sleep and acetaminophen for headache. Her family believed that the patient had "qi-gong deviation syndrome," in which her breathing exer-cise had led her qi to follow the wrong channels. The families asked permis-sion to consult a qi-gong master who could evaluate her situation and provide qi-gong therapy to get her qi back to the right channels and places. Medical treatment included administering lorazepam, monitoring her behaviors, and having a qi-gong master provide therapy to her for 1 hour every day. The pa-tient improved within a week. She was able to sleep better, and her hand movements, auditory hallucinations of noises, episodes of trance, and faint-ing spells stopped. She was able to read newspapers, watch TV, and focus on tasks in occupational therapy groups. The patient was discharged with refer-ral information for community mental health clinics if necessary and with the recommendation that she practice qi-gong under the guidance of a master.

Overcoming Stigma

The stigma of having a mental illness is the most significant obstacle prevent-ing Asian Americans from seeking help. Religious and cultural beliefs associ-ate mental illness with guilt and shame that affect the patient and the whole family. Mental patients are afraid of being rejected by siblings and relatives, as well as by the community. The family's reputation is protected by denial and concealment (Gee and Mutsumi 1997). Overcoming stigma is difficult and challenging. Clinically, a biological explanation of mental illness helps to dis-pel part of the stigma of guilt and shame, particularly when the patient and family understand that mental illness is caused by neurotransmitter imbal-ances. Close cooperation among social services, health clinics, primary care providers, and psychiatric clinics is very important in providing psychoedu-cation about the benefits of early evaluation and treatment of mental illness in Asian American communities. Referral to support groups where the family can obtain help and information from others who experience similar struggles in coping with their mental illness is very helpful to lessen their feelings of be-ing an outcast.

Ensuring Adherence With Medication and Appointments

Adherence with medication and treatment is another challenge in working with Asian Americans. Often, patients expect an immediate "cure." They have the tendency to reduce their medication dose when they encounter side effects or when their symptoms have improved (Kinzie et al. 1987; K.M. Lin and Cheung 1999; K.M. Lin and Shen 1991). They may drop out of therapy when they feel that the therapist does not understand them.

Kleinman (1980) suggested an explanatory model for understanding patients from different cultures and engaging them in treatment. Initially, the therapist should listen empathically and acknowledge the patient's and family's cultural health beliefs about the illness, then tactfully compare the similarities and differences between the patient's belief models and the therapist's clinical models. The first step in healing is to let patients tell their stories of mental illness according to their health beliefs. A treatment plan that includes a compromise between the differences of health beliefs will improve the patient's commitment to therapy. The physician should be a cultural broker, negotiating differences and addressing commonalities to create a compromise or a bridge between two cultures.

Most Asian American patients stay with their families. The family can be helpful in monitoring the patient's side effects, adherence with treatment, and appointments.

In the community, Asian Americans utilize mental health services more when they are able to participate in ethnic-specific programs in their own communities (Sue and McKinney 1975). They will stay in therapy longer and are less likely to drop out if they are matched with ethnically similar therapists or with therapists who speak their primary language (Gamst et al. 2003; Sue et al. 1991).

Conclusion

Working with Asian Americans is a fascinating challenge that provides ample opportunities to learn their cultures, health beliefs, and philosophies of life. An empathic, nonconfrontational approach that allows for compromises to resolve cultural differences in evaluation and therapy is crucial to understanding Asian American patients' dynamics and therefore improving the potential to engage them in treatment. Therapists should pay more attention to vulnerable Asian American groups such as children, women, elderly, and refugees. Particular attention should be paid when prescribing medication to Asian Americans because of their sensitivity to psychotropic medications. Knowledge of mental health needs, diagnostic issues, and methods of treatment of Asian American groups is essential to ensure appropriate, culturally competent approaches in therapy, treatment, prevention, and services.

Reading List

A short, selective list of suggested books for further reading on Asian American issues:

Gaw AC (ed): Culture, Ethnicity, and Mental Illness. Washington, DC, American Psychiatric Press, 1993

Gaw AC: Concise Guide to Cross-Cultural Psychiatry. Washington, DC, American Psychiatric Publishing, 2001

Gibbs JT, Huang L: Children of Color: Psychological Interventions With Culturally Diverse Youth. San Francisco, CA, Jossey-Bass, 1998

Group for the Advancement of Psychiatry Committee on Cultural Psychiatry: Cultural Assessment in Clinical Psychiatry. Washington, DC, American Psychiatric Publishing, 2002

Herrera JM, Lawson WB, Sramek JJ: Cross Cultural Psychiatry. New York, Wiley, 1999

Holtzman WH, Bornemann TH: Mental Health of Immigrants and Refugees. Austin, TX, Hogg Foundation for Mental Health, 1990

Kleinman A: Rethinking Psychiatry: From Cultural Category to Personal Experience. New York, Free Press, 1988

Kleinman A, Lin TY (eds): Normal and Abnormal Behavior in Chinese Culture. Boston, MA, Reidel, 1981

Kleinman A, Kunstader P, Russel EA, et al: Culture and Healing in Asian Societies: Anthropological, Psychiatric and Public Health Studies. Boston, GK Hall, 1978

Lee E (ed): Working With Asian Americans: A Guide for Clinicians. New York, Guilford, 1997

Lin KM, Poland RE, Nakasaki G (eds): Psychopharmacology and Psychobiology of Ethnicity. Washington, DC, American Psychiatric Press, 1993

Locke DC: Increasing Multicultural Understanding, Thousand Oaks, CA, Sage, 1992

Mezzich JE, Kleinman A, Fabrega H, et al (eds): Culture and Psychiatric Diagnosis: A DSM-IV Perspective. Washington, DC, American Psychiatric Press, 1996

Powell GJ: The Psychosocial Development of Minority Group Children. New York, Brunner/Mazel, 1983

Simons RC, Hughes CC: The Culture-Bound Syndromes: Folk Illnesses of Psychiatric and Anthropological Interest. Boston, MA, D Reidel, 1985

Takaki RT: Strangers From a Different Shore: A History of Asian Americans. Boston, MA, Little Brown, 1998

Tseng W-S: Handbook of Cultural Psychiatry. San Diego, CA, Academic Press, 2001

Tseng W-S, Streltzer J (eds): Culture and Psychotherapy: A Guide to Clinical Practice. Washington, DC, American Psychiatric Press, 2001

Tseng W-S, Streltzer J (eds): Cultural Competence in Clinical Psychiatry. Washington, DC, American Psychiatric Publishing, 2004

Westermeyer J: Psychiatric Care of Migrants: A Clinical Guide. Washington, DC, American Psychiatric Press, 1989

References

Akhtar S: Four culture-bound psychiatric syndromes in India. Int J Soc Psychiatry 34:70–74, 1988

American Psychiatric Association: Appendix I: Outline for cultural formulation and glossary of culture-bound syndromes, in Diagnostic and Statistical Manual of Mental Disorders, 4th Edition, Text Revision. Washington, DC, American Psychiatric Association, 2000, pp 897–903

Aoki BK: Gay and lesbian Asian Americans in psychotherapy, in Working With Asian Americans: A Guide for Clinicians. Edited by Lee E. New York, Guilford, 1997, pp 411–419

Arameta EG: Psychiatric care for Pilipino Americans, in Culture, Ethnicity, and Mental Illness. Edited by Gaw AC, Washington, DC, American Psychiatric Press, 1993, pp 377–412

Aronson L: Traditional Cambodian health beliefs and practices. R I Med J 70:73–78, 1987

Barry DT, Mizrahi TC: Guarded self-disclosure predicts psychological distress and willingness to use psychological services among East Asian immigrants in the United States. J Nerv Ment Dis 193:535–539, 2005

Bernstein RL, Gaw AC: Koro: proposed classification for DSM-IV. Am J Psychiatry 147:1670–1674, 1990

Caiyun W et al, Neuropsychology Department of Suzhou Medical College: Spontaneous dynamic Qi gong (SDQ) (involuntary motion in Qi gong) and psychological medicine, in Joint Meeting of the American Psychiatric Association and the Chinese Medical Association: Advances in Psychiatry: Chinese and American (Chinese Part). Beijing, China, 1988, pp 122–124

Canda ER, Phaobtong T: Buddhism as a support system for Southeast Asian refugees. Soc Work 37:61–67, 1992

Chang DF, Myers HF, Yeung A, et al: Shenjing shuairuo and the DSM-IV: diagnosis, distress, and disability in a Chinese primary care setting. Transcult Psychiatry 42:204–218, 2005

Chen PN: A study of Chinese American elderly residing in a hotel room. Soc Casework 60:89–95, 1976

Chung W: Asian American children, in Working With Asian Americans: A Guide for Clinicians. Edited by Lee E. New York, Guilford, 1997, pp 165–174

Cima RJ: Vietnam, A Country Study. Washington, DC, Library of Congress, Federal Research Division, 1989

Comas-Diaz L, Jacobsen FM: Ethnocultural transference and countertransference in the therapeutic dyad. Am J Orthopsychiatry 61:392–402, 1991

Conrad MM, DF Pacquiao: Manifestation, attribution, and coping with depression among Asian Indians from the perspectives of health care practitioners. J Transcult Nurs 16:32–40, 2005

Cook J: Samoan patterns in seeking health services. Hawaii Med J 42(6):138–142, 1983

Crohn J: Asian intermarriage: love versus tradition, in Working With Asian Americans: A Guide for Clinicians. Edited by Lee E. New York, Guilford, 1997, pp 428–438

Du N, Lu FG: Assessment and treatment of posttraumatic stress disorder among Asian Americans, in Working With Asian Americans: A Guide for Clinicians. Edited by Lee E. New York, Guilford, 1997, pp 275–294

Gamst G, Aguilar-Kitibutr A, Herdina A, et al: Effects of racial match on Asian American mental health consumer satisfaction. Ment Health Serv Res 5(4):197–208, 2003

Gaw AC: Psychiatric care for Chinese Americans, in Culture, Ethnicity, and Mental Illness. Edited by Gaw AC. Washington, DC, American Psychiatric Press, 1993, pp 245–280

Gee KK, Mutsumi IM: Assessment and treatment of schizophrenia among Asian Americans, in Working With Asian Americans: A Guide for Clinicians. Edited by Lee E. New York, Guilford, 1997, pp 227–251

Gellis SS, Feingold M: Pseudobattering in Vietnamese children. Am J Dis Child 130:857–858, 1976

Group for the Advancement of Psychiatry Committee on Cultural Psychiatry: Cultural Assessment in Clinical Psychiatry. Washington DC, American Psychiatric Publishing, 2002

Homma-True R: Asian American women, in Working With Asian Americans: A Guide for Clinicians. Edited by Lee E. New York, Guilford, 1997, pp 420–427

Hsu E, Davies CA, Hansen, DJ: Understanding mental health needs of Southeast Asian refugees: historical, cultural, and contextual challenges. Clin Psychol Rev 24:193–213, 2004

Hsu J, Tseng WS: Intercultural psychotherapy. Arch Gen Psychiatry 27:700–705, 1972

Huaihai S et al, Shanghai Mental Health Center: A clinico-phenomenological study on mental disorder caused by breathing exercise, in Joint Meeting of the American Psychiatric Association and the Chinese Medical Association: Advances in Psychiatry: Chinese and American (Chinese Part), Beijing, China, 1988, pp 1–2

Huang DD, Charter RA: The origin and formulation of Chinese character: an introduction to Confucianism and its influence on Chinese behavior patterns. Cult Divers Ment Health 2:35–42, 1996

Huang LN: Asian American adolescents, in Working With Asian Americans: A Guide for Clinicians. Edited by Lee E. New York, Guilford, 1997, pp 175–195

Hughes CC, Littlewood R, Wintrob RM, et al: Culture-bound syndromes, in Culture and Psychiatric Diagnosis: A DSM-IV Perspective. Edited by Mezzich JE, Kleinman A, Fabrega H, et al. Washington, DC, American Psychiatric Press, 1996, pp 289–323

Ja DY, Aoki B: Substance abuse treatment: cultural barriers in the Asian-American community. J Psychoactive Drugs 25:61–71, 1993

Juthani NV: Immigrant mental health: conflicts and concerns of Indian immigrants in the U.S.A. Psychol Dev Soc J 4:133–148, 1992

Kao RSK, Lam ML: Asian American elderly, in Working With Asian Americans: A Guide for Clinicians. Edited by Lee E. New York, Guilford, 1997, pp 208–223

Kim LIC: Psychiatric care for Korean Americans, in Culture, Ethnicity, and Mental Illness. Edited by Gaw AC. Washington, DC, American Psychiatric Press, 1993, pp 347–376

Kim SC: Ericksonian hypnotic framework for Asian Americans. Am J Clin Hypn 25:235–241, 1983

Kinzie JD: Lessons from cross-cultural psychotherapy. Am J Psychother 32:510–520, 1978

Kinzie JD, Fleck J: Psychotherapy with severe traumatized refugees. Am J Psychother 41:82–94, 1987

Kinzie JD, Tran KA, Breckenridge A, et al: An Indochinese refugee psychiatric clinic: culturally accepted treatment approaches. Am J Psychiatry 137:1429–1432, 1980

Kinzie JD, Sack WH, Angell RH: The psychiatric effects of massive trauma on Cambodian children. J Am Acad Child Adolesc Psychiatry 25:370–376, 1986

Kinzie JD, Leung P, Boehnlein JK, et al: Antidepressant blood levels in Southeast Asians: clinical and cultural implications. J Nerv Ment Dis 175:480–485, 1987

Kinzie JD, Sack W, Angell R, et al: A three-year follow-up of Cambodian young people traumatized as children. J Am Acad Child Adolesc Psychiatry 28:501–504, 1989

Kleinman AM: Patients and Healers in the Context of Culture: An Exploration of the Borderland Between Anthropology, Medicine, and Psychiatry. Berkeley, CA, University of California Press, 1980

Kleinman A: Social Origins of Distress and Disease: Depression, Neurasthenia, and Pain in Modern China. New Haven, CT, Yale University Press, 1986

Landre R, Miller M, Porter D: Asian gangs, in Gangs: A Handbook for Community Awareness. Edited by Landre R, Miller M, Porter D. New York, Facts on File, 1997, pp 82–85

Le T: Delinquency among Asian/Pacific Islanders: review of literature and research. The Justice Professional 15:57–70, 2002

Lee E: Asian American families: an overview, in Ethnicity and Family Therapy, 2nd Edition. Edited by McGoldrick M, Giordano J, Pearce JK. New York, Guilford, 1996, pp 227–248

Lee E: Cross-cultural communication: therapeutic use of interpreters, in Working With Asian Americans: A Guide for Clinicians. Edited by Lee E. New York, Guilford, 1997a, pp 477–489

Lee E: Overview: the assessment and treatment of Asian American families, in Working With Asian Americans: A Guide for Clinicians. Edited by Lee E. New York, Guilford, 1997b, pp 3–36

Lee SM: Asian Americans: diverse and growing. Popul Bull 53:1–40, 1998

Leong FT, Lau AS: Barriers to providing effective mental health services to Asian Americans. Ment Health Serv Res 3:201–214, 2001

Lin EHB, Carter WB, Kleinman AM: An exploration of somatization among Asian refugees and immigrants in primary care. Am J Public Health 75:1080–1084, 1985

Lin KM: Hwa-byung: a Korean culture-bound syndrome? Am J Psychiatry 140:105–107, 1983

Lin KM, Cheung F: Mental health issues for Asian Americans. Psychiatr Serv 50:774–780, 1999

Lin KM, Finder E: Neuroleptic dosage for Asians. Am J Psychiatry 140:490–491, 1983

Lin KM, Shen WW: Pharmacotherapy for Southeast Asian psychiatric patients. J Nerv Ment Dis 179:346–350, 1991

Lin KM, Poland RE, Nuccio I, et al: A longitudinal assessment of haloperidol doses and serum concentration in Asian and Caucasian schizophrenic patients. Am J Psychiatry 146:1307–1311, 1989

Lin KM, Lau JK, Yamamoto J, et al: Hwa-byung: a community study of Korean Americans. J Nerv Ment Dis 180:386–391, 1992

Lin KM, Poland RE, and Nakasaki G (eds): Psychopharmacology and Psychobiology of Ethnicity. Washington, DC, American Psychiatric Press, 1993

Lin KM, Cheung F, Smith M, et al: The use of psychotropic medications in working with Asian patients, in Working With Asian Americans: A Guide for Clinicians. Edited by Lee E. New York, Guilford, 1997, pp 388–399

Lin TY: Neurasthenia revisited: its place in modern psychiatry. Psychiatr Ann 22:173–175, 177–187, 1992

Lin TY, Lin MC: Love, denial, and rejection: responses of Chinese families to mental illness, in Normal and Abnormal Behavior in Chinese Culture. Edited by Kleinman A, Lin TY. Boston, MA, D Riedel, 1980, pp 387–401

Lu FG, Lim RF, Mezzich JE: Issues in the assessment and diagnosis of culturally diverse individuals, in American Psychiatric Press Review of Psychiatry, Vol 14. Edited by Oldham JM, Riba MB. Washington, DC, American Psychiatric Press, 1995, pp 477–510

Mak WW, Zane NW: The phenomenon of somatization among community Chinese Americans. Soc Psychiatry Psychiatr Epidemiol 39:967–974, 2004

Marsella AJ: Counseling and psychotherapy with Japanese Americans: cross-cultural considerations. Am J Orthopsychiatry 63:200–208, 1993

Masaki B, Wong L: Domestic violence in Asian community, in Working With Asian Americans: A Guide for Clinicians. Edited by Lee E. New York, Guilford, 1997, pp 439–451

Mollica RF, Lavelle J: Southeast Asian refugees, in Clinical guidelines in Cross-Cultural Mental Health. Edited by Comas-Diaz L, Griffith EHE. New York, Wiley, 1988, pp 262–304

Moore LJ, Boehnlein JK: Treating psychiatric disorders among Mien refugees from Highland Laos. Soc Sci Med 32:1029–1036, 1991

Nagata DK: Transgenerational impact of the Japanese-American internment: clinical issues in working with children of former internees. Psychotherapy 28:121–128, 1991

Nakajima GA, Chan YH, Lee K: Mental health issues for gay and lesbian Asian Americans, in Textbook of Homosexuality and Mental Health. Edited by Cabaj RP, Stein TS. Washington, DC, American Psychiatric Press, 1996, pp 563–582

Nemoto T, Aoki B, Huang K, et al: Drug use behaviors among Asian drug users in San Francisco. Addict Behav 24:823–838, 1999

Ng BY: Qigong-induced mental disorders. Aust N Z J Psychiatry 33:197–206, 1999

Nguyen SD: Psychiatric and psychosomatic problems among Southeast Asian refugees. Psychiatr J Univ Ottawa 7:163–172, 1982

O'Brien DJ, Fugita S: The Japanese American Experience. Bloomington, Indiana University Press, 1991

Petry NM, Armentano C, Kuoch T, et al: Gambling participation and problems among South East Asian refugees to the United States. Psychiatr Serv 54:1142–1148, 2003

Prathikanti S: East Indian American families, in Working With Asian Americans: A Guide for Clinicians. Edited by Lee E. New York, Guilford, 1997, pp 79–100

Reid D: The Complete Book of Chinese Health and Healing. New York, Barnes and Noble, 1994

Reid J, Silove D, Tam R: The development of the New South Wales Service for the Treatment and Rehabilitation of Torture and Trauma Survivors (STARTTS): the first year. Aust N Z J Psychiatry 24:486–495, 1990

Ross RR: Cambodia: A Country Study, 3rd Edition. Washington, DC, Library of Congress, Federal Research Division, 1990

Rozee PD, Van Boemel G: The psychological effects of war trauma and abuse on older Cambodian refugee women. Women Ther 8:23–50, 1989

Russell JG: Anxiety disorders in Japan: a review of the Japanese literature on shinkeishitsu and taijinkyofusho. Cult Med Psychiatry 13:391–403, 1989

Sack WH, Clarke GN: Multiple forms of stress in Cambodian adolescent refugees. Child Dev 67:107–116, 1996

Savada AM: Laos: A Country Study, 3rd Edition. Washington, DC, Library of Congress, Federal Research Division, 1995

Sue S, McKinney H: Asian Americans in the community mental health care system. Am J Orthopsychiatry 45:111–118, 1975

Sue S, Fujino D, Hu LT, et al: Community mental health service for ethnic minority groups: a test of cultural responsiveness hypothesis. J Consult Clin Psychol 59:533–540, 1991

Takaki RT: Strangers From a Different Shore: A History of Asian Americans (updated and revised edition). Boston, MA, Little, Brown, 1998

Tang NM: Psychoanalytic psychotherapy with Chinese Americans, in Working With Asian Americans: A Guide for Clinicians. Edited by Lee E. New York, Guilford, 1997, pp 323–341

Tracy TJ, Leong FTL, Gildden C: Help-seeking and problem perception among Asian Americans. J Couns Psychol 33:331–336, 1986

Tseng W-S: Amok (indiscriminate mass homicide attacks), in Handbook of Cultural Psychiatry. San Diego, CA, Academic Press, 2001a, pp 230–233

Tseng W-S: Latah (startle-induced dissociative reaction), in Handbook of Cultural Psychiatry. San Diego, CA, Academic Press, 2001b, pp 245–250

Tseng W-S, Mo KM, Hsu J, et al: A sociocultural study of koro epidemics in Guangdong, China. Am J Psychiatry 145:1538–1543, 1988

U.S. Census Bureau: The Native Hawaiian and Other Pacific Islander Population: 2000. Census 2000 Brief. Prepared by Grieco EM. December 2001. Available at: http://www.census.gov/population/www/cen2000/brief.html. Accessed January 25, 2006.

U.S. Census Bureau: The Asian Population: 2000. Census 2000 Brief. Prepared by Barnes JS, Bennett CE. February 2002. Available at: http://www.census.gov/population/www/cen2000/brriefs.html. Accessed January 25, 2006.

U.S. Census Bureau: Income in the United States: 2002, in Current Population Reports. Prepared by Denavas-Walt C, Cleveland R, Webster B Jr. September 2003. Available at: http://www.census.gov/hhes/www/income/income02.html, pp 60–221. Accessed January 25, 2006.

U.S. Census Bureau: We the People: Asians in the United States. Census 2000 Special Reports. Prepared by Reeves TJ, Bennett TJ. December 2004. Available at: http://www.census.gov/prod/2004pubs/censr-17.pdf. Accessed January 25, 2006.

U.S. Department of Health and Human Services: Mental Health: Culture, Race, and Ethnicity. A Supplement to Mental Health: A Report of the Surgeon General. Rockville, MD, U.S. Department of Health and Human Services, Public Health Service, Office of the Surgeon General, 2001. Available at: http://www.surgeongeneral.gov/library/mentalhealth/cre

Westermeyer J: On the epidemicity of Amok violence. Arch Gen Psychiatry 28:873–876, 1973

Westermeyer J: Folk medicine in Laos: a comparison between two ethnic groups. Soc Sci Med 27:769–778, 1988

Westermeyer J, Vang TF, Neider J: Refugees who do and do not seek psychiatric care: an analysis of premigratory and postmigratory characteristics. J Nerv Ment Dis 171:86–91, 1983

Wong L, Mock MR: Asian American young adults, in Working With Asian Americans: A Guide for Clinicians. Edited by Lee E. New York, Guilford, 1997, pp 196–207

Yamamoto J: Psychiatric diagnosis and neurasthenia. Psychiatr Ann 22:171–172, 1992

Yeatman GW, Shaw C, Barlow MJ, et al: Pseudobattering in Vietnamese children. Pediatrics 58:616–618, 1976

Ying YW, Miller LS: Help-seeking behavior and attitude of Chinese Americans regarding psychological problems. Am J Community Psychol 20:549–556, 1992

4

Latino Patients

Amaro J. Laria, Ph.D.

Roberto Lewis-Fernández, M.D.

Hispanic or Latino groups include individuals from different countries who share substantial cultural and ethnic bonds through a common Spanish language and Latino/Hispanic ancestry.[1] While sharing common bonds, Latinos also comprise a heterogeneous group with richly diverse histories, customs, and cultural characteristics. An adequate understanding of issues pertinent to the psychiatric assessment and treatment of Latino patients in the United States requires a deep appreciation of the commonalities as well as the differences among individuals from these diverse groups. In the process of generalizing, we run the risk of oversimplifying complex cultural traits into gross stereotypes.

---

[1] It should be noted that the terms *Latino* and *Hispanic* are used interchangeably throughout this chapter. Neither is a perfect choice because *Latino* implies Latin descent and *Hispanic* gives priority to Spanish origins or language. These terms will be discussed in greater detail later in this chapter.

Appreciating the influence of culture on a particular individual's values and behavior requires walking the fine line between the pitfalls of "overculturalizing" (attributing an observed individual characteristic inaccurately to cultural factors) and "underculturalizing" (failing to recognize the influence of culture on an observed behavior or trait). For example, failing to appreciate the divergent views of gender relations that may be held by a young Argentinean immigrant woman who was raised in an affluent suburb of Buenos Aires from those of an older woman from rural El Salvador could result in simplistic stereotyping and overgeneralizing with little practical clinical value. On the other hand, dismissing existing commonalities between them because of their different social backgrounds also could cause important cultural information to be missed. Shared values toward family orientation, such as the need to preserve family cohesiveness at all costs, may represent a similar aspect of these women's experiences shaped by their common Latino cultural heritage.

Social Demographics and History of U.S. Migration Patterns

According to the U.S. Census 2004 Current Population Survey, there are approximately 40.4 million Hispanics in the United States, constituting about 14% of the total population (U.S. Census Bureau 2004). This figure represents almost a 50% increase since 1990 (22 million), and projections estimate this number to rise to 97 million, or about 25% of the U.S. population, by 2050. Ironically, although Spanish is not the official national language, the United States has the fifth largest Spanish-speaking population in the world (preceded only by Mexico, Colombia, Spain, and Argentina). Latinos in the United States are a relatively young group, with a median age of 26.8 years, compared with 35.9 years for the overall population (U.S. Census Bureau 2004). Thirty-four percent of Hispanics are age 18 years or younger, compared with 23% for the national population. In addition, it was estimated in 2004 that 60% of Hispanics living in the United States were U.S. born, contradicting the popular misconception of Hispanics as a population of immigrants (U.S. Census Bureau 2002a). However, there is controversy as to the precise proportion of U.S.-born to foreign-born Latinos due to a potential marked undercount of Hispanic migrants in the U.S. Census Bureau data. One source estimates a more conservative figure of 40%–60% for each group (Alegría et al. 2004).

Persons of Mexican background are the largest Latino group in the United States, comprising 65.9% of the total Latino population (U.S. Census Bureau 2004). They are followed by Puerto Ricans (9.5%), Cubans (4.0%), and Dominicans (2.6%). The rest of the U.S. Latino population is composed of Central Americans (7.8%), South Americans (5.2%), and a category composed of Spaniards and others who self-label as "Spanish," "Spanish American," or "other Hispanic or Latino" (7.6%) (U.S. Census Bureau 2004).

There are seven states with more than 1 million Hispanics: California, Texas, New York, Florida, Illinois, Arizona, and New Jersey (ranked in order of total Latino population). The states with the largest concentration of Latinos, in terms of percentage of total population, are New Mexico (42%), California (32%), Texas (32%), and Arizona (25%) (U.S. Census Bureau 2004). In addition, Latinos are spreading to regions of the United States that have not previously been associated with large numbers of Latinos.

As a rule, Latinos have lower educational and socioeconomic levels than the national average. Only 58% of Latinos over age 25 have graduated from high school—compared with 90% of the total non-Hispanic white population—and only 12% have a college degree—compared with 31% of non-Hispanic whites (U.S. Census Bureau 2004). However, the various Latino groups differ from one another in this respect, with Cubans generally having achieved a higher educational level than Mexicans and Puerto Ricans (U.S. Census Bureau 2004). Hispanics in the United States also have a significantly lower socioeconomic status than the U.S. average, as revealed by various indices such as median family income ($34,275 vs. $59,937 among non-Hispanic whites in 2003) (U.S. Census Bureau 2004), proportion of individuals below the poverty line (23% for Latinos vs. 8% for non-Hispanic whites), and unemployment rates (8% for Latinos vs. 6% for non-Hispanic whites) (U.S. Census Bureau 2004). As in the case of education, marked intergroup differences exist (Table 4–1).

Latinos have migrated to this country for more than two centuries. It must be noted, however, that many Hispanics were never immigrants, since they inhabited regions of the country that were originally part of Spain and Mexico (i.e., Texas, California, New Mexico, Florida, Arizona, Colorado, Nevada) before the arrival of Anglo colonists, who came to these areas mainly during the nineteenth century (Parrillo 2005). This presents obvious ironies because many of their descendants may be inaccurately regarded in contem-

Table 4–1. Educational, financial, and employment status of Hispanics in the United States, 2002

Group	Educational level (%)[a]					Income level		
	Less than 9th grade	Some high school	High school diploma	Some college	College degree[b]	Median family income ($)[c]	Below poverty line (%)	Unemployed (%)[d]
Non-Hispanic white	3.3	6.7	32.8	26.6	30.6	59,937	8.2	5.7
All Hispanic	25.1	16.5	27.7	18.6	12.1	34,275	22.5	7.5
Mexican	29.8	18.3	26.8	17.2	7.9	32,263	24.1	8.3
Puerto Rican	11.0	17.2	34.3	23.4	14.1	34,519	23.7	8.2
Cuban	19.5	8.4	30.3	17.8	24.0	44,847	14.4	4.0

[a]Data for adults age 25 years or older.
[b]Bachelor's or advanced degree.
[c]Income in 2003.
[d]Based on persons in the civilian labor force.
Source. U.S. Census Bureau 2004.

porary U.S. society as immigrants. The Spaniards were the first Europeans to settle in the Americas, arriving in 1492, 115 years before the founding of Jamestown in 1607. Ponce de León, the former governor of Puerto Rico, was the first European to set foot in Florida, in 1513, and Saint Augustine, the first city established by European colonists in North America, was founded by the Spaniards in 1565. At the time the 13 colonies declared independence from Great Britain in 1776, Spain maintained control of most present-day U.S. territory west of the Mississippi River.

Subsequent to the early Spanish presence in the Americas, diverse historical and political events influenced the course of major migration trends from different Latin American countries. We will describe some of these migratory patterns, as well as salient characteristics of Latino cultural groups, by classifying the groups into four geographic subcategories: Mexicans, Caribbean Islanders, Central Americans, and South Americans.

Mexicans

Mexico is the most populous Spanish-speaking country and the only one that shares a border with the United States. Therefore, it is not surprising that Mexicans constitute the largest Latino cultural group in the United States, estimated at 26.6 million in 2004 (U.S. Census Bureau 2004). A large number of Mexicans lived in parts of Mexico that later became U.S. territories (i.e., California, Texas, New Mexico, Arizona, Oklahoma, Nevada, and Colorado). They gradually became an ethnic and cultural minority after the United States formally occupied these territories following the Mexican-American War (1846–1848). Ironically, those whose families had lived in the region for generations were suddenly regarded as foreign farmworkers in their own homeland. Subsequently, the Mexican Revolution (1910–1917) brought substantial social, economic, and political instability to Mexico, which triggered a massive migration to the United States (Parrillo 2005). The migratory flow increased after World War II and has persisted to the present day. In addition, large numbers of Mexican migrant workers come to the United States as temporary or seasonal rural laborers, returning to Mexico after limited periods of employment. Patterns of migration from Mexico have been influenced by economic conditions in the United States and in Mexico, as well as by changing political relationships between the two countries. For example, the United States has recruited Mexicans at times of need for cheap labor (e.g., during the construction of the railroad system in the 1880s) while organizing massive deportation efforts during periods of lower economic activity (e.g., the Great Depression) (Portes et al. 1996).

Although migration waves from Mexico have fluctuated according to socioeconomic factors both in Mexico and the United States, there has been a steady increase of Mexican immigrants in recent years. The estimated unauthorized resident population from Mexico increased from about 2.0 million in 1990 to 4.8 million in January 2000 (U.S. Immigration and Naturalization Service 2003), when it was estimated that Mexicans represented 69% of the total unauthorized resident population in the United States. Yet despite the large number of undocumented Mexicans, a large proportion (40%–60%) of those now living in the United States were born in this country (Alegría et al. 2004; U.S. Census Bureau 2004), constituting the largest number of U.S.-born Latinos. The majority of Mexicans in the United States work as either service laborers or rural farmworkers.

Most of the nearly 27 million Mexicans in this country remain a largely marginalized ethnic minority group. Factors leading to this situation include the harsh socioeconomic conditions in Mexico, the history of antagonism between the two countries, and the general tendency of U.S. dominant culture to discriminate against poor, dark-skinned or "colored" immigrants and resist their assimilation into U.S. society. Despite the antagonistic circumstances faced by many Mexican immigrants, their numbers continue to increase exponentially, and their migration patterns are diversifying across the United States.

Caribbean Islanders

There are three officially Spanish-speaking countries in the Caribbean: Cuba, the Dominican Republic, and Puerto Rico. Despite significant cultural characteristics shared by these "*caribeños*" resulting from their geographic proximity and common ethnic and historical roots, unique sociopolitical circumstances have resulted in divergent U.S. migration patterns. Because they represent the three largest groups of Latino immigrants in the United States after the Mexicans, we will describe each group separately.

Puerto Ricans

The first sizeable Puerto Rican communities in the United States formed in New York City around 1868, when many Puerto Ricans and Cubans migrated to organize revolutionary activities against Spanish domination (Rodriguez 1991). Puerto Ricans began to migrate in larger numbers after World War II in search of employment and better economic opportunities. Approximately 30% of Puerto Ricans living on the U.S. mainland reside in New York City, making it the largest Puerto Rican community in the United States. There are other large concentrations of Puerto Ricans residing in New Jersey, Connecticut, Florida, Illinois, Massachusetts, and Pennsylvania (U.S. Census Bureau 2004).

An important fact that sets Puerto Ricans apart from all other Latino groups is the island's political status as a U.S. Commonwealth, officially labeled an *estado libre asociado* ("associated free state"). By virtue of this political arrangement, extant since 1952, Puerto Rico is not an independent nation; despite some relatively autonomous elements of government, it still functions as a U.S. colony. Puerto Ricans have been U.S. citizens since 1917, making it easier for them to relocate to and work in the United States. Coupled with the relative geographic proximity of the island, this facilitates a continuous flow of Puerto Ricans back and forth from the island to the U.S. mainland, a process known as "circular migration." Aided by routing and marketing decisions of the airline industry, many Puerto Ricans in the United States are able to maintain close ties with their culture of origin. Approximately 3.8 million Puerto Ricans live on the U.S. mainland, and another 3.8 million reside on the island. Of those living in the United States, 54% were mainland born in 1990 (U.S. Census Bureau 1990).

An interesting dilemma about Puerto Ricans living on the mainland is whether or not to regard them as immigrants, given their status as U.S. citizens. Despite their greater social and political ties with the United States, many Puerto Ricans still face substantial difficulty adapting to U.S. mainstream society, much like other Latino groups. In fact, they currently remain one of the most marginalized groups in the country.

Similar to most Mexican immigrants, the majority of Puerto Ricans on the mainland live in poverty and face discrimination and prejudice, sometimes resulting from historical and political hostility from U.S. mainstream society. However, there has been a marked increase in the number of Puerto Rican college students and professionals migrating from the island in more recent decades. Many Puerto Ricans living on the U.S. mainland contextualize their current marginalization in light of the prolonged colonial relationship between the two societies. The United States annexed Puerto Rico in 1898 after the Spanish-American War, imposing the English language and "Americanization" on the islanders and manipulating economic development to suit mainland priorities. Despite these efforts, the island has maintained its Hispanic heritage.

Many Puerto Ricans, regardless of their political persuasion, view the United States with mistrust and are wary of the political and economic hegemony of their northern neighbor. However, Puerto Ricans vary widely in their political position toward relations with the United States, advocating political agendas that range from full independence to statehood. Although many resent their lack of autonomy from the United States, a large number see it as a strategic compromise.

Cubans

Cubans are the third largest Latino group in the United States, numbering approximately 1.6 million (U.S. Census Bureau 2004). They are also one of the most highly concentrated groups, with the vast majority living in Southeast Florida, primarily in Miami-Dade County. Other states with large numbers of Cubans include New Jersey, New York, and California. Many Cuban revolutionaries who engaged in the struggle for independence from Spain migrated to the United States around 1868, establishing small communities in Florida and New York (Parrillo 2005). Skilled Cuban cigar makers were recruited by the growing U.S. cigar industry during the late nineteenth and early twentieth centuries, establishing communities in Tampa, Key West, New York City, and New Orleans. However, the largest exodus of Cubans to the United States began after the Cuban socialist revolution of 1959, and primarily after 1961 when leader Fidel Castro established a communist political and economic system in Cuba and broke relations with the United States. Thus, unlike most other Latino immigrant groups, early Cuban arrivals in the United States were not poor socioeconomic immigrants, but rather political refugees. These exiles tended to be wealthier, better educated, and characterized by their strong anti-Castro and anticommunist political stance; but subsequent migrations of *balseros* ("rafters") have included Cubans from all social strata (Portes et al. 1996). Another major exodus of Cubans took place during the 1980 Mariel boatlift, when a large group of predominantly working-class Cubans came to the United States. More recent Cuban immigrants appear to be motivated to migrate by socioeconomic as well as political factors.

An important difference between Cubans and the other two largest Latino groups in the United States, Mexicans and Puerto Ricans, is that Cubans, in general, maintain a more pro-U.S. political attitude. This should not be surprising. Many migrating Mexicans and Puerto Ricans view the history of relations between the United States and their countries of origin as a protracted resistance against northern economic and political encroachment. By contrast, many Cuban exiles regard the United States as their most strategic ally in their political opposition to Fidel Castro's communist government. Some prevailing misconceptions about Cuban exiles should be addressed. They are often stereotyped as an elite group among Latinos, with the erroneous implicit assumption that Cubans brought with them wealth that facilitated their adaptation to U.S. society and the attainment of high-status positions. Although some economic indices are better for Cubans compared with the Hispanic population at large, the economic position of Cubans is still substantially lower than that of the mainstream non-Hispanic white population. Rather than wealth, many Cuban immigrants brought job skills that facilitated their adaptation process, as a logical result of the urban, professional, and entrepreneurial sectors many of them represented in Cuba. Another factor is their establishment of an economic enclave, promoted through the solidarity and geographic concentration created by the group's political struggle. A second common misconception about Cubans is that their pro-U.S. stance reflects an assimilationist attitude. In fact, as a rule Cubans maintain a strong sense of ethnic identity and show low levels of cultural incorporation of U.S. mainstream values (Rogg and Cooney 1980). In addition, only 31.5% of Cubans living in the United States are U.S. born, compared with higher proportions of Mexicans and Puerto Ricans (U.S. Census Bureau 2004). Cubans also experience substantial prejudice and discrimination in this country and political tension with other Latinos and non-Latinos, who often stereotype them as political conservatives. However, the political views of most Cubans seem to have little to do with traditional U.S. political dichotomies of "liberal" versus "conservative" and more to do with what is most at stake for them, a "pro-Castro" versus an "anti-Castro" political stance.

Dominicans

Migrants from the Dominican Republic have entered the United States more recently, with the largest influx beginning in the 1970s. In the year 2000, there were nearly 800,000 Dominicans in the United States (U.S. Census Bureau 2004), concentrated mostly in New York City, where approximately 65% live, with other large communities in Massachusetts, New Jersey, and Florida (U.S. Census Bureau 2001). In the 1960s, following decades of U.S.-supported authoritarian rule, including the Trujillo dictatorship from 1930 to 1961, the Dominican Republic suffered deteriorating economic conditions, such as a marked decline in agricultural production and a subsequent rise in unemployment (Portes et al. 1996). These factors triggered a massive exodus of migrants to Puerto Rico and the United States. Many Dominicans enter the United States as undocumented migrants via Puerto Rico. In that respect they differ markedly from Puerto Ricans and the earlier waves of Cuban exiles who migrated legally. However, Dominicans are becoming more settled in the United States, and in 1990 approximately 27.8% of those living in the United States were U.S. born (U.S. Census Bureau 1990).

Like many Puerto Rican migrants, most Dominicans in the United States come from rural areas and low socioeconomic backgrounds and have a grade school education. This causes them to be the target of significant prejudice and discrimination from mainstream U.S. society. The fact that many Dominicans are dark-skinned, given their mixed African, Amerindian, and European background, makes them additionally vulnerable to U.S. racist attitudes (Portes et al. 1996). Another similarity to Puerto Ricans is the rise of a circular migratory pattern due to geographic proximity and the relative ease of air travel between the Dominican Republic and the East Coast of the United States. As a result, Dominicans engage in repeated back-and-forth cycles in an attempt to strengthen family, cultural, and economic ties between the two countries. Dominicans reside alongside Puerto Ricans in many communities, partly because of their cultural and socioeconomic commonalities (Parrillo 2005). Intermarriage between the two groups is increasing, although the degree of cultural intermixing varies by region and each group typically displays a strong sense of cultural identity.

Most Dominicans in the United States remain marginalized, despite their individual dedication and hard work, for reasons similar to those faced by Puerto Ricans, Mexicans, and other poor rural Latino migrants. Ironically, the low social status held by many Dominicans in the United States contrasts sharply with the positive image created by the success of the numerous Dominican professional baseball players who have become idols to thousands in this country. It remains to be seen whether the dramatic concentration of the Dominican migration in a small number of ethnic enclaves (e.g., the Washington Heights area of New York City) will result over time in relative economic success similar to that of the Cuban exiles, despite the more limited number of migrants with professional-level skills.

Central Americans

Central America includes seven countries: Guatemala, Belize, El Salvador, Honduras, Nicaragua, Costa Rica, and Panama. Belize, a British colony until 1981, is the only non-Spanish-speaking Central American nation; therefore, Belizeans are not typically referred to as Latinos. Of the other countries, El Salvador, Guatemala, Honduras, and Nicaragua have sent the largest number of immigrants to the United States. An estimated 3.2 million Central Americans reside in the United States (U.S. Census Bureau 2004). Emigrants from these countries have left primarily for political and socioeconomic reasons. In fact, it is often difficult to discern factors related to poverty from those connected to political violence, given their close interdependence. Many Central American immigrants, especially Salvadorans but also Nicaraguans and Guatemalans, have experienced intensely traumatic experiences as victims of political violence, including imprisonment, torture, and widespread witnessing of killings. This exposure sets certain groups like the Salvadoran refugees apart from other Latino immigrants in terms of mental health, particularly because of the higher prevalence of posttraumatic reactions (Farias 1994). Because of the harsh socioeconomic conditions in their countries of origin, Central American immigrants tend to be poor, from rural areas, and with low levels of education. An exception to this rule is the migration of some wealthier Nicaraguan refugees who escaped the Sandinista revolution of 1979, many of whom settled in the Miami area.

The racial ancestry of Central Americans also varies substantially across the countries in the region, with important consequences for the adaptation of particular groups to U.S. society. For example, a high proportion of the population of Panama and Honduras is of African descent, leading to the settling of many dark-skinned Panamanians and Hondurans in traditionally segregated black neighborhoods in the United States. *Mestizos* (primarily a mix of Spanish Caucasian and native indigenous groups) predominate among Salvadorans, Guatemalans, Nicaraguans, and Costa Ricans. In general, as with most other Latino groups, the social, economic, educational, and racial characteristics of Central Americans, in the context of a traditionally racist and segregationist host society, explain their general social and economic deprivation at the margins of U.S. society.

South Americans

South America is composed of 13 nations. With the exception of Brazil (official language Portuguese), French Guiana (official language French), Guyana (official language English), and Suriname (official language Dutch), the other nine countries—Venezuela, Colombia, Ecuador, Perú, Bolivia, Chile, Argentina, Paraguay, and Uruguay—are officially Spanish-speaking. However, there are many indigenous languages and dialects that are widely spoken throughout the continent. In 2004, there were an estimated 2.1 million South American immigrants living in the United States (U.S. Census Bureau 2004). The largest groups of South American immigrants (listed according to group size) are Colombians, Ecuadorians, Peruvians, Argentineans, and Venezuelans (U.S. Census Bureau 2001). There has also been a substantial migration from Brazil in recent years. Although Brazilians share many cultural characteristics with other Latin Americans and are sometimes catalogued as "Latinos," they are usually distinguished from Hispanic groups in the United States because of their Portuguese, as opposed to Spanish, heritage. (We will expand our discussion of the usage of the terms *Latino* and *Hispanic* in a later section.)

Despite definite cultural differences across the various South American groups, there are certain commonalities that help explain their migration patterns to the United States. Many South American immigrants bring with them greater financial resources and higher levels of education than Mexicans, Dominicans, and some Central Americans (U.S. Census Bureau 2004). This is due, in part, to their greater geographic distance from the United States, which makes it more difficult for individuals with very scarce resources to migrate. Yet although some South Americans arrive in the United States legally with tourist visas, others enter undocumented, primarily via Mexico. There are also important differences in the social and economic backgrounds of the various South American groups. In general, immigrants from Argentina, Chile, and Venezuela tend to come from more affluent backgrounds and to be more educated, more urban, and lighter-skinned than most Ecuadorians, Colombians, and Peruvians. It is important to note that these differences may be more reflective of the characteristics of the particular subgroups within those countries that are likely to migrate than of general cross-national differences. For example, the fact that some Argentinean and Chilean immigrants appear more educated than other Latinos in the United States may cause some to overgeneralize and wrongly assume that these groups, at large, are more educated or sophisticated.

Another important difference among South Americans is their racial composition. Whereas some groups, like Ecuadorians, Colombians, Peruvians, Venezuelans, and Bolivians have a large *mestizo* racial representation, others, like Argentineans and Chileans, have a substantially larger European ancestry. These differences determine to a large extent the level of prejudice and discrimination that members of these groups are likely to face in the United States, as well as help explain some of the prejudices held by some members of these Latino groups against other Latinos.

In the following sections, we will apply the DSM-IV-TR Outline for Cultural Formulation (American Psychiatric Association 2000) and show how it can be used to diagnose and treat Latino patients.

Applying the DMS-IV-TR Outline for Cultural Formulation

A. Cultural Identity of the Individual

Cultural/Ethnic/Racial Identities

Assessing a patient's cultural and ethnic identity is a complex process. It is essential for clinicians to make this evaluation based on information provided by the patient rather than on the evaluator's unsubstantiated assumptions. The clinician should ask patients to describe the culture with which they identify. Patients' descriptions of their social and family practices as well as other values and behaviors can provide a wealth of data about their level of involvement with their culture of origin. Interesting dilemmas may arise when patients' subjective identifications do not converge with more objective cultural assessments of their values and behaviors. For example, a patient may describe her cultural identity as "Latina," despite no knowledge of Spanish, no participation in practices characteristic of Latino cultures, and clear endorsement of values typical of Anglo-American mainstream culture. Nonetheless, her self-representation as a Latina provides useful information about how she likes to be categorized, even if this is more indicative of a desire to belong to that culture than of the direct influence of Latino culture on her values and behaviors.

In another potential scenario, a teenage boy born in this country to Latino immigrant parents may defensively respond to inquiries about cultural identity by saying: "I'm American," thus resisting any categorization as Latino. Yet this teenager may speak fluent Spanish at home, live in a primarily Latino neighborhood, and engage in numerous Latino cultural practices. Similar to the previous example, his response provides valuable information about his subjective self-representation and wish for mainstream group membership. However, taking his response at face value, without further inquiry and attention to other data related to observable cultural practices, could result in missing information that might be useful in developing an effective intervention strategy.

Cultures are not static entities, and most Latinos in the United States, by definition, live in a multicultural context that causes ongoing modifications in their cultural identity. Intermixing with other ethnocultural groups is common, and Latino individuals and communities vary greatly in the degree to which they are affected by surrounding cultural influences. For example, the emergence of a hybrid Latino–U.S. African American culture in some large urban centers, the development of a local "Nuyorican" identity as an adaptive response by Puerto Rican migrants to the idiosyncrasies of New York life, and the evolution of a "Chicano" cultural identity among Mexican immigrants in California, Texas, and other U.S. southwestern states are cases in point.

Another important aspect of identity among Latinos is their perceptions of racial identity. Latin America is one of the most richly diverse regions in the world with regard to racial intermixing. Therefore, most Latin American societies have developed complex categorizations along a racial continuum with subtle gradations of "Europeanness," "Africanness," and "Indianness" that have little in common with more dichotomous/dichromatic U.S. concepts based on the legacy of the "one-drop rule." This is not to suggest that Latin American societies are devoid of racism. Yet the physical cues that distinguish "whites" from "blacks" in the United States lack the same significance in many Latin American countries. For example, an individual who is regarded as white or *mestizo* in a Caribbean country may be classified as black in the United States. Coming to terms with a dichotomous conception of race is one of the hardships associated with migration for many Latinos. As a result, they typically resist U.S. "white/black" classifications. In the 2000 U.S. Census, Hispanics described their race as follows: 48% chose "white," 42% "some other race," 6% mix of "two or more races," 2% "black or African American," 1% "American Indian or Alaska Native," 0.3% "Asian," and 0.1% "Native Hawaiian and other Pacific Islander" (U.S. Census Bureau 2002). In general, Latinos have a stronger sense of group affiliation according to their cultural or ethnic identity than to their racial identity; this can cause difficulties adapting to the United States, where racial identity precedes all other social categorization.

Preferred Terms

The term *Hispanic* refers to persons who share a common language (Spanish) and a common cultural and ethnic heritage associated with either Spain or Spanish colonization. *Latino,* on the other hand, is generally used in the United States to refer to individuals who trace their heritage to one of the Spanish-speaking Latin American countries. However, the term can also be used to refer to those whose language has Latin roots, including not just Spain, but also Portugal, France, Italy, and their colonies. This vagueness makes the use of the term *Latino* somewhat inconsistent, since it is not clear, for example, whether it excludes Spaniards but includes Brazilians on the basis of geography, or vice versa, on the basis of language. A preference for *Latino* over *Hispanic* exists among some in the United States for two main reasons: 1) a sociopolitical position advocating use of a Spanish term popularized by the group members themselves, and 2) a desire to dissociate the group from the former Spanish colonizers and acknowledge the essential contribution of non-European ethnic and cultural elements to the formation of Latin American peoples.[2] Other terms have been proposed, such as *hispanos* (Spanish for *Hispanics*), and *americanos* (Spanish for *Americans*), as a statement that Latin Americans residing in Latin America are also Americans as

---

[2] Ironically, the term *Latin America* was deliberately coined by the French in the mid-nineteenth century in an attempt to naturalize the expansion of Napoleon's empire to Latin American by highlighting the "common" "Latin" roots of the French with the Spanish- and Portuguese-speaking peoples who inhabited the region.

residents of the American continent, as well as to reflect a sense of belonging to a particular U.S. Latino subpopulation. Despite the lack of consensus, *Latino* and *Hispanic* are still the most common terms used in the United States by both Anglo and Hispanic Americans.

Cultural Factors in Development

Family Structure. Latino cultures tend to be family oriented, in the sense that most cultural activities center on the family unit, a high value is placed on family cohesiveness and interdependence, and family goals often supersede individual ones. This tendency has been described as *familismo* or "familism" in social science research (Sabogal et al. 1987). Although a stronger bond typically exists within the nuclear family, the extended family also tends to play a central role in many Latino family dynamics. The concept of extended family may also go beyond grandparents, uncles, aunts, cousins, and in-laws. In many Latino groups, there is a strong family bond of *compadrazgo,* which signifies the relationship between parents and godparents, or *compadres.* Grandparents, especially, tend to occupy a central role in many Latino families, often becoming closely involved in raising grandchildren. Grandparents are also typically valued and respected as sources of advice and "old wisdom."

Family cohesiveness among Latino immigrants tends to be enhanced with the migration process: greater family interdependence is common because of the loss of their extended family network. Moreover, the cohesiveness and solidarity that are common among oppressed groups in a society may reinforce these tendencies even further. An interesting aspect of family cohesiveness and interdependence is that these dynamics can serve both as sources of support and causes of marked distress. This duality is relevant to the assessment of mental health problems in Latino patients, because very frequently these problems are rooted in disruptions within the family system. Taking an individuocentric approach to psychiatric assessments with Latino patients may result in the clinician's missing key information with significant diagnostic, etiological, and treatment relevance.

Developmental Issues. A substantial portion of the Latino population in the United States complete most of their development in this country (40%–60% are U.S. born, and 34% are 18 years or younger), which should lead clinicians to consider the developmental impact of growing up and living as a

Latino in U.S. society. The potential negative consequences of ethnic minority status for child development—such as low self-esteem, low motivation and aspirations, and higher vulnerability to antisocial and disruptive behaviors—have been clearly documented (Phinney and Kohatsu 1997). Clinicians must carefully consider the influence of psychosocial developmental processes on any observed psychopathology.

Dependency-related behaviors are commonly evaluated in psychiatric assessments to determine the presence of psychopathology or behavioral problems associated with developmental factors. Cultural factors influence the level of interdependence considered appropriate or "normal" among members of a particular group. The U.S. values of independence and autonomy, deeply rooted in European American Protestant traditions, contrast sharply with Latino cultural values of collectivism and group orientation (Marín and Triandis 1985). What may be regarded as normal levels of interdependence among Latino patients may be inaccurately assessed as overdependence by Anglo-American clinicians. For example, it is quite common for many young Latino adults to live with their parents until they get married, or during college, while demonstrating culturally appropriate levels of independence and autonomy. Such behaviors, if assessed through a U.S. mainstream cultural lens, may be misinterpreted as indicative of overdependent personality styles.

Behaviors that are adaptive in a given cultural context may also become dysfunctional in a different setting. Expanding on the previous example, a young Latino adult raised in the United States who is in the process of deciding whether to move away from home to attend college may experience distress in attempting to reconcile internalized U.S. mainstream values of independence and autonomy with strong feelings of loyalty to preserving family closeness. In this case, the clinician should accurately assess the problem as stemming from a cross-cultural conflict rather than from pathological overdependence. Treatment can then focus on validating both conflicting tendencies and helping the patient reach an acceptable and functional compromise, rather than steering the patient toward resolving misattributed overdependency needs.

Latinos tend to value and respect the elderly, who traditionally are seen as knowledgeable and wise. This often contrasts sharply with the "senior citizen" image commonly portrayed in many industrialized societies, such as U.S. urban settings, where citizens who are out of the workforce are regarded as weak, vulnerable, and unable to care for themselves. A case in point is the negotiation of nursing home placement for the elderly. Although increasingly common in some Latin American countries, nursing home placements are generally considered a last resort for many Latinos and, when pursued, tend to generate guilt, shame, and family distress. A more common practice among Latinos is for family members to take responsibility for the care of the elderly. However, as a result of adaptation to more typical U.S. lifestyles, many Latinos feel increasingly pressured to institutionalize their sick, elderly relatives. Clinicians should approach such situations with sensitivity, being mindful that these decisions tend to generate much distress for many Latino patients. Moreover, clinicians should avoid imposing their own cultural values regarding these decisions on their patients.

Gender Roles and Gender Relations

Gender roles tend to be clearly delineated in Latino cultures. The differentiation of gender roles in the prototypical traditional Latino family includes a heterosexual couple in which the woman is primarily involved in the functions of childcare and homecare and the man has the role of primary breadwinner. The mother's role as a daily caregiver and nurturer makes the family "matrifocal," counterbalancing the "patrilineal" character of authority.

Undoubtedly, many Latinos conform to these traditional gender roles to some degree. However, Latino gender relations have been the object of much stereotyping. The usual caricature describes an all-submissive female and an oppressive and aggressive male or *macho.* These stereotypes ignore the difference between pathological extremes of submission and aggression, on the one hand, and the diversification of gender roles that may serve an adaptive function within particular sociocultural contexts, on the other. Highly hierarchical societies with traditionally agricultural economies, such as those from which many Latino migrants originate, have been associated with more differentiated gender roles than is expected in postindustrial urban power centers.

Two terms to describe prototypical gender values among Latinos that have been widely used in the United States social science literature are *machismo* and *marianismo. Machismo,* which refers to men's attitudes and behaviors associated with sexual dominance and aggressive behavior, has been promoted in the United States almost as the quintessential trait of Latino men. The fact that this Spanish term has entered contemporary English language usage may reinforce the implicit notion that male oppressiveness is a particular trait of Latinos. Clearly, male dominance and aggressive behavior toward women exist in Latino cultures, as well as in most cultures, including U.S. mainstream society. However, the original notion of the term *macho* includes more than its inarguably negative aspects. It involves other adaptive features of culturally determined masculinity in Latino societies, such as personal responsibility, strength and bravery in the face of adversity, and being a good husband, father, provider, and protector of the family's honor at all times (Morales 1996).

The term *marianismo* is often regarded as a sort of cultural complement to *machismo*. It refers to qualities of culturally determined femininity presumably modeled after the Virgin Mary, such as submissiveness to men, acceptance of domestic chores and family responsibilities, and taking on an unconditional nurturing and self-sacrificing role as mother and wife. While the term *machismo* has been popularized in Latino and U.S. mainstream cultures, *marianismo* has seldom been used except in the U.S. social science literature. As with its male counterpart, *marianismo* tends to describe prototypical features of traditional female gender roles in most hierarchical societies of Mediterranean and Catholic background. The clinician is urged to explore meanings beyond the stereotypical terms *marianismo* and *machismo*. This exploration also should include a careful assessment of the patient's possible genuine disagreement and discomfort with these values and practices.

Spirituality and Religion

Roman Catholicism has been the dominant religion of all Hispanic countries. Nevertheless, Latinos also display a diversity of spiritual and religious traditions that reflects the heterogeneity of cultural and ethnic influences in Latin America. A comprehensive analysis of elements of Catholicism that have permeated the values and behaviors of Latino cultures goes beyond the scope of this chapter. Some often cited and largely stereotyped examples of such values include *marianismo* (described above) and the expectation that female virginity will be maintained before marriage. However, other more positive aspects of Catholicism, such as the strong value placed on humility and selflessness tend to be underemphasized, especially when critically examined through the lens of Protestant-dominant societies.

Diverse Protestant and other Christian traditions have grown in importance in recent years throughout Latin America and among U.S. Latinos.

Common church affiliations of many Latinos in the United States include Pentecostal, Evangelical, Jehovah's Witness, and Seventh Day Adventist, among others. About 23% of Latinos in the United States (9.5 million) identify themselves as Protestants or "other Christians" (Espinosa et al. 2005). Judaism is also practiced by many Latinos, especially from countries that received a large influx of European Jewish immigrants, such as Argentina and Chile. In addition to the religious traditions brought from Latin America, many Latinos have adopted new religions while living in the United States, including Islam, Buddhism, and spiritual practices associated with nontraditional or alternative philosophies and movements.

Given the mix of Amerindian, African, and European ethnicities in Latin America, a variety of religious and spiritual practices reflecting the intermingling of these traditions have also evolved. One set of traditions derives from the syncretism of African and Catholic practices, with a lesser influx of Amerindian elements. These include *santería* and *palo mayombe* among Cubans (Cabrera 1995) and *brujería* and *gagá* among Dominicans (Rosenberg 1979). Among these, *santería* is the most widespread among Latinos in the United States. This religious practice is a syncretism of African, primarily Yoruban, traditions and Catholicism. It involves an elaborate pantheon of deities called *orichas* or *santos* (saints) who exert influence over all elements of life. Most frequently, *orichas* are called on to intervene in matters related to health, wealth, and social relations, especially those of a romantic nature. The practice of *santería* has spread from Cuba to other Latin American areas, such as Puerto Rico and the Dominican Republic, as well as to major U.S. cities, where it includes converts from diverse Latino as well as non-Latino groups.

Another set of indigenous traditions is usually subsumed under the generic label *curanderismo* and is characterized by a variety of folk healing practices primarily of Amerindian origin (Harwood 1981). *Curanderos* (indigenous folk healers) of various sorts are commonly employed as part of their help-seeking regimen by many Latinos, especially of Mexican, Central American, and South American origin. Another spiritual practice that is popular among some U.S. Latinos is *espiritismo* ("spiritism") (Harwood 1987). The roots of *espiritismo* can be traced to the combination of nineteenth-century European spiritualistic movements with syncretic folk healing practices in Latin America. Some of the countries and areas that received a significant influence of spiritism are Argentina, Brazil, Cuba, Puerto Rico, and Venezuela.

These practices have been stigmatized as nonscientific and primitive both in Latino cultures and in the United States, resulting in reluctance among their practitioners to openly discuss their beliefs and involvement, especially with those outside their cultural group. These topics will be generally avoided in encounters with clinicians and researchers, who are assumed not to be accepting of these traditions. Clinicians should be cautious not to let the unfamiliar or exotic appearance of these practices lead to their pathologization, since they often provide supportive and healing functions for those who practice them. The actual prevalence of these practices among U.S. Latinos remains unknown, given inconsistent results from various surveys (Hohmann et al. 1990; U.S. Department of Health and Human Services 2001). Although they are used by some, one must avoid overgeneralizing about the prevalence of these practices among Latinos.

B. Cultural Explanations of the Individual's Illness

General Health-Related Concepts and Practices

There is great heterogeneity in health-related concepts and practices among Latinos, both in Latin America and in the United States. Reasons for this include individual differences and cultural variations related to diversity in national and regional origin, urban or rural background, education, and socioeconomic status. In general, Latinos with greater access to wealth and education favor evidence-based biomedical practices over indigenous forms of care. However, spiritual notions of health and emotional well-being are also common among Latinos across diverse socioeconomic strata, considerably broadening the appeal of indigenous healing practices that are based on spiritual traditions.

The role of spirituality is reflected in ideas about the supernatural causation of illness, the power of prayer, faith, and certain folk healing practices (e.g., special baths with spiritually endowed natural compounds). Most spiritual forms of therapy among Latinos, however, are seen as adjunctive rather than alternative treatments; as a rule, conventional medical interventions are neither thought of as contraindicated nor routinely discouraged. For example, a person may believe that his or her cancer is caused by negative spiritual influence, and consequently engage in fervent prayer, yet at the same time carefully follow medically prescribed chemotherapy.

For mental health disorders, however, several factors complicate popular acceptance of psychiatric diagnoses and treatments among many Latinos. These include the absence of concrete confirmatory diagnostic tests, the stigma attached to psychiatric labels and medications, and the perception that mental health disorders are just exaggerated versions of common coping difficulties in the face of adverse circumstances. As such, help for mental disorder may be sought within the family, community, or church. However, many Latinos from societies with long psychotherapy traditions, like Argentina, may display more openness to particular forms of psychiatric treatment, such as psychoanalysis. In addition, the mind-body-social split is less pronounced among many Latinos than in mainstream Anglo-American culture, leading to more unified understandings of physical, emotional, and social (biopsychosocial) etiologies, symptoms, and treatments.

Predominant Idioms of Distress and Local Illness Categories

Indigenous views about health and illness contribute to shaping pathological emotional/behavioral expressions among Latinos. The notion of *nervios* (nerves) is common to many Latino groups. This general idiom of distress is based on the cultural view that the nervous system, including the anatomical nerves, is "altered" in unspecified ways by the impact of stressful life events, resulting in a diversity of pathological states. The severity of the impact is mediated by the person's vulnerability, which is believed to have both bodily (e.g., inherited, temperamental) and social/interpersonal aspects. On the one hand, this tends to normalize the pathology as an appropriate reaction to adverse circumstances, unless it exceeds popular norms for symptom expression (e.g., violent or suicidal outbursts). On the other hand, the view that *nervios* is connected to at least transient "alterations" of the nervous system opens the door to the possibility of biomedical evaluation and treatment. Much of the cultural work involved in the determination of whether a person is actually suffering from *nervios* has to do with assessment of the relative relationship of stressors and vulnerabilities, the extent to which the person should be held responsible for controlling their distress, and the perceived risk of chronic and severe psychopathology.

Acute exacerbations of *nervios* may be labeled *ataques de nervios* (attacks of nerves) by some Latino groups, notably those of Caribbean origin, and are supposed to arise from overwhelming suffering, especially if unexpected. Labeled a "culture-bound syndrome" or locally identified symptom complex in DSM-IV-TR (American Psychiatric Association 2000), *ataque de nervios* refers to dramatic episodes of loss of control, accompanied by distressing, fit-like expressions of emotionality and physical symptoms. According to DSM-IV-TR:

> Commonly reported symptoms include uncontrollable shouting, attacks of crying, trembling, heat in the chest rising into the head, and verbal or physical aggression. Dissociative experiences, seizurelike or fainting episodes, and suicidal gestures are prominent in some attacks but absent in others....People may experience amnesia for what occurred during the ataque de nervios, but they otherwise return rapidly to their usual level of functioning. (p. 899)

Ataques do not have a one-to-one relationship with psychiatric disorders. In community epidemiological studies in Puerto Rico, they were found to be significantly more likely in persons with major depression, dysthymia, panic disorder, posttraumatic stress disorder, and generalized anxiety disorder than in persons without these disorders (Guarnaccia 1993). The presence of *ataques* therefore does not signal a specific psychiatric disorder but rather seems to be associated with the experience of being overwhelmed, which cuts across many forms of psychopathology. The episodes are supposed to call forth the person's support network, but they may be ineffective in situations of very limited resources, overly frequent distress, or cultural change, when the implied message may be misunderstood or unattended.

Another idiom of distress that is common across several Latino groups has been labeled somatization, a tendency to report medically unexplained physical symptoms in the context of emotional distress (Escobar 1987). There is an inherent assumption, deeply rooted in biomedical culture and widespread among clinicians, that the tendency to somatize represents a more primitive or less adaptive mode of symptomatic expression. The verbal expression of emotional distress (often referred to as *psychologization*) is assumed to be more adaptive, as well as implicitly associated with a higher level of sophistication. However, the greater adaptive value of psychologization over somatization has yet to be proven. In fact, the universality of somatization challenges these assumptions (Kirmayer 1998; Kleinman 1980).

Moreover, the tendency to express distress via somatic idioms should not be construed as an inability to express or even label emotional states. It seems to derive instead from the less pronounced nature of the mind-body-social split, as mentioned earlier. A.J. Laria and A. Calvillo ("Echoes of Migration: Medically Unexplained Symptoms Among Latino Immigrant Patients Attending a U.S. Primary Care Clinic," unpublished manuscript, 2006) found that most of the Latino primary care patients they studied who reported medically unexplained physical symptoms expressed clear ideas about the relationship between social, psychological, and physiological events. Rather than lacking verbal-psychological expressions to channel their emotional distress, these patients expressed it through a combination of verbal-psychological *and* somatic idioms. In fact, the apparent integration of "somatic" and "mental" forms of emotion may derive less from Latino cultural peculiarities than from historical commitments of the culture of biomedicine, which splits mental, physical, and social problems into separate entities. Ironically, although the health-related views of many Latinos seem quite compatible with the current biopsychosocial paradigm of health, clinical interventions that adequately address relationships among biological, psychological, and social factors are scarce. New applied models and interventions are needed that can effectively target these biopsychosocial relationships in an integrative fashion.

Another important idiom of distress common to several Latino groups is that of reporting distressing perceptual alterations as signs of psychopathology. These perceptual changes include visual, auditory, and tactile/haptic experiences, with both illusory and hallucinatory phenomenology. Typical examples include seeing a shadow or a glimpse (*celaje*); hearing one's name called when alone; other auditory experiences, such as noises or mumbling sounds; and feeling the presence of someone nearby when alone. These experiences are often attributed to spiritual influences that are becoming manifest and distressing because of the weakened physioemotional state induced by the person's suffering. Although such phenomena are sometimes described by psychotic persons, most of these reports occur in persons with other forms of psychopathology or as nonpathological experiences. Lewis-Fernández and colleagues (2003a) have found that these experiences are more frequent among psychiatric outpatients with posttraumatic stress disorder and major depression than with social phobia and can occur independently of any clearly psychotic symptoms. These reports are very prevalent in primary care settings, where they are more common in Latino than non-Latino respondents and are associated with more severe distress, including greater suicidality and psychosocial impairment (Olfson et al. 2002). Although often resulting from emotional distress, these experiences can easily mislead clinicians to diagnose a psychotic disorder where none is present, with the attendant risks of neuroleptic medication and missed attention to more salient psychosocial interventions. There is also evidence that these experiences can occur in the absence of any associated psychopathology. Labeling such nonordinary perceptual experiences "normal dissociative experiences," Laria (1998) identified high levels of intensity and frequency among a group of Cuban *mediums espiritistas* (spiritist mediums) who did not show any psychopathology or emotional distress. These findings further support the role of cultural factors in shaping these perceptual experiences.

Many other idioms and local illness categories are present among Latinos. Some of these are described in Appendix I of DSM-IV-TR in the Glossary of Culture-Bound Syndromes (American Psychiatric Association 2000). Notable among them is *susto* (literally, "fright"), a syndrome especially common among Central Americans, Mexicans, and some South Americans. *Susto* typically follows a frightening event, which may or may not be of traumatic proportion, and is characterized by a mix of depressive, anxiety, and somatic symptoms. In the original Amerindian perspective, following the belief that fright causes the soul to leave the body, treatment consists of calling back the soul through a series of ritualistic events and cleansing the person to restore bodily and spiritual balance. Other Latino cultural categories of illness include *cólera* (literally, "rage"), also known as *bilis* or *muina,* and *mal de ojo* (evil eye), which are described briefly in DSM-IV-TR.

Clinicians should appreciate that these syndromes are intricately embedded in the patient's sociocultural world. A parallel integrative nosological approach, using both Western and culturally congruent concepts, should be used in evaluating and treating these conditions, paying attention simultaneously to biomedical, psychological, and cultural factors relevant to illness and treatment.

Cultural Factors in Help-Seeking

Studies have shown that Latinos in the United States underutilize mental health services relative to non-Latino whites and to their own mental health need (U.S. Department of Health and Human Services 2001; Vega et al. 1999; Wells et al. 1987). Several studies have shown that Latino underutilization extends not only to lower rates of initial entry into mental health care compared with non-Latino whites, but also to poorer treatment retention once care has been accessed (Padgett et al. 1994; Sue 1977; Temkin-Greener and Clark 1988).

Structural and Cultural Barriers to Utilization of Mental Health Services. Various factors may account for Latino underutilization of mental health services. Structural barriers, such as low rates of insurance or the lack of bilingual, bicultural providers in low-income and rural areas where many Latinos reside, clearly impede overall access to care for Latinos (Dworkin and Adams 1987; J. Miranda et al. 1996). Financial limitations and inflexible job demands affect the ability to arrange for transportation, childcare, and time off work.

Several studies have emphasized the key role that cultural factors play in creating barriers to care (Vega et al. 1999; Wells et al. 1987). The substantial social stigma of carrying a mental health diagnosis and seeking mental health treatment among Latinos discourages many from seeking appropriate services, even when these are available. Latinos defined as more "traditional"— as measured by nativity, immigration status, language fluency, and degree of acculturation—consistently show significantly lower utilization than those with greater connection to mainstream U.S. society, even after controlling for differences in sociodemographic and economic status, physical and mental health status, and type of insurance (M.R. Miranda et al. 1976; Vega et al. 1999; Wells et al. 1987). The 2001 supplement to the Surgeon General's report on mental health singled out Latino immigrants as being particularly underserved with regard to mental health services (U.S. Department of Health and Human Services 2001).

Cultural Congruence.   The importance of migration and acculturation status in underutilization underlines the key role that cultural congruence plays in the process of health care access and retention. *Cultural congruence* refers to the degree to which the characteristics of the health care system match the cultural expectations of treatment in the target community. These expectations extend to the language in which the clinical encounter occurs, the nature of the workup and interpretation of symptoms, the treatments offered, and the outcomes envisioned. In addition, other important factors are the attitude toward including social support networks, such as folk healers and other spiritual religious practitioners, in recovery, and the ways in which the perceived stigma of mental illness is addressed (Cheung and Snowden 1990; Guarnaccia and

Rodríguez 1996; Kleinman 1980). Investigators have repeatedly noted that Latinos are typically responding to culturally syntonic norms regarding these issues (Rogler 1996; U.S. Department of Health and Human Services 2001). Therefore, the clinician should be aware of the cultural norms of the patient and, when appropriate, enlist the aid of a *cultural broker* (someone with appropriate cultural knowledge whom the clinician can consult about the impact of cultural factors on assessment and treatment). The following case vignette illustrates the role of cultural factors in shaping how patients experience and describe psychiatric symptoms as well as their help-seeking expectations.

Mrs. T is a 56-year-old woman from Puerto Rico who migrated to New York City at the age of 27. Her husband died of a heart attack 3 years ago. She has one daughter, age 32, who lives close by, and a son, age 29, living in Florida. Mrs. T was referred to a mental health clinic by her primary care clinician because of multiple chronic somatic complaints, including chest pain, headaches, fatigue, and pain in her legs. Mrs. T reported that her symptoms began shortly after her husband passed away. She also experiences frequent crying spells whenever she thinks of her husband.

Several follow-up medical examinations revealed no apparent organic basis for her symptoms, resulting in a diagnostic impression of psychogenic factors underlying her condition and a referral to mental health. The referral note indicated "mixed depression and anxiety with somatization—no organic basis for her physical complaints."

At the mental health clinic, Mrs. T saw a psychiatrist for a psychopharmacological evaluation and a psychologist for psychotherapy. She received a diagnosis of chronic depressive disorder with subsyndromal anxiety and somatization. Her evaluators also concluded that she was having a "protracted pathological grief reaction," supported by the fact that her symptoms exceeded the 1-year limit typically expected for a "normal" grief process. Her pathological grief reaction was assumed to be caused by a combination of her cognitive style and her neurochemical makeup. A selective serotonin reuptake inhibitor antidepressant was prescribed, and she was referred for individual cognitive-behavioral therapy (CBT) for depression.

Mrs. T initially showed some resistance to mental health treatment, insisting that her physical symptoms were "real" and "not in my head." Although she acknowledged feelings of depression and anxiety, she explained that these were to be expected, given her being in mourning after her husband's death. Moreover, she associated these symptoms to feeling estranged from her children, yet she said she did not want to impose on their lives, claiming that they were too busy with their own families. She expressed strong doubts that antidepressant medication would help her with her physical symptoms (her original chief complaint) and argued that her thinking style had nothing to do with her feeling sad about missing her husband, to whom she was very close. When the mental health clinicians tried to explain to her that normal grief reactions typically last about 1 year, she responded, "sometimes you can feel very sad and depressed about someone you loved for your whole life." Mrs. T showed minimal response to the combination of antidepressant medication and CBT, and shortly thereafter she dropped out of treatment.

This case illustrates several points in the process of negotiating between a psychiatric evaluation and a Latina patient's explanatory model of illness. First, the primary care clinician's referral to mental health exemplifies conventional medical practice, which reflects a mind-body-social split that distinguishes between physical and psychological symptoms and separates them into distinct specialty systems of care. Despite the prevailing biopsychosocial model of health, social-contextual factors tend to be underemphasized in practice, as illustrated in this case, where the major social factors associated with Mrs. T's distress—her husband's death and her estrangement from her children—were underemphasized in the treatment regimen. Instead, treatment focused on the neurochemical and cognitive aspects of her condition. This approach clashed with her understandings and expectations about her condition, and she interpreted the fact that her physical symptoms provoked a referral to mental health as indicative that her symptoms were regarded as "mental," and therefore not physically "real."

Care was predicated on the cultural assumption that a normal grief process should not exceed 1 year. Following from this assumption, Mrs. T's symptoms could not be attributed solely to a normal grief reaction. This clinical formulation contrasted sharply with the patient's explanatory model, which allowed for a more flexible and lengthy mourning process. Although she acknowledged that her physical symptoms were originally triggered by the stressful impact of her husband's sudden death, she still insisted that there were physical factors involved in her symptoms.

Therapeutic failure in this case may be attributed to the inability to reconcile conventional medical and psychiatric formulations with the patient's explanatory model of illness. A more culturally congruent and potentially effective way of designing an intervention for Mrs. T could have involved an attempt to negotiate between the two models from a truly integrative perspective. Working from a sociopsychosomatic model, the primary care clinician could have collaborated closely with the mental health clinicians as an integrative team working jointly to treat Mrs. T's symptoms. Moreover, accepting the cultural limitations of our biomedical assumptions could have allowed clinicians the flexibility to consider Mrs. T's symptoms as part of a culturally shaped normative grief process. Such recognition could have led to a greater emphasis of the need to incorporate factors related to her grief process into her treatment.

Greater attention to the importance of social factors in her condition could have resulted in prioritizing the theme of her estrangement from her children in the treatment. Greater flexibility on the part of the clinicians to consider her explanatory model of illness would have also conveyed a sense of sociocultural validation. This might have facilitated Mrs. T's openness to try other tools, such as antidepressants and culturally modified CBT, which were initially outside of her explanatory model. Thus, using culturally congruent integrated biopsychosocial treatment could have represented a satisfactory compromise between the explanatory models of patient and clinicians, leading to a greater likelihood of treatment adherence and effectiveness.

C. Cultural Factors Related to Psychosocial Environment and Levels of Functioning

Social Context

In general, Latinos living in the United States are poorer, have darker skin, and are less educated, more lacking in marketable job skills, and less socially esteemed than white Anglo members of the U.S. mainstream. Often, Latinos are the victims of substantial prejudice, discrimination, social neglect, and other forms of institutionalized violence. It is essential to recognize that the consequences of these social ills do not constitute cultural characteristics of Latino groups, but rather cultural characteristics of U.S. society as a whole. Misrepresenting the negative consequences of social violence as individual or group psychopathology can serve to obscure the roots of these social problems and "blame the victims." To be treated effectively, socially rooted psychopathologies require interventions that recognize and address the social nature of these conditions, such as racism, classism, and stereotyping.

Higher rates of mood and anxiety disorder, substance abuse, and overall psychiatric disorders are reported among U.S.-born Mexican Americans compared with immigrants born in Mexico (Escobar et al. 2000; Kessler et al. 1994; Vega et al. 1999). Moreover, the rates for recent migrants are similar to those obtained in Mexico City, and the rates for U.S.-born Mexican Americans are virtually identical to those of the U.S. mainstream population as assessed in the National Comorbidity Survey (Kessler et al. 1994), anchoring the prevalence rates in national estimates at both ends of the migration continuum (Vega et al. 1999). In addition, for Mexican migrants, a longer length of stay in the United States is associated with increased psychopathology (Vega et al. 1999). Higher rates of lifetime depression have also been found among Puerto Ricans in New York City compared with those living in Puerto Rico (Canino et al. 1987; Moscicki et al. 1987). The rates of substance-related disorders are alarmingly higher for U.S.-born Mexican Americans compared with Mexican immigrants—seven times higher for women and two times higher for men (Vega et al. 1999). Factors associated with living in, and especially growing up in, the United States seem to have a detrimental effect on the general mental health of Latinos (Hernández and Charney 1998). The apparent paradox of these findings is that declining mental health often coincides with increased access to financial programs and health care services. Social indices by themselves do not explain these findings, and it is likely that cultural differences in lifestyle factors, expectations of mainstream culture integration, social roles, and loss of cultural protective factors play important roles.

Developmental Issues

Several studies have confirmed that Latino children and adolescents living in the United States have higher rates of depression and anxiety-related behavioral problems than mainstream non-Hispanic white children (Achenbach et al. 1990; Glover et al. 1999). Similar to the case of adults, U.S.-born Latino children fare worse than immigrant children born in Latin America. Mexican American children, for example, report higher rates of depression, suicide, and drug use than Mexican children (Swanson et al. 1992). An alarming finding is that although U.S. Latinos in general have a lower suicide rate than the U.S. mainstream population, U.S. Latino adolescents report higher suicidal ideation and suicidal attempts than either white or African American children (Centers for Disease Control and Prevention 1998). Given that more than one-third of Latinos in the United States are younger than 18 and that the majority of Latino youth are U.S. born, these findings suggest an extraordinary epidemic of mental health problems among Latino children and adolescents. Another area of concern is the extremely high rates of law-related behavioral and mental health problems among U.S. Latinos. Latino prison inmates outnumber non-Latino whites by three to one (9% vs. 3%) (U.S. Bureau of Justice Statistics 1999). Further, Latinos are four times more likely than non-Latino whites to be imprisoned at some point in their lives, and Latino youth have much higher delinquency rates (Vazsonyi and Flannery 1997). In turn, incarcerated individuals have higher rates of mental health problems than community residents (Teplin 1994).

Social Support: Protective Factors

Some characteristics of Latino cultures appear to function as protective factors against mental health problems. For example, one suggested explanation for the lower suicide rate among Latinos, as compared with non-Latino whites (Oquendo et al. 2001), is their high reliance on spirituality, which promotes a sense of hope and acceptance in the face of adversity. Another protective factor appears to be immigrant status. Immigrants may be protected through a sense of hardiness and hope in the future, especially when compared with the economic hardships they suffered "back home" (Suárez-Orozco and Suárez-Orozco 1995). Conversely, the healthier outcomes among Latino immigrants may have more to do with the mere absence of the increased vulnerability that U.S.-born Latinos experience due to their ethnic minority status in U.S. society and the differential treatment and detrimental effects that result from it.

Social orientation also appears to be a protective factor among Latinos. In light of the importance of social support in promoting mental health, the more sociocentric orientation of Latinos compared with a more individualistic U.S. mainstream culture may foster greater family and community support. An illustration of this in terms of the positive role of the extended family is the lower rates of foster home placement for Latino children and of nursing home referrals among Latino elderly, who tend to be cared for at home (Angel 1998; Santiago-Rivera et al. 2002).

The following case vignette illustrates the influence of the psychosocial context of U.S. Latinos on an individual's psychopathology and level of functioning.

Miguel is an 11-year-old Mexican American boy who was referred for psychiatric evaluation by his school counselor because of his increasing distractibility in school and his inconsistent pattern of academic performance. Psychiatric assessment identified attention difficulties and yielded a diagnosis of attention-deficit/hyperactivity disorder (ADHD). A combination of psychopharmacological management and behavioral therapy for his inattentiveness and hyperactivity was prescribed. Miguel's mother requested permission to leave work early once a week to take Miguel to his weekly psychotherapy appointment. Besides the financial stress that resulted from this, the parents also struggled to afford Miguel's medications, which were not covered by his insurance. Miguel showed only minimal responsiveness after 6 months, at which point his parents decided to discontinue his treatments. The clinicians working with Miguel argued that the parents did not allow the intervention sufficient time for him to show any significant progress and claimed that they had acted irresponsibly given that their son's condition required treatment.

A closer look at Miguel's psychosocial life reveals a Mexican immigrant family struggling with substantial financial stress to provide for a family of nine. Both parents had to work; consequently, the children spent a large amount of time on their own. Miguel would typically be supervised by one of his older siblings. His 17-year-old brother Pacho had been hospitalized a month earlier after being shot and seriously wounded in a street gang fight. This incident was very upsetting for the entire family, especially for Miguel, who was very close to Pacho. In addition, there had been several other recent incidents of relatives and neighborhood acquaintances who had been involved in violent incidents, including some fatal cases. Further, the family had received several threats from gang members involved in Pacho's shooting. Their home had been broken into on two occasions, resulting in loss of valuable personal belongings. Another of Miguel's siblings had been arrested on drug-related charges and was spending time in a correctional institution. The parents were very concerned about violence in their neighborhood and about their increasing loss of control over their children. However, they were unable to afford a move into a safer neighborhood because of their tenuous financial situation.

Cases of ADHD in the United States have risen to almost epidemic proportion in recent years, especially among children. Although there is support for a neurochemical basis of ADHD, difficulties in attention can also be associated with high levels of psychological stress. A closer examination of Miguel's psychosocial experience reveals information relevant to assessing his level of functioning. Going beyond an exclusively biomedical etiology to conduct a more comprehensive assessment would reveal the value of contextualizing Miguel's attentional dysfunction within the elevated psychosocial stress that characterizes his life. Medication management and behavioral therapy focused on his attention problem could have been better integrated into a more psychosocially relevant treatment. This more integrated approach would have taken into account the psychosocial stressors that most likely played an important role in the etiology and maintenance of his condition, resulting in a more effective treatment.

D. Cultural Elements of the Relationship Between the Individual and the Clinician

Expectations of Mental Health Practitioners

In general, Latinos tend to regard clinicians as experts, and to expect authoritative opinions and advice. They also expect providers to show genuine caring and concern for their patients, which, for Latinos, is communicated overtly via personal warmth in direct personal interactions. The formal, personally detached, and neutral professional stance that is quite normative among many health care providers in the United States is often interpreted by Latino patients as indicative of a cold, impersonal, and therefore uncaring clinician. In addition, as ethnic minority group members, many Latino patients have experienced significant prejudice and discrimination in the United States, which may predispose some initial distrust and guardedness, especially with Anglo-American clinicians. This should be understood as a generalized defensive reaction with some adaptive value, offering protection against real experiences of prejudice. In general, as increased contact yields evidence of the clinician's genuine concern, most Latinos will be able to establish a trusting therapeutic relationship regardless of differences in cultural, ethnic, or racial backgrounds. In contrast, empathic failures on the part of clinicians who behave in a rude, condescending, or excessively impersonal manner may confirm patients' negative expectations, leading to distrust and impeding a therapeutic alliance. Given the cultural value placed on politeness, many Latino patients may not express their disgust openly toward these clinicians, yet they may resist treatment recommendations, cancel appointments, or drop out of treatment. Clinicians may feel confused when they misinterpret a polite attitude as acceptance of their recommendations and prescribed treatments.

Styles of Communication

Verbal Communication. As in every country or large geographic area sharing a common language, there is a wide range of national and regional accents and colloquial forms of Spanish that clearly distinguish Latinos from diverse countries and regions. Language is also an important way of communicating social class, educational level, and urban or rural origin. Often, there is a confounding of social and national differences, given the specific class, geographic, or educational characteristics of particular groups who migrate from the various Latin American countries. For example, the verbal style of many Argentinean or Chilean immigrants may reveal more advantaged educational and class backgrounds, compared with many Puerto Rican or Mexican migrants, who are of working-class origin.

In addition, language can reflect the level of acculturation of a Latino individual. Most Latinos in the United States are bilingual to some degree, but with different levels of proficiency in Spanish and English. A common mistake among clinicians is to assume that cross-cultural factors are not relevant in working with English-proficient Latino patients. Latinos who are predominantly English-speaking may still display a strong affiliation with a Latin American or U.S. Latino culture.

Another mistake commonly made by clinicians is to assume that because a Latino individual speaks English with a particular accent, he or she is more fluent in Spanish, thus confusing a regional or subcultural accent (e.g., the typical *Nuyorican* or *Chicano* patterns of speech) with lack of English proficiency. Such individuals may be inappropriately referred to Spanish-speaking clinicians on the assumption that they will be able to communicate better in Spanish. Therefore, clinicians must be cautious in making assumptions that lead to cultural and linguistic matching; the best practice is always to ask patients directly about their preferences. A patient's preferred language can also be a way of making an important personal statement. For example, Latino individuals who are fluent in English yet prefer to communicate in Spanish with other Latinos are typically expressing their level of cultural pride and their comfort with adopting a Latino cultural identity in the United States.

Finally, the language used during the clinical interview may affect the level of psychopathology perceived by the clinician. There is some evidence to suggest that Spanish-dominant individuals may appear either more or less pathological during a psychiatric evaluation carried out in English. Some research supports the notion that the greater difficulty of communicating in an unfamiliar language may cause the patient to exert greater care in self-presentation and decrease spontaneous speech, thereby reducing the florid expression of psychopathology (Price and Cuéllar 1981). By contrast, other studies suggest that the additional communication barrier caused by the use of English makes patients appear more pathological than they really are, particularly with regard to the evaluation of thought process, which is usually done through observation of language production (Marcos et al. 1973).

Nonverbal Communication.   Like all cultural groups, Latinos from various national origins display particular nonverbal styles of communication. Many Latinos show a preference for direct and personal interactions and place less emphasis on formality and social distance. This may emerge in a clinical situation as a more interactive style, personally revealing stories, and informal and humorous comments. Latinos generally place a strong value on politeness, which is typically communicated through behaviors such as handshakes, as well as through social agreeability and more receptive attitudes. Some Latinos may interpret the mainstream Anglo-American value of displaying an assertive personality, which is often communicated through an individualistic "critical consumer" stance, as rude and impolite. Similarly, some Anglo-Americans may misinterpret the overt politeness displayed by many Latinos as a lack of assertiveness, when actually it may be a highly valued sign of social competence in Latino culture. Anglo-American clinicians frequently misinterpret the level of agreement expressed by a Latino patient as signifying the patient's acceptance of treatment recommendations and likelihood of adherence to them, only to be confused when the patient shows poor adherence in following their recommendations.

Social distance and physical touch are two potential areas of confusion and misinterpretation in clinical situations. Appropriate social distance among Latinos tends to be closer than the typical norm for Anglo-American culture, and physical touch is more common. Handshakes are expected during most introductions or greetings, and kissing is very common. The appropriateness of kissing is also subculture-specific and class-specific, as well as generational. For many Latinos, especially younger adults from urban areas, kissing on the cheek is typical when either greeting an acquaintance or being introduced to someone in a social situation. Hugging tends to be a sign of closer affection and is usually reserved for relatives and close friends.

Some of the ways in which confusion may arise in a clinical setting due to differences in nonverbal communication can be illustrated with a scenario encountered by one of the authors (A.L.).

> The 6-year-old daughter of a recently migrated Argentinean couple was referred to an outpatient community mental health clinic for evaluation of a possible anxiety disorder. After several meetings, the girl naturally began to approach the therapist to greet him with a kiss on the cheek. As treatment also involved family sessions, the father would always shake hands with the therapist on greeting him, and over time the mother's greeting naturally evolved from a handshake to a kiss on the cheek. The clinician interpreted these behaviors as culturally appropriate, especially in the context of forming a close personal relationship. Having been raised in a Latino culture, yet also acculturated into professional norms typical of psychotherapy training in the United States, the therapist experienced a cross-cultural ethical dilemma. Being observed by colleagues greeting patients with a kiss would undoubtedly be interpreted as a clear violation of professional boundaries. On the other hand, they would likely see refusing the socially appropriate greeting from the mother and daughter as a sign of coldness and rejection. Reaching a compromise was challenging, and there was significant disagreement, even among Latino therapists working at the clinic, about how to behave appropriately. After peer consultation, the therapist chose to continue to reciprocate the culturally determined behavior.

The solution to a given dilemma will depend on the particular circumstances of each case, as well as on the clinician's degree of comfort with adjusting his or her behavior in the service of the patient-clinician relationship. Obviously, Latino patients may also exhibit inappropriate behaviors. As with any other behavioral assessment, if unclear in the interpretation of a given situation, a clinician will need supplemental information, further inquiry and observation, and possibly consultation from cultural experts. In the case discussed above, a non-Latino clinician might not have felt the same level of comfort in reciprocating the patient's and mother's behaviors. However, the key issue was making an accurate assessment of the behavior in terms of the adequate cultural frame of reference; in this case, kissing as an appropriate sign of social appreciation. The non-Latino clinician could have replaced the kiss with a culturally equivalent sign of appreciation, such as a handshake or a verbal comment, or could have openly discussed his or her discomfort with kissing patients, while acknowledging this as a cross-cultural difference. Cultural sensitivity would have been communicated in either case.

Therapy Issues and Stereotypes

There are two cultural agents present in every therapeutic dyad. In addition to a focus on the patient's cultural traits, attention must be paid to the ways in which the cultural characteristics of the clinician influence the therapeutic relationship as well as the patient's behavior. This process of "contextualization" of the patient in the clinical dyad can be seen as a two-step approach. First, the clinician may focus on the patient and ask two basic questions: 1) How does the patient's cultural background influence her/his and my behavior? and 2) What culturally related assumptions may the patient be making about me? Second, the clinician should ask 1) How does my cultural background influence my behavior as well as the patient's? and 2) What culturally related assumptions am I making about the patient?

The importance of such bidirectional analytic processes that allow for the clinician's self-assessment should not be underestimated. Clinicians must be open to recognizing that having preconceived assumptions and biases about other individuals and groups is a universal human trait; the forming of attributions and stereotypes are normative cognitive mechanisms essential to our survival. However, deeply ingrained and emotionally driven ethnic, racial, and cultural biases and prejudices have a more self-serving function, such as the release or displacement of frustration and aggression onto others. A clinician's self-reflection and self-assessment are essential in order to decrease the potential negative impact from prejudicial biases and overgeneralized assumptions on his or her assessment and intervention with Latino patients. A serious commitment to the promotion of culturally sensitive clinical competence skills may eventually lead to reducing some of the marked disparities in health care that have been identified with Latinos, as well as with members of other ethnic minority groups in the United States.

Transference and Countertransference: Working With Latino Patients

In analyzing any therapeutic relationship, it is important to discern the displaced or projective nature of transference and countertransference reactions from appropriate responses to actual attitudes that are accurately perceived by either patient or therapist. In other words, not all prejudiced reactions from an Anglo therapist, or guardedness from a Latino patient, should be considered transferential or countertransferential. Transference reactions that are particular to a given patient must also be discerned from defensive attitudes that may be shared by members of a group given their collective social experience. An example of such shared experiences is the "cultural paranoia" or generalized mistrust toward majority group members that is often observed among members of groups that are victimized in a society, such as ethnic minority groups in the United States, and that may in fact have functional adaptive value (Whaley 2001).

An example of a transference reaction that may be displayed by some Latino patients is that of idealizing an Anglo-American therapist in order to ensure the therapist's approval, as an indirect way of seeking acceptance in U.S. mainstream society. Given the general lack of social validation that Latinos receive in U.S. society, such idealization may serve a compensatory function. The patient may go so far as to devalue or underemphasize his or her own cultural values (a type of "ethnic flight") as a way of securing the unequivocal acceptance of the therapist and the mainstream culture. In such cases, the level of agreeability that is displayed by the patient may cause clinicians to inaccurately assess that the patient has established a genuine trusting relationship. However, a patient can also have a true corrective experience through the development of a genuine validating therapeutic relationship, which may result from accurately perceived, as opposed to projected, qualities of the therapist. In the latter case, the patient's therapeutic experience is likely to effect positive changes in his or her life (e.g., improved sense of self-esteem, enhanced social functioning). By contrast, in the former case, if the transference reaction goes unrecognized, the therapist may be puzzled by the patient's lack of progress despite an apparent positive therapeutic experience. In addition to the patient's idealization of the therapist, the patient may also projectively identify with the therapist and adopt behaviors or attitudes modeled after the therapist. One way of interpreting such transference reactions is as a way of "identifying with the aggressor," thus compensating for the general powerlessness an oppressed patient may experience in U.S. society. A related interpretation may be that the patient seeks to identify with feelings of superiority that are projected onto the therapist, thus attempting to compensate for internalized feelings of low social esteem or self-esteem.

The possible transferential and countertransferential reactions that may emerge with therapists from diverse cultural backgrounds working with Latino patients can be quite varied and complex. Rather than attempting to learn about all possible clinical scenarios, it is the best practice for therapists to become sensitive to exploring the intricate ways in which social and cultural factors may interface with individual elements in the development of transferential reactions by patients. Most important, therapists must develop an honest, self-reflective openness to exploring their own countertransferential reactions. These reactions may either interfere with the therapeutic process or be utilized for therapeutic growth depending on the therapist's ability to recognize them, analyze them accurately, and manipulate them in accordance with the established therapeutic goals.

Ethnocultural transference and countertransference issues have been discussed in detail in Chapter 1. The following vignette illustrates a possible scenario that may emerge with a Latino patient.

Sergio is an 18-year-old college student who emigrated from Ecuador to the United States with his family at age 12. At his roommate's suggestion, he sought help at the college counseling center because of a recent marked decrease in motivation, difficulty sleeping, and loss of appetite with resulting weight loss. In addition, his academic performance had markedly decreased and he had become increasingly isolated. He was evaluated at the counseling center, where he received an antidepressant prescription and was assigned to an Anglo-American psychotherapist for treatment of symptoms of depression.

During his initial visits, Sergio spent most of his time describing the difficulty that his parents experienced when he left home and moved out of state to attend college. He made constant references to the cross-cultural differences between his parents and him, contrasting what he considered the old-fashioned, overprotective, and overdependent style of his Ecuadorian parents with his more "American" values of independence and autonomy. Sergio's manner of relating to the therapist clearly suggested that he felt the therapist could really understand his conflict, given their "shared American perspective." For example, once while describing his conflict with his parents, he said: "As you and I well know, here in the United States, we see things very differently. We're not as dependent on each other, like my parents and my relatives in Ecuador, who think that children should always stay close to home to take care of their parents. Here, we're much more independent, and we strongly believe in pursuing our goals, even if it means moving away from family." In addition, he made frequent derogatory jokes caricaturing his parents' culture. The therapist's initial impression was that although Sergio was an immigrant, he displayed a high degree of assimilation to U.S. culture. This afforded the therapist the sense that he clearly understood his patient's perspective. The therapist regarded these shared values as instrumental in facilitating the formation of a close therapeutic alliance. In an attempt to be empathetic to his patient the therapist expressed his understanding of Sergio's cross-cultural conflict with his parents, and encouraged him to assert his independence and openly express his divergent views to them. Although Sergio continued to act out an empathic identification with the therapist, the therapist became puzzled at Sergio's lack of progress after several months of psychotherapy and psychopharmacological treatment.

One possible way of making sense of the therapeutic impasse is by considering cross-cultural transferential and countertransferential identifications. Sergio's depression may have been partly rooted in an internal cross-cultural conflict resulting from his bicultural experience. As an unconscious strategy to attain an apparent resolution of this conflict, Sergio may have split his ambivalence and projected the part of him that felt conflicted about his decision to move away from home—which violated Ecuadorian cultural norms—onto his parents. Forming a transferential projective identification with his therapist, who represented his more "American" side, facilitated this. However, in doing so, Sergio may have split off the internal core conflict that underlay his depression. The therapist, in a countertransferential reaction triggered both by his need to develop a bond with his patient and be perceived as an effective healer and to assert the validity of his own cultural values, encouraged Sergio's "American values" of autonomy and independence. It is possible that the therapist, in moving quickly to a familiar and comfortable cultural position, may have denied Sergio the opportunity to explore his own ambivalent feelings related to his internal cross-cultural conflict, which would have been necessary to resolve his depression.

Other Important Considerations in the Interaction Between Clinician and Patient

Various cultural values have been emphasized in the social science literature on Latinos, among them *simpatía, personalismo, respeto,* and *dignidad,* all discussed below. Clinicians should be aware that essentializing Latino cultures into this set of values runs the risk of reductionistic and overly simplistic cultural stereotyping. Nevertheless, critical discussion of these constructs serves to illustrate certain interpersonal dynamics that clinicians commonly encounter in dealing with Latino patients.

Simpatía translates literally as "sympathy"; however, in Spanish it refers to an expression of likability and agreeability. When a person is *simpático* or *simpática,* he or she demonstrates competent and pleasing social skills and is typically well liked. The expression of this social skill is highly valued by most Latino cultures. In a U.S. mainstream cultural setting, however, behaviors that are associated with being *simpático* may often be interpreted as indicative of an overly agreeable and thus nonassertive person. Latinos tend to associate lack of assertiveness not with high agreeability, but with shyness, introversion, and limited social skills. Similarly, not being *simpático* in a social situation may be interpreted as rudeness and even lack of generosity. These cultural differences may cause misunderstandings by both clinicians and patients. For example, a Latino patient who behaves in a culturally appropriate pleasant and friendly manner may be wrongly regarded by a U.S. mainstream clinician as lacking assertiveness. Similarly, a Latino patient may misinterpret a U.S. Anglo clinician's attitude of seriousness and "matter-of-factness" as reflective of a rude, cold, or uncaring individual.

Somewhat related to *simpatía,* the term *personalismo* refers to a preference among many Latinos for direct personal interactions over more indirect practices. Thus, the neutral and reserved stance adopted by some U.S. clinicians may be perceived by some Latino patients as reflective of an excessively cold and aloof individual, hindering the formation of a close therapeutic alliance. In contrast, a Latino patient's use of handshakes, personal touch, and expressive gestures may be misinterpreted as indicative of someone with poor interpersonal boundaries and inappropriate social distance, as illustrated in the earlier example of culturally appropriate kissing in social situations. Some practices commonly used by clinicians, such as sending letters to remind patients of their appointments, leaving recorded telephone messages, or handing out written educational literature may seem too formal and impersonal, and consequently not be as effective with Latinos as more direct forms of personal communication (e.g., face-to-face personal communication, having a "live" telephone conversation).

Respeto translates into English as "respect." Yet in Latino cultures it generally has a connotation of much stronger personal significance and emotional weight, characterizing an individual's pride and sense of self-dignity. Consequently, disrespecting someone is typically regarded as a very serious interpersonal violation in Latino cultures; a sort of violation of one's honor. For example, some Latino parents who find out that their adolescent daughter has engaged in sexual relations may regard this event as a *falta de respeto* (literally, "breach of respect") or serious violation of the family's honor. This situation may provoke intense feelings of anger and retaliative behaviors directed toward the daughter's sexual partner (who is seen as a "perpetrator"), as well as strong feelings of disgust and rejection toward the daughter. A more subtle illustration of the importance of *respeto* or the related value of *dignidad* (self-dignity) may be the case of Latino patients who feel devalued on sensing from their clinician that assumptions are being made about their limited educational background and lack of intellectual sophistication (e.g., explaining medical procedures in an overly simplistic fashion; requesting an interpreter after noticing an accent, without adequate assessment of the patient's level of English fluency). These patients, although feeling shamed and disrespected by their clinicians, may engage with them in a culturally appropriate polite and pleasant manner, yet not return for further appointments.

E. Overall Cultural Assessment for Diagnosis and Care

General Considerations in Assessing Psychopathology Among Latinos

Four basic questions can help clinicians assess for the presence and severity of psychopathology, as well as its etiology, in patients with cultural backgrounds different from those of the clinician or mainstream U.S. society:

1. Are the reported or observed experiences and behaviors considered pathological in the individual's culture of origin?
2. Are they considered pathological in the current social context, including mainstream U.S. society?
3. Are they clearly associated with marked distress or functional impairment?
4. Is the existing distress or impairment caused by individual psychopathology or, rather, by the presence of divergent values and interpretations between the patient, his or her culture, and the host culture?

Four possible scenarios arise from addressing these questions. First, an individual may report behaviors that are considered pathological both in the culture of origin and in the new context, and which cause significant functional impairment.

Second, an individual may report a behavior that is considered pathological in the current social context but not in the culture of origin, and there is no evidence of any associated functional impairment. This could be the case of Latinos who report hearing voices or having visions that do not appear to be associated with distress or functional impairment. They may explain these in culturally syntonic terms as stemming from a special spiritual faculty, such as *espiritista* mediumship, which allows them to be in contact with spirits of the deceased. Such individuals should neither be diagnosed as having a psychiatric (e.g., psychotic or dissociative) disorder, nor treated for these experiences, unless it can be clearly established that these are directly causing clinically significant distress or functional impairment.

Third, a situation may arise in which a behavior that is not considered pathological in the culture of origin of the patient is seen as such in the new social context, but there is clear evidence of resulting dysfunction in the new setting. Illustrating this are cases of some Latino parents who use frequent spanking, belting, or other corporal punishment to discipline their children in line with cultural norms, yet their behavior is clearly defined in the United States as physical abuse. Such parents may be reported to the Department of Social Services and the child eventually removed from the home, a process that causes a significant disruption in the family unit and is typically experienced as extremely distressing for both parents and child. Regardless of what ethical or moral position one takes on corporal punishment, it is clear that the resulting dysfunction in this case arises primarily from a divergence in the value systems of the parents and the host culture. This important distinction can lead to very different interventions, such as treatment focused on providing parenting education to caring and well-meaning parents about alternative forms of disciplining their children, rather than subjecting them to inappropriate clinical or forensic approaches targeted for malicious perpetrators of physical abuse.

A fourth scenario is that of an individual who displays a behavior regarded as pathological in the culture of origin but viewed as normal in the new social setting, yet the individual experiences significant distress as a result of this condition. Examples of this are the cases of a Latino man raised in a very traditional environment who experiences homosexual feelings yet chooses not to openly express them and a Latino woman who feels oppressed in her marriage and decides to suppress her wishes to leave her husband. In both cases, a clinician with more liberal U.S. values may attempt to normalize these individuals' distress and encourage them to act out their feelings. However, the clinician's priority in such cases should be to validate the patients' genuine distress and assess any pathology or dysfunction resulting from this conflict. Rather than assessing these problems as stemming from internal psychopathology or solely from sociocultural prejudice, a culturally sensitive clinical formulation should account for the sociocultural roots of the problem and emphasize the conflict between individual feelings and cultural values. Intervention should then be directed toward seeking a resolution of this cross-cultural conflict that is satisfactory to the patient, rather than toward fixing a defective individual or cultural value or satisfying the clinician's own personal and moral agenda.

Misdiagnosis

Latinos are commonly the objects of misdiagnosis. Members of the U.S. mainstream often regard Latinos, as well as many persons from Mediterranean cultures, as overly dramatic and emotional. This should not be surprising, given marked differences in cultural styles of emotional expressiveness observed when comparing Latin and Mediterranean cultures with cultures heavily influenced by white Anglo-Saxon Protestant traditions, like the United States. However, such purely cross-cultural differences with little relevance to psychopathology may affect diagnostic practice, particularly the valid assessment of affect intensity, and lead to inaccurate assessments of pathological levels of affectivity such as those found in histrionic and borderline personality disorders (Buffenstein 1997; Castillo 1997). Moreover, the typical gender role–based behaviors of many Latinos and Latinas may be regarded as overly sexually provocative by U.S. mainstream members, and such behaviors may be further confounded with symptoms typical of these character pathologies. For example, it has been noted that certain male behaviors normative in Latino cultures, such as those often associated with the notion of *machismo,* may be confounded with traits of histrionic or narcissistic personality disorder (Castillo 1997; Paniagua 2000).

Differences in culturally shaped affective communication styles, often expressed in children through high levels of physical activity, can also lead to the inaccurate assessment of some Latino children as having disruptive behavioral problems or pathological levels of hyperactivity and attentional problems, such as those commonly found in ADHD. Although some cases of hyperactivity and disruptive behaviors may be related to greater psychosocial stress among Latino families and children, the diagnosis of ADHD may also result from changing cultural norms about the containment of emotion and behavior. In either case—pathology caused by psychosocial stress or misdiagnosed culturally patterned behavior—sociocultural factors must be considered in order to achieve an accurate assessment. There is also evidence that Latino children are at a higher risk than Anglo children for misdiagnosis of academic difficulties related to limited English proficiency as a learning problem or disability (McCray and Garcia 2002).

Latino children and adults also appear to be at higher risk of overdiagnosis for "antisocial" tendencies typical of conduct disorder and antisocial personality disorder. Certain behaviors with high protective and adaptive value for vulnerable ethnic minority individuals, such as inner-city youth living in settings characterized by poverty, high criminality, and institutionalized social violence, may be inaccurately assessed as pathological in a decontextualized fashion (Buffenstein 1997; Castillo 1997). Normative Latino family dynamics may also be regarded as overdependent, codependent, or enmeshed from the perspective of U.S. mainstream culture, leading to inaccurate assessments of pathological overdependence (Santiago-Rivera et al. 2002). A final example of potential misdiagnosis was mentioned earlier with respect to the misinterpretation and overpathologization of culturally normative perceptual alterations as signs of psychosis, particularly, schizophrenia and psychotic depression (Laria 1998; Lewis-Fernandez 2003b).

In light of these potential clinical misappraisals, it is essential for clinicians to avoid misdiagnosis by becoming aware of the sociocultural aspects affecting the presentation of experience and behavior among Latinos. In particular, valid diagnoses should rely on evidence of distress or impairment as well as accurate clinical attribution of etiology, including the interplay of internal and social factors.

Use of Testing and Assessment Tools With Latinos

The application of standard psychological testing and assessment tools to Latinos raises specialized questions regarding potential misdiagnosis. This topic has been the subject of much controversy and criticism. An extensive review of this area is beyond the scope of this chapter; some general issues have been covered in Chapter 1. However, it may be useful to familiarize clinicians with a few of the major issues involved.

Two major problems in using assessment tools with Latinos are 1) the scarcity of instruments developed specifically to be used with Latino populations and 2) the lack of adequate cross-cultural validation (not just cross-linguistic or semantic equivalence) of many of the standard instruments used with the U.S. mainstream population. Therefore, in the assessment of Latino patients, clinicians are encouraged to use cautiously any information provided by assessment tools and measures that have not been normed specifically with U.S. Latinos, and to rely on supplemental clinical information in making important diagnostic and other clinical decisions.

We will discuss one test, the Thematic Apperception Test (TAT), as an example of how culture can bias test results, and another test that addresses these biases, the TEMAS ("Tell Me A Story"). The TAT is a widely used projective test in which subjects are instructed to create a narrative story in response to pictures that depict subjects interacting in a variety of scenes. The TAT is hypothesized to provide clinically relevant information about a subject's personality traits, such as individual needs, as well as other relational traits. The TAT has been criticized for its cultural and racial bias given the culturally and racially specific characteristics of the individuals, objects, and scenarios that are depicted. In an attempt to challenge the test's validity, a "bottom-up" approach (developing an instrument specifically for a group, rather than adapting an existing instrument to a group different from the one for which it was originally developed) was used in the development of the TEMAS (Costantino et al. 1988). TEMAS depicts scenes with Latino characters using cultural themes in urban settings that are more relevant to U.S. Latinos. Studies comparing the TAT with the TEMAS show that Latinos display greater responsiveness and verbal fluency when given the TEMAS. These traits are interpreted as suggestive of greater sophistication and maturity in interpersonal relations. Another interesting finding is that bilingual subjects tend to create stories in English with the TAT and to switch from English to Spanish with the TEMAS (Costantino et al. 1982), which evidences the complexity involved in using these measures with Latinos.

A variety of psychiatric symptom rating scales have been translated into Spanish and used extensively with Latino patients, such as the Hopkins Symptom Checklist–90 (SCL-90) and its shorter version, the Brief Symptom Inventory (Sánchez-Lacay et al. 2001); the Beck Depression Inventory (Bonilla et al. 2004); the Brief Psychiatric Rating Scale (Hafkesheid 1991); the Patient Health Questionnaire (Wulsin et al. 2002); and the Psychiatric Research Interview for Substance and Mental Disorders (PRISM) (Torrens et al. 2004). Although there is some support for their applicability with Latinos, clinicians are encouraged to use these instruments with caution, given that they were originally derived for mainstream U.S. samples.

Empirically Tested Psychosocial Interventions

There is little research on the efficacy of specific mental health interventions with Latinos. Limited preliminary efficacy has been found for CBT, interpersonal psychotherapy, and behavior therapy with depressed Latino women (Comas-Díaz 1981; J. Miranda et al. 2003; Rosselló and Bernal 1999). However, most of these studies have been conducted primarily with women of Puerto Rican or Mexican origin. Some studies have focused on family therapy with Latinos. One study found that behavioral family management—a highly structured type of family therapy—in Latino schizophrenic patients led to a worsening of symptoms in the less acculturated families compared with less structured case management (Telles et al. 1995). Canino and Canino (1982) used an ecostructural family therapy approach and a systems-oriented family therapy approach with low-income Puerto Rican migrants and found these modalities to be both culturally syntonic and effective with this population. Szapocznik and colleagues (1989) tested cultural adaptations of both strategic family therapy and structural family therapy, and found these interventions to be highly effective with Latino adolescents suffering from drug-related behavioral and emotional problems.

Other studies have suggested a variety of culturally relevant strategies that can be effectively implemented with Latinos. These include *cuento* therapy (storytelling using native cultural stories and characters) (Costantino et al. 1986); using *dichos* (sayings) and *refranes* (proverbs) as central points in therapy (Aviera 1996); culturally relevant modeling therapy (Malgady et al. 1990a); using folk heroes as experience-near behavioral models (Malgady et al. 1990b); culturally relevant images (Bracero 1998); and focusing therapy on the relationship between cultural idioms of distress and politically rooted psychosocial factors, such as anger and injustice (Rogler et al. 1994). These strategies constitute promising approaches to culturally relevant forms of therapy and should be tested further using more rigorous research designs. In conclusion, clinicians must rely on cultural knowledge, culturally sensitive assessment procedures, flexibility with existing protocols, and creativity in designing and carrying out culturally relevant mental health interventions with

Latinos. For example, the treatment for patients meeting DSM-IV-TR criteria for *ataques* should focus on helping the patient to manage the distressing situations that provoked the episodes as well as on treating the associated psychopathology, which may be distinct in each case.

Conclusion

Understanding Latinos requires an appreciation of the group's commonalities as well as the wide range of individual and group variations observed among members of the various Latino cultures. Clearly, seeking treatment adherence and effective intervention with Latino patients requires the provision of mental health services that have relevance to them. Culturally sensitive assessment and presentation of therapeutic options are essential in this process, such as what can be obtained by consistent use of the DSM-IV-TR Outline for Cultural Formulation model. Patients are not likely to engage in lengthy mental health interventions that lack practical relevance and run counter to their culturally informed understandings and expectations of how illness should be assessed and treated.

We have offered other suggestions for how to avoid various pitfalls in the treatment of Latino patients, such as avoiding simplistic stereotypes and *a priori* or precipitous assumptions, as well as exercising caution with the potential misinterpretation of culturally normative behaviors.

Direct personal relatedness and perceived clinician warmth emerge as key variables in promoting the therapeutic alliance and participation of Latino patients. In addition, given the centrality of the family in Latino cultures, attention to family matters is essential for an accurate assessment of a patient's problems. Active engagement of family members in treatment, when appropriate, can be a very effective intervention.

Practical barriers to treatment, such as financial limitations and transportation or work-related difficulties, also need to be addressed and discerned from lack of motivation for treatment. Whenever these are present, efforts should be made to help patients attempt to resolve them. Clinicians are encouraged to rely as much as possible on cultural knowledge, flexibility, and creativity in adapting existing therapeutic models with Latino patients. They should also take into account some of the significant differences in cultural concepts, values, and normative behaviors discussed. It is to be hoped that future research will provide us with much-needed knowledge of empirically supported interventions that work effectively with Latinos. In the meanwhile, attention to three basic elements that underlie the cultural formulation model, namely awareness of, sensitivity to, and appreciation of cultural differences, can guide clinicians in designing competent strategies that yield effective results with their Latino patients.

References

Achenbach TM, Bird HR, Canino G, et al: Epidemiological comparisons of Puerto Rican and U.S. mainland children: parent, teacher, and self-reports. J Am Acad Child Adolesc Psychiatry 29:84–93, 1990

Alegría M, Takeuchi D, Canino G, et al: Considering context, place, and culture: the National Latino and Asian American Study. Int J Methods Psychiatr Res 13:208–220, 2004

American Psychiatric Association: Appendix I: Outline for cultural formulation and glossary of culture-bound syndromes, in Diagnostic and Statistical Manual of Mental Disorders, 4th Edition, Text Revision. Washington, DC, American Psychiatric Association, 2000, pp 897–903

Angel J: Nuestros padres: elder care in Hispanic families. Hispanic 11:18–23, 1998

Aviera A: "Dichos" therapy group: a therapeutic use of Spanish language proverbs with hospitalized Spanish-speaking psychiatric patients. Cult Divers Ment Health 2:73–78, 1996

Bonilla J, Bernal G, Santos A, et al: A revised Spanish version of the Beck Depression Inventory: psychometric properties with a Puerto Rican sample of college students. J Clin Psychol 60:119–130, 2004

Bracero W: Intimidades: confianza, gender, and hierarchy in the construction of Latino-Latina therapeutic relationships. Cult Divers Ment Health 4:264–277, 1998

Buffenstein A: Personality disorders, in Culture and Psychopathology: A Guide to Clinical Assessment. Edited by Tseng, W, Streltzer J. New York, Brunner/Mazel, 1997, pp 190–205

Cabrera L: El monte, igbo, finda, ewe orisha, vititi nfinda: notas sobre las religiones, la magia, las supersticiones y el folklore de los negros criollos y el pueblo de Cuba. Miami, FL, Ediciones Universal, 1992

Canino GJ, Canino IA: Culturally syntonic family therapy for migrant Puerto Ricans. Hosp Community Psychiatry 33:299–303, 1982

Canino GJ, Bird HR, Shrout PE, et al: The prevalence of specific psychiatric disorders in Puerto Rico. Arch Gen Psychiatry 44:727–735, 1987

Castillo RJ: Culture and Mental Illness: A Client-Centered Approach. Pacific Grove, CA, Brooks/Cole, 1997

Centers for Disease Control and Prevention: CDC surveillance summaries: youth risk behavior surveillance: United States, 1997. MMWR 47:1–89, 1998

Cheung FK, Snowden LR: Community mental health and ethnic minority populations. Community Ment Health J 26:277–291, 1990

Comas-Díaz L: Effects of cognitive and behavioral group treatment on the depressive symptomatology of Puerto Rican women. J Consult Clin Psychol 49:627–632, 1981

Costantino G, Malgady R, Vazquez C: A comparison of the Murray-TAT and a new Thematic Apperception Test for urban Hispanic children. Hisp J Behav Sci 3:291–300, 1982

Costantino G, Malgady R, Rogler L: Cuento therapy: a culturally sensitive modality for Puerto Rican children. J Consult Clin Psychol 54:639–645, 1986

Costantino G, Malgady R, Rogler L: Technical Manual: TEMAS Thematic Apperception Test. Los Angeles, CA, Western Psychological Services, 1988

Dworkin RJ, Adams GL: Retention of Hispanics in public sector mental health services. Community Ment Health J 23:204–216, 1987

Escobar JI: Cross-cultural aspects of the somatization trait. Hosp Community Psychiatry 38:174–180, 1987

Escobar JI, Hoyos Nervi C, Gara MA: Immigration and mental health: Mexican Americans in the United States. Harv Rev Psychiatry 8:64–72, 2000

Espinosa G, Elizondo V, Miranda J: Latino Religions and Civic Activism in the United States. New York, Oxford University Press, 2005

Farias P: Central and South American refugees: some mental health challenges, in Amidst Peril and Pain: The Mental Health and Well-Being of the World's Refugees. Edited by Marsella AJ, Bornemann T, Ekblad S, et al. Washington, DC, American Psychological Association, 1994, pp 101–113

Glover SH, Pumariega AJ, Holzer CE, et al: Anxiety symptomatology in Mexican American adolescents. J Child Fam Stud 8:47–57, 1999

Guarnaccia PJ: The prevalence of ataques de nervios in the Puerto Rico Disaster Study: the role of culture in psychiatric epidemiology. J Nerv Ment Dis 181:157–165, 1993

Guarnaccia PJ, Rodríguez O: Concepts of culture and their role in the development of culturally competent mental health services. Hisp J Behav Sci 18:419–443, 1996

Hafkesheid A: Psychometric evaluation of a standardized and expanded Brief Psychiatric Rating Scale. Acta Psychiatr Scand 84:284–300, 1991

Harwood A (ed): Ethnicity and Medical Care. Cambridge, MA, Harvard University Press, 1981

Harwood A: Rx: Spiritist as Needed: A Study of a Puerto Rican Community Mental Health Resource. Ithaca, NY, Cornell University Press, 1987.

Hernández DJ, Charney E: From Generation to Generation: The Health and Well-being of Children in Immigrant Families. Washington DC, National Academy Press, 1998

Hohmann AA, Richeport M, Marriott BM, et al: Spiritism in Puerto Rico: results of an island-wide community study. Br J Psychiatry 156:328–335, 1990

Kessler RC, McGonagle KA, Zhao S, et al: Lifetime and 12-month prevalence of DSM-III-R psychiatric disorders in the United States. Arch Gen Psychiatry 51:8–19, 1994

Kirmayer LJ: Culture and somatization: clinical, epidemiological, and ethnographic perspectives. Psychosom Med 60:420–430, 1998

Kleinman A: Patients and Healers in the Context of Culture. Berkeley, University of California Press, 1980

Laria AJ: Dissociative experiences among Cuban mental health patients and spiritist mediums. Doctoral dissertation, University of Massachusetts, Boston, MA, 1998

Lewis MW, Wigen KE: The Myth of Continents: A Critique of Metageography. Berkeley, University of California Press, 1977

Lewis-Fernández R: Mental health disparities in the Hispanic population. Paper presented at CME conference, University of Arizona College of Medicine, 2003b

Lewis-Fernández R, Blanco C, Schmidt A, et al: Assessing psychosis screeners among underserved urban primary care patients. Paper presented at the annual meeting of NARSAD (National Association for Research on Schizophrenia and Depression), New York, NY, October 18, 2003a

Malgady RG, Rogler LH, Costantino G: Culturally sensitive psychotherapy for Puerto Rican children and adolescents: a program of treatment outcome research. J Consult Clin Psychol 58:704–712, 1990a

Malgady RG, Rogler LH, Costantino G: Hero/heroine modeling for Puerto Rican adolescents: a preventive mental health intervention J Consult Clin Psychol 58:469–474, 1990b

Marcos LR, Uruyo L, Kesselman M, et al: The language barrier in evaluating Spanish-American patients. Arch Gen Pscyhiatry 29: 655–659, 1973

Marín G, Triandis HC: Allocentrism as an important characteristic of the behavior of Latin Americans and Hispanics, in Cross-Cultural and National Studies in Social Psychology. Edited by Díaz-Guerrero R. Amsterdam, North-Holland, 1985, pp 85–104

McCray AD, Garcia SB: The stories we must tell: developing a research agenda for multicultural and bilingual special education. In Multicultural and Bilingual Special Education: A Case for Socioculture Contexts and Voices in Research and Practice (special issue). International Journal of Qualitative Studies in Education 15:599–612, 2002

Miranda J, Azocar F, Organista KC, et al: Recruiting and retaining low-income Latinos in psychotherapy research. J Consult Clin Psychol 64:868–874, 1996

Miranda J, Chung J, Green B, et al: Treating depression in predominantly low-income young minority women: a randomized controlled trial. JAMA 290:57–65, 2003

Miranda MR, Andujo E, Guerrero CC, et al: Mexican American dropouts in psychotherapy as related to level of acculturation, in Psychotherapy With Spanish-Speaking: Issues in Research and Service Delivery. Edited by Miranda MR. Los Angeles, University of California Press, 1976, pp 35–50

Morales E: Gender roles among Latino gay and bisexual men: implications for family and couple relationships, in Lesbians and Gays in Couples and Families: A Handbook for Therapists. Edited by Laird J, Green RJ. San Francisco, CA, Jossey-Bass, 1996, pp 272–297

Moscicki EK, Rae D, Regier DA, et al: The Hispanic Health and Nutrition Examination Survey: depression among Mexican Americans, Cuban Americans, Puerto Ricans, in Health and Behavior: Research Agenda for Hispanics. Edited by Gaviria M, Arana JD. Chicago, Publication Services of the University of Illinois, 1987

Olfson M, Lewis-Fernández R, Weissman MM, et al: Psychotic symptoms in an urban general medicine practice. Am J Psychiatry 159:1412–1419, 2002

Oquendo MA, Ellis SP, Greenwald S, et al: Ethnic and sex differences in suicide rates relative to major depression in the United States. Am J Psychiatry 158:1652–1658, 2001

Padgett DK, Patrick C, Burns BJ, et al: Ethnicity and the use of outpatient mental health services in a national insured population. Am J Public Health 84:222–226, 1994

Paniagua FA: Culture-bound syndromes, cultural variations, and psychopathology, in Handbook of Multicultural Mental Health (monograph). Edited by Cuéllar I, Paniagua FA. San Diego, CA, Academic Press, 2000, pp 139–169

Parrillo VN: Strangers to These Shores: Race and Ethnic Relations in the United States, 8th Edition. Boston, MA, Allyn & Bacon, 2005

Phinney JS, Kohatsu EL: Ethnic and racial identity development and mental health, in Health Risks and Developmental Transitions During Adolescence. Edited by Schulenberg J, Maggs JL. New York, Cambridge University Press, 1997, pp 420–443

Portes A, Rumbaut RG: Immigrant America: A Portrait. Berkeley, University of California Press, 1996

Price CS, Cuéllar I: Effects of language and related variables on the expression of psychopathology in Mexican-American psychiatric patients. Hisp J Behav Sci 3:145–160, 1981

Rodríguez CE: Puerto Ricans: Born in the USA. Boulder, CO, Westview Press, 1991

Rogg EM, Cooney RS: Adaptation and Adjustment of Cubans: West New York, New Jersey. Monograph No 5.101. Bronx, NY, Hispanic Research Center, Fordham University, 1980

Rogler LH: Research on mental health services for Hispanics: targets of convergence. Cult Divers Ment Health 2:145–156, 1996

Rogler LH, Cortés DE, Malgady RG: The mental health relevance of idioms of distress: anger and perceptions of injustice among New York Puerto Ricans. J Nerv Ment Dis 182:327–330, 1994

Rosenberg JC: El Gagá: religión y sociedad de un culto dominicano. Un estudio comparativo. Santo Domingo, Dominican Republic, Universidad Autónoma de Santo Domingo, 1979

Rosselló J, Bernal GL: The efficacy of cognitive-behavioral and interpersonal treatments for depression in Puerto Rican adolescents. J Consult Clin Psychol 67:734–745, 1999

Sabogal F, Marín G, Otero-Sabogal R, et al: Hispanic familism and acculturation: what changes and what doesn't? Hisp J Behav Sci 9:397–412, 1987

Sánchez-Lacay JA, Lewis-Fernández R, Goetz D, et al: Open trial of nefazodone among Hispanics with major depression: efficacy, tolerability, and adherence issues. Depress Anxiety 13:118–124, 2001

Santiago-Rivera AL, Arredondo P, Gallardo-Cooper M: Counseling Latinos and La Familia: A Practical Guide. Thousand Oaks, CA, Sage, 2002

Suárez-Orozco C, Suárez-Orozco MM: Transformations: Immigration, Family Life, and Achievement Motivation Among Latino Adolescents. Stanford, CA, Stanford University Press, 1995

Sue S: Community mental health services to minority groups: some optimism, some pessimism. Am Psychol 32:616–624, 1977

Swanson JW, Linskey AO, Quintero-Salinas R, et al: A binational school survey of depressive symptoms, drug use, and suicidal ideation. J Am Acad Child Adolesc Psychiatry 31:669–678, 1992

Szapocznik J, Río A, Murray E, et al: Structural family versus psychodynamic child therapy for problematic Hispanic boys. J Consult Clin Psychol 57:571–578, 1989

Telles C, Karno M, Mintz J, et al: Immigrant families coping with schizophrenia: behavioural family intervention v. case management with a low-income Spanish-speaking population. Br J Psychiatry 167:473–479, 1995

Temkin-Greener H, Clark KT: Ethnicity, gender, and utilization of mental health services in a Medicaid population. Soc Sci Med 26:989–996, 1988

Teplin LA: Psychiatric and substance abuse disorders among male urban jail detainees. Am J Public Health 84:290–293, 1994

Torrens M, Serrano D, Astals M, et al: Diagnosing comorbid psychiatric disorders in substance abusers: validity of the Spanish versions of the Psychiatric Research Interview for Substance and Mental Disorders and the Structured Clinical Interview for DSM-IV. Am J Psychiatry 161:1231–1237, 2004

U.S. Bureau of Justice Statistics: Correctional Populations in the United States, 1996. Washington, DC, Bureau of Justice Statistics, 1999

U. S. Census Bureau: 1990 Census Population. Washington, DC, U.S. Government Printing Office, 1990

U.S. Census Bureau: The Hispanic Population in the United States: March 2002. Detailed Tables (PPL-165). Washington, DC, U.S. Census Bureau, 2002b. http://www.census.gov/population/www/socdemo/hispanic/ppl-165.html. Accessed September 16, 2005.

U.S. Census Bureau: The Hispanic Population in the United States: Population Characteristics: March 2004. Population Division, Ethnic and Hispanic Statistics Branch. Available at: http://www.census.gov/population/www/socdemo/hispanic/cps2004.html

U.S. Department of Health and Human Services: Mental Health: Culture, Race, and Ethnicity. A Supplement to Mental Health: A Report of the Surgeon General. Rockville, MD, U.S. Department of Health and Human Services, Public Health Service, Office of the Surgeon General, 2001. Available at: http://www.surgeongeneral.gov/library/mentalhealth/cre

U.S. Immigration and Naturalization Service: January 31, 2003, Executive Summary: Estimates of the Unauthorized Immigrant Population Residing in the United States: 1990 to 2000. Available at: http://www.bcis.gov/graphics/shared/aboutus/statistics/2000ExecSumm.pdf. Accessed September 16, 2005.

Vazsonyi AT, Flannery D: Early adolescent delinquent behaviors: associations with family and school domains. J Early Adolesc 17:271–293, 1997

Vega WA, Kolody B, Aguilar-Gaxiola S, et al: Gaps in service utilization by Mexican Americans with mental health problems. Am J Psychiatry 156:928–934, 1999

Wells KB, Hough RL, Golding JM, et al: Which Mexican-Americans underutilize health services? Am J Psychiatry 144:918–922, 1987

Whaley AL: Cultural mistrust: an important psychological construct for diagnosis and treatment of African Americans. Prof Psychol Res Pr 32:555–562, 2001

Wulsin L, Somoza E, Heck J: The feasibility of using the Spanish PHQ-9 to screen for depression in primary care in Honduras. Prim Care Companion J Clin Psychiatry 4:191–195, 2002

5

American Indian and Alaska Native Patients

Candace M. Fleming, Ph.D.

T he non-Native mental health clinician sat down at his work computer at the start of his day. He noted that his first patient was affiliated with one tribal nation recognized by the U.S. federal government and a second tribe recognized by a neighboring state. His response was high interest mixed with apprehension. He had recently completed his agency's cultural competence training for the quarter, but those particular tribes were not featured in any of the specific examples. He clicked to the paraprofessional's intake summary, where he reviewed her summary of the Native Assessment of Functioning. The tool assessed the strengths and challenges of a Native person in five realms of living: physical, emotional, intellectual, spiritual, and social. What emerged from the descriptions across domains gave the clinician an initial idea of how this Native individual might be negotiating the various Native and non-Native circumstances of life in the region.

The intake information suggested the patient was fairly bicultural and was open to both mainstream and Native-specific approaches to mental health intervention. The clinician wondered what evidence-based practices have been shown to work with the tribal nations with whom this patient was affiliated. A quick query of the evidence-based database revealed that mental health and substance use research has not yet been completed with the cultural groups of the two tribal nations, but there were several published articles written by providers working in Native communities that described promising practices. The clinician smiled to himself. He would enter the therapeutic relationship with this Native person very aware of the high complexity of the patient's experiences. The immediate need to know more was in sharp contrast with his slowly growing knowledge about Natives. However, the paraprofessional, scientists, and practitioners working with Natives provided some valuable information that would help him convey respect and understanding to this new patient. "Another chance to learn," he told himself as he got up to greet his first patient of the day.

The vignette above is presented as if it were in the past, but the advances in assessment, intervention, service system development, and training suggested by the brief story are very much in the future for North America's indigenous populations. Reliable knowledge about these populations and their distinctive place in American life is difficult to come by. The mental health services provider in the United States typically does not have personal or professional connections with indigenous populations and obtains information from books, films, television programming, and the occasional newspaper article. Sadly, indigenous perspectives on life views, philosophy, history, and contemporary issues are missing from these typical venues of information. Thus, it is usually left to the patient to bring his or her individual, family, and cultural perspectives to the mental health setting. Indian patients, while quite aware of the various stereotypical characterizations that are held by non-Indians about Indians, may not be accustomed to describing the various individual, family, clan, tribal, and pan-Indian perspectives and distinguishing them from each other. Therefore, this chapter will provide the clinician with basic social and historical information on which to build his or her understanding of Indian patients and partnership with cultural consultants.

Information and perspectives are offered here to show the impact of cultural issues on assessment, diagnosis, and intervention with American Indians and Alaska Natives who have behavioral health disorders, or in words that resonate more with the Native person, are in a state of distress or imbalance within the intrapersonal realm (thought, emotion, behavior), within one or more interpersonal relationships, or within a spiritual relationship with spiritual deities or other parts of creation.

The DSM-IV-TR Outline for Cultural Formulation (American Psychiatric Association 2000) provides the framework for summarizing what has been said by mental health and substance abuse treatment providers, prevention specialists, researchers, community development specialists, policy makers, and Indian/Native community members about the provision of effective and culturally relevant mental health services to Indians and Natives. The chapter also will highlight where knowledge development needs to be done in basic science, epidemiology and needs assessment, intervention research and evaluation, and the sharing of promising practices across Indian and Native communities.

Current Status

In the 2000 U.S. Census, 4.1 million citizens identified themselves as American Indian or Alaska Native; this is less than 1.5% of the total U.S. population (U.S. Census Bureau 2001), but it represents an exceptional increase for this population from previous census enumerations. The growth is due to several major factors: better data collection by the Census Bureau, greater willingness to report Native ancestry, higher birth rate, and reduced infant mortality. "Indian Country" is generally believed to be the West, and indeed, the data bear this out: most Indians live in Western states, mainly in California, Arizona, New Mexico, South Dakota, Alaska, and Montana, and 42% reside in rural areas (Rural Policy Research Institute 1997). Many reservations and trust lands (areas with boundaries established by treaty, statute, and executive or court order) exist for Indian nations, but currently only one in five Indians live in these areas. The majority (62%) reside in urban, suburban, or rural nonreservation areas (U.S. Census Bureau 1993), and most maintain close family and political ties with reservation and trust land communities.

From the beginning of contact with Europeans, the original peoples of North America were almost exclusively viewed as homogeneous, and this stereotype prevails today; in the minds of many Americans, high cheekbones and tepee dwellings are the hallmarks of every indigenous person. Trimble and Thurman (2002) present a compelling explanation for the 400-year transformation of North America's original populations from multiple groups of peoples with little in common to one of the United States' four officially recognized ethnic groups. As with other racial/ethnic populations, the Indian group has considerable heterogeneity.

Much of the heterogeneity is owed to the several environments that indigenous peoples have lived in and adapted to over the centuries. Indigenous groups that shared environments tended to develop similar skills, knowledge, beliefs, and customs. The different geographic regions have defined North American Indian cultural areas that are unique and complex: Arctic, Subarctic, Plateau, Northwest Coast, California, Great Basin, Southwest, Plains, Northeast, and Southeast (Waldman 1985). Indian language families (Algonquian, Athapascan, Siouan, Iroquoian, and Eskimo-Aleut) are another hallmark of diversity. Scholars estimate that at the beginning of European colonization of North America, there were between 200 and 300 distinct Native languages spoken. Sadly, more than half of these languages are now extinct and another large set is nearly extinct. The transmission of the nuances of cultural beliefs and ways is severely compromised when a native language is known by only a few people within an Indian community, and the recognition of this has led to the establishment of literacy in Native language as a high priority for contemporary tribal nations.

With the formation of the United States, the federal government began to establish treaties with individual tribes and groups of tribes, but the uniqueness of each tribal nation was underplayed when it came to federal policies that largely considered American Indians as a single entity. Sovereign nation status has been given to more than 550 tribal entities by the U.S. federal government (National Congress of American Indians 2004), and hundreds more are recognized by state governments. Sovereignty for each tribal group and the right of each group to be treated as having unique strengths and challenges are central issues that today pervade every aspect of tribal life, including health and mental health.

There are many terms of reference for the indigenous populations of North America, including *American Indians, Alaska Natives, Native Americans, Native Indians, Native American Indians, Indians, Natives,* and *First Nations.* Each term is useful, depending on the historical, societal, and political nature of the setting. The terms *Indian* and *Native* are used in this chapter for expedience, but it is far more preferable to use an individual's specific tribal or village name as a group reference.

Historical Issues That Relate to Mental Health

Many historical events affect our relationships with Native American patients—warfare between grossly unmatched opponents, massacres of entire villages, disease epidemics, trickery in treaty making, forced removal from ancestral lands, and shrinking land base due to theft, land runs, and sales by impoverished and ill Indian wards of the federal government. This is just a partial list of major historical traumas and losses endured by Indians and Natives. It is vital to know the history from the Native point of view; one readable and well-documented resource is *The Complete Idiot's Guide to Native American History* (Fleming 2003). The concept of the "Vanishing Red Man" was close to becoming a reality in the early 1990s, the point when Indians and Natives numbered only 5% of their estimated population of 400 years earlier (Thornton 1987). Today this group is growing fast, and in some ways thriving. The incredible resiliency of Indian people and tribes must be acknowledged and celebrated.

Subjugation of Indian and Native beliefs and practices that could have assisted with recovery from traumas, losses, and rapid societal change was thorough and happened through a variety of means, beginning with the isolation and neglect of Indians on reservations and other trust lands. The beginning of the reservation system coincided with the California Gold Rush of the 1840s and 1850s, when wagon trains crossed Indian lands, increasing hostility toward Western tribes. Peacemaking was attempted with treaties in which tribal territories were defined, but the defining process resulted in the loss of millions of acres of Indian lands to the U.S. government. The redefined territories, called reservations, were not lands given to Indians by the non-Indian government but lands that Indians were allowed to retain. Often the lands were not well understood by the Indians, and virtually no technical support was given to build up tribal human resources to effectively adapt to the natural resources within the reservation boundaries. Violence against Native traditions in the form of enforced bans on traditional Indian objects and ways were commonplace. It is no wonder that cycles of poverty, societal disorder, and ill health have resulted from the reservation system. On the other hand, the reservation was a cradle for nurturing intense belonging to the tribal unit and connection to the beloved homeland.

Educational systems, most notably those established by religious institutions and the federal government, were another means for drastically eroding

Indian cultures. Education of Indian youth was considered a solution to the "Indian problem," with the goal being to Christianize and civilize Indians. The federal boarding school system (often off-reservation) began in 1879, and for decades, children were taken from their families for months or years at a time. Their outward appearance (hairstyle and clothing) was changed to meet the standards of the day, and, to diminish their psychological, emotional, and spiritual identity with their tribal people, they were punished for speaking their Native languages. It was hoped that in time, the educated Indians would blend in with the white world; in large part, this hope was not realized, and as a whole, Indian and Native children and their families experienced trauma and losses of great magnitude. Horejsi and colleagues (1992) cited evidence that many Indian children were sexually abused while attending boarding schools. Few Indian boarding schools exist today, but many believe that the sequelae of Indian children having been placed in the boarding school system continue in the form of family and educational stress (Kleinfeld 1973; Kleinfeld and Bloom 1977; Special Subcommittee on Indian Education 1969).

As if boarding Indian children in schools far away from home and for long periods of time were not stress enough, Indian families were greatly weakened by aggressive out-of-home placements by the child welfare system. It is estimated that in the decades prior to 1975, 25%–30% of Indian and Native children were placed in foster care or adopted out to non-Indian families (Cross et al. 2000). The Indian Child Welfare Act passed by the U.S. Congress in 1978 stopped this practice and has since provided support for the tribe's role in Indian family preservation. The children who experienced this dislocation from their families, communities, and cultures are now adults. Although their needs have not been systematically studied, one can surmise that their mental health needs are complex (K. Nelson et al. 1996; Roll 1998). It is estimated that 9% of American Indian and Alaska Native children have a serious emotional disturbance, which is two to three times the national average (K. Nelson et al. 1996; Roll 1998).

Mental and emotional disturbance among American Indian and Alaska Native children and adults is best understood in the context of the multigenerational trauma that Native people have experienced (Duran and Duran 1995). These psychological patterns of colonization may be transmitted through family dynamics even while rapid social change is occurring (Yellow Horse Brave Heart and DeBruyn 1998). The trauma dates back to colonial and military subjugation that contributed to the loss of connection to tribal lands, separation of family members, and the disappearance of tribal languages. This trauma is closely associated with high rates of alcohol and drug use, interpersonal violence, and suicide among American Indian and Alaska Native people.

Mental Health Needs and Service System Issues

Focus on American Indians and Alaska Natives has increased in the mental health field during the past decade, but few large-sample epidemiological studies identifying rates of mental disorder have been published. Empirically derived data are still lacking in most areas related to mental health. Even so, existing data suggest that Indian and Native persons across the life span suffer a disproportionate burden of mental health and substance use problems compared with other Americans. High suicide rates serve as a very strong indicator of need (Beals et al. 2005a, 2005b; Blum et al. 1992; Gessner 1997; Kettle and Bixler 1991; May 1990; Mock et al. 1996).

Comorbid conditions, especially alcohol problems and mental health disorders, are of great concern in Indian and Native communities (Beals et al. 2002; Kinzie and Manson 1987; Westermeyer 1982; Westermeyer and Peake 1983; Whittaker 1982). Robin and colleagues (1997) studied over 600 members of three large Indian families and found that more than 70% qualified for a lifetime diagnosis of alcohol disorders. Men and women who were alcohol dependent or who were binge drinkers were more likely to have psychiatric disorders than family members who did not have alcohol use problems. Emerging evidence suggests that Indian adolescents with serious drinking problems are likely to be at risk for mental health problems as well (Beals et al. 2002).

American Indians are the most underserved ethnic group in the United States. Congressional appropriations for the Indian Health Service (IHS), the primary provider of care to American Indian and Alaska Native people, grew by 8% from 1994 to 1998, but after adjustments for inflation and population growth, the funding had actually declined by 18% (Dixon et al. 2001). In 1998, the IHS established the Level of Need Funded (LNF) Workgroup, which compared the IHS's per capita spending level with the Federal Employees Health Benefits Program. The study concluded that "the current Indian

Table 5–1.   Preparing to see a Native patient

- When you know the particular tribe, learn about the tribe's family structure, age and gender roles, and characteristics of typical nonverbal and paralinguistic behavior.
- What are the tribe's beliefs about how problems should be resolved?
- What is the meaning attributed to illness or disability?
- What are the traditional healing practices?
- What are the natural support systems?
- What are the developmental stress points?
- What are the coping strategies?

Health Service budget for personal health care services falls short of parity with other Americans by an estimated 46%" (LNF Workgroup 1999). The IHS is able to address only 43% of the known need for mental health services (Dixon et al. 2001). The ratio of mental health service providers to American Indian and Alaska Native children at the beginning of the new millennium was an astonishing 1 to 25,000. The issues that are most salient in examining the mental health service system for Indians and Natives are the need for culturally sensitive providers, greater geographic and economic accessibility of services, outreach to special populations and settings within the community, and intervention in primary care settings (U.S. Department of Health and Humans Services 2001). Table 5–1 provides an overview of the questions that may be asked during the first session to start the culturally appropriate assessment of the Native American patient.

Applying the DSM-IV-TR Outline for Cultural Formulation

A case example of a young Indian child who was referred for a mental health evaluation by one of her schoolteachers illustrates the application of the DSM-IV-TR Outline for Cultural Formulation to American Indians and Alaska Natives.

Susie, age 10 years, was referred to the school-based health clinic at a public school on a Northern Plains tribal reservation by her fifth-grade teacher. Susie was a midyear transfer student from a much smaller school located in a remote part of the reservation. Her records contained a history of excellent academic and social achievement, but after she had 2 months of sporadic attendance at the new school, a lack of involvement in classroom activities, and episodes of inattention, the teacher requested a psychosocial evaluation of Susie. The teacher highlighted the recent death of Susie's teenage male cousin in a car accident as a possible source of preoccupation and sadness for Susie.

A. Cultural Identity of the Individual

Susie was a member of a Lakota tribe in South Dakota through her mother. She was born in the IHS hospital in the agency town where the tribal seat of governance and various federal Indian offices were located, but she was raised in the mountainous part of the reservation. Susie's father is Ute. He took part in her life during her infancy but stopped doing so after he moved to his home reservation in Utah. Susie's Lakota relatives are numerous and provided active and instrumental support of Susie and of her mother, who remained single. Susie was doted on by her extended family, and spiritual leaders believed that she was gifted with a special connection to the spirits. The bilingual education of Susie's Head Start and elementary schools plus her proximity to Lakota-speaking relatives contributed to her moderate level of proficiency in understanding and speaking the Lakota language. Her English skills were very good. Prior to the move to the new school and setting, Susie had liked school very much.

Cultural Reference Group(s)

Often, identifying information at intake will reveal whether a new mental health client has a connection to an Indian tribe or tribes, and if that is the case, it is natural for the clinician to ask about this early in the relationship. From the patient's point of view, he or she expects to be asked about tribal affiliation as one of the beginning topics. Indeed, when one Indian or Native meets another Indian or Native, one of the first actions of the protocol is to identify where each belongs. "What tribe are you?" is a common question that acknowledges the high value of belonging to a tribal group. The answer can be global (Cheyenne) or specific (Northern Cheyenne).

"Belonging" can be interpreted as formal enrollment as a member, but it can also imply blood affiliation to more than one tribe. Indians and Natives typically are very glad to speak of maternal and paternal Indian ancestry to explain belonging to more than one tribal group. In fact, asking patients to start their sharing about tribal affiliation by speaking about their parents and grandparents may be very comfortable for many. Note, however, that some tribal teachings do not allow a deceased person's name to be spoken, and thus the patient may use only the general relationship terms.

Mainstream U.S. culture is well acquainted with the terms "full blood," "half blood," "half-breed," and "breed," in large part through the film and print media. The question "Do you know your blood quantum?" would likely create tension for most Indian/Native patients and thus is best avoided. Many Indians and Natives do know their blood quantum (calculated by knowing one's Indian ancestors) because it is a criterion for proving Indian ethnicity to tribes, states, and the U.S. federal government. However, many Indians now are ambivalent about the calculation of blood quantum, viewing it as a colonial concept imposed when treaties were signed with the U.S. government. Further, it is thought to breed intragroup oppression in the form of "bloodism," insinuating that having less Indian blood means one is less acceptable or less legitimate.

There are roughly 562 federally recognized tribes in the United States, with a total membership of about 1.7 million (National Congress of American Indians 2004). In addition, there are several hundred groups seeking recognition, a process that often takes decades to complete. As there are hundreds of tribes, the typical clinician cannot be expected to be familiar with every tribal designation. Further complicating the situation, several tribes have recently changed their legal names from those given them by non-Indians or other tribes to the names for themselves in their tribal languages. Thus, the group of Indians named the Winnebago by the French now prefers to be referenced as the *HoChunk,* and those known as Navajo prefer *Diné.* Alaska Natives did not establish treaties with the U.S. government, but they did develop corporations for groups of villages located in Alaska regions. Communal identity for the Alaska Native is most likely first with a specific village or region (e.g., Yukon-Tanana region, with the village of Tanana as the hub of several villages) and second with a native corporation (e.g., Tanana Chiefs Conference).

Escobar and Vega (2000) recommend using open-ended questions that obtain information about 1) education, 2) wage employment, 3) urbanization, 4) media influence, 5) political participation, 6) religion, 7) daily life, 8) social relations, and 9) perception of past significant events (illnesses, traumas, and tragedies) and their causes.

There are other levels of belonging to tribal groups that relate to psychological, spiritual, and social connections. Indians who live or have lived in metropolitan areas are likely to have strong affiliations with Indians from tribes other than their tribes by blood. Also, through intermarriage to non-Indians, many Indians have European, African, Latino, and/or Asian ancestry. Understanding the patient's sense of belonging to Indian and other racial or ethnic groups is vital to a complete and multifaceted assessment of needs and strengths.

Language

Is English your first language? Do you speak any Native languages? How has communicating in English been for you? These are important questions that address language. Tribal language is central to the modern renaissance and survival of Indian and Native cultures. The five major indigenous language families in North America each contains scores of languages within. However, only the few of the oldest generation of Indians/Natives can still understand and speak their native language fluently. The literacy rate in these languages for succeeding generations is extremely low, creating a cultural crisis for most Indian/Native nations. Many believe that spiritual and social ceremonies would be rendered useless or less effective if conducted in a non-Indian language. Others believe that the spiritual and social forces and powers can transcend language, thus allowing for the desired positive outcomes of a ceremony even if a non-Indian language is used. No matter what an Indian or Native believes about this issue, most feel it as a great loss that literacy rates are not high. Nations and villages that have instituted language classes or immersion projects need great support to continue programming, since Indian and Native communities are losing native speakers at a much higher rate than they are gaining literate persons.

Fluent Native language speakers thus are few in number in many Indian communities. Mental health services are usually conducted in English, and it is not likely that a clinician will need translation services. However, proficiency in the use of English is likely to vary greatly across Indian patients—especially when communicating about emotional states and beliefs about wellness and illness. Therefore, having a family member or friend accompany an Indian patient who is not comfortable with his or her English skills is an important choice to offer. It should be noted that trained interpreters with Native language fluency are rarely available within mental health systems, even in Indian communities. When needed, community members are pressed into service. In such cases, following guidelines that protect confidentiality and preserve healthy clinician-patient relationship boundaries is extremely important.

Cultural Factors in Development

Tribes have various ways of addressing developmental stages from the prenatal period to the end of life. A patient who has been an active participant in tribal life is subject to primary expectations regarding these stages, and there are important transitions and ceremonies for marking them. Any of these aspects can be centrally related to the patient's presentation of wellness and illness. Thus, it is important to ask the patient the following: What are valued qualities for a [tribal name] person during this phase of life? What are the necessary accomplishments for the person in this phase of life? What role does the family have in helping the person become what he or she needs to be in this phase of life? What role does the Indian community have in helping the person go through this phase in a good way? What might happen if a person does not do what he or she needs to do during this time? Is there any cultural way to reverse a negative outcome or make it less of a problem?

Involvement in the Culture of Origin

Obviously, if the patient is living within the boundaries of or close to a tribal community, there will be multiple opportunities to participate in tribal-specific and general events for individuals and families. Although these are more difficult to access, many cities have Indian-serving organizations that sponsor events such as Indian dances, craft fairs, health fairs, culture classes, sports programs, meal programs for elders, and social get-togethers. Sometimes a cultural practice from another tribe is available, and it is important to know if participation presents a conflict within the patient's family or circle of friends.

Involvement With Host Culture

Like other distinct American ethnic groups, Indians and Natives have achieved great familiarity with American culture largely by means of television, movies, and print media. The youth, in particular, have access to cultural perspectives from around the world through educational venues and the Internet. There are some individuals who lack comfort in non-Indian settings, but many move in and out of mainstream circumstances with ease.

Some carry substantial distrust of other cultures—much of this wariness justified by life experiences of prejudice and oppression. Others cultivate understanding of other cultures as a way to take the best of all worlds while continuing to nurture Indian beliefs and practices. Many Indian and Native elders rely on family members to serve as cultural mediators or negotiators. How comfortable are these roles for the patient and his/her family? How does the patient deal with ambivalence about non-Indian cultures? How does the patient deal with stereotypes about Indian and Native cultures?

Gender and Sexual Orientation

Mainstream American concepts of gender tend to revolve around being male or female; likewise, sexuality tends to be categorized as "straight" or "gay." By contrast, at least 168 Native languages have terms for people who are not considered either male or female. Additionally, many Native cultures prescribed important roles within the tribal unit for individuals who were not male or female (Balsam et al. 2004). Most of these roles were eliminated or diminished in the colonization process, and many contemporary Native communities struggle with strong bias against anything other than heterosexual male and female roles. Such bias often prevents a Native person from full access to family and community social support, spiritual coping, and participation in traditional ceremonies and health practices. Native males suffered greatly when cultural change reduced the options for providing for the family and tribal units through warrior and hunter roles. Today, conflicts between sexual/gender identities and ethnic identities can result in great challenges to one's balance and can compromise the mobilization of personal and cultural resources. In response to limited gender roles and to homophobia, the term "two-spirited" or "two-spirited people" was introduced and has been a helpful self-attribution for many Natives. Two-spirited indicates that someone possesses both a male and a female spirit. This term often carries a sense of positive acceptance or even celebration within many Native communities (Tafoya 2003).

Nonverbal Communication

Native American patients tend to avoid eye contact, to speak only in a low tone of voice, and to have limp handshakes. An approach that may work to show respect for a patient's communication style is to take the lead from the patient; note the patient's behaviors (tone of voice, pace of speech, and degree of eye contact) and match them subtly.

B. Cultural Explanations of the Individual's Illness

Susie, her older teen brother, and her mother moved to the agency town a week before Susie's cousin died in the accident. The transition of the mother enrolling in the tribal college and the children in their respective schools was less smooth than desired because they went back to attend the wake and funeral in their outlying town, rituals that lasted 3 days. Susie did worry very much about her brother's safety because he was a frequent companion of the cousin who passed away. Worry about others is normative in this tribal society, even for young children, where the value is to have concern for the family and community network. Because of the move, Susie did not receive as many assurances from her family about her own safety and the safety of her brother as she would have otherwise. Her mother viewed Susie's preoccupation about her brother as normal until she realized that the balance of assurances was not present in the situation.

Further complicating the situation was Susie's report of hearing "spirits." *Seeing* the spirit of a deceased person during the grieving period of several months after the death is not uncommon in this tribal community. Susie did not experience this, but her teacher thought this was happening and thus encouraged Susie to speak of it. Hearing the singing of spirits was an occasional experience for Susie and was attributed to her special gift. The family believed that speaking about this gift needed to be kept within the privacy of the family because Susie was young and the gift was still emerging. An increase in hearing the singing after her cousin's death was considered by her family's spiritual leaders to be positive and comforting, but to be a matter for the family only.

American Indians and Alaska Natives have implemented effective, holistic diagnostic methods and maintained multiaxial diagnostic knowledge about the human body and human behavior for hundreds of years (Trimble and Thurman 2002). In most Native diagnostic systems, there is belief that this body of knowledge was a gift from the Creator and that it continues to be valuable in contemporary thinking. Although many Indian communities have lost much of this indigenous knowledge, there are elders and culture bearers who can provide advice, guidance, and intervention based on Indian-honored perspectives. Some are willing to share across tribal boundaries, and many consider their system a private matter with a patient and his or her family.

Predominant Idioms of Distress and Local Illness Categories

Many scholars, particularly those contributing to ethnographic work, believe that some Indians and Natives express emotional distress and conceive of ill health in ways that do not match the diagnostic nosology of DSM-IV-TR. Idioms of distress and local illness categories in this population have been described (Manson 1994; Manson et al. 1985; S. Nelson and Manson 2000; Trimble et al. 1984). Frequently cited examples are *ghost sickness* or *windigo* (a preoccupation with death and the deceased, identified in Northern Algonquian peoples [Marano 1985]), *pibloktoq* or *Arctic hysteria* (abrupt episodes of extreme excitement), and *wicinko* (a Siouan-language term referring to a form of cultural "time-out," used for coping when the patient believes family members are placing too much of a burden on him or her).

Many of the indigenous illness and wellness categories are related to spiritual conditions. Jilek-Aall (1976) reminds us that the question of how spiritual matters may or may not affect the patient's current situation has to be raised at a time when the patient has confidence in the therapeutic process. One prudent approach would be to ask the patient to tell her life story and let her reveal what she believes is appropriate. When the patient brings it up, it is important to be nonjudgmental about the belief system and share observations of the positive outcomes that many people have had by embracing and practicing traditional ways.

The understanding of mainstream diagnostic classification is very limited in Indian and Native communities, but most Indians and Natives have been exposed to the same layman's terms for the common disorders in actions, cognitions, and emotions as other English-speaking citizens of the United States. Many Indians and Natives today associate stigma with many of these disorders even though there might have been less stigma or none in times prior to modern diagnosis from Western medicine. Understandably, the process of labeling is highly suspect for many Indians and Natives.

Meaning and Severity of Symptoms in Relation to Cultural Norms

It may be an Indian/Native cultural norm that physical symptoms and medical diagnoses such as arthritis are easier to talk about than emotional pain or distress, but little empirical research is available on this. Somervell and colleagues (1993) analyzed responses to the Center for Epidemiologic Studies Depression Scale. Somatic complaints and emotional distress were not well differentiated from each other in the adult sample from a Northwest Coast tribe. It is important to ask about the relative importance of symptoms to the patient, since cultural norms may not place the same degree of emphasis on symptoms that they receive in the DSM-IV-TR diagnostic system. An example of an Indian person who appears depressed and without energy illustrates this. The person may not actually be in a hopeless state and may believe that solutions will emerge in their own time. This state of expectation may be misinterpreted through a Western perspective as passivity and lack of initiative (Blue and Blue 1983).

Perceived Causes and Explanatory Models

Indian and Native beliefs about why and how illness develops differ widely across North America; spiritual elements are common in explanatory models. This is also true of why and how wellness is achieved and maintained. The range of explanations includes 1) a wrong act against another person, part of creation, or the Creator; 2) not performing an act when it is warranted; 3) being the victim of spiritual hexing perpetrated by another person; 4) being out of balance or harmony; and 5) being influenced or affected by spiritual entities. A good way to assess for this is to ask: "Families and communities have ideas about why and how experiences such as the one you are describing come about. If a trusted elder from your community were here, what would he or she say was the reason you are experiencing this?"

Help-Seeking Experiences and Plans

One in five Indians and Natives report that they have access to health services provided by the IHS to those living on or near reservations and trust lands (Brown et al. 2000). Because of chronic underfunding of the agency, mental health services, if present at all, are often extremely limited. Indians and Natives are largely uninsured or underinsured and thus do not have access to mainstream mental health service in the public and private sectors. Often there is great mistrust of formal health care systems, and it is important to learn the patient's history with regard to available mental health services, whether through the IHS, a tribally administered health department, Medicaid, Medicare, or another system.

Many contemporary Indian/Native communities are fortunate enough to have long-standing traditional healing and support for personal and family development. By and large, family leaders arrange access to this healing. The medicinal use of plants and roots is common in some Indian communities. Several targeted studies suggest that American Indians and Alaska Natives use alternative therapies at rates that are equal to or greater than the rates for whites (Buchwald et al. 2000; Gurley et al. 2001; Kim and Kwok 1998; Marbella et al. 1998). In these studies, native healing generally was used in addition to mainstream health services, not as a substitute for them. Care must be taken not to be intrusive in questioning about traditional healing. The clinician could say, "Since seeking traditional healing may be a private matter for you and your family, I will understand if you choose not to share details about it. It will be helpful for me to at least know the different ways you and your family are getting help for your situation." Indians and Natives who do not have access to traditional healing may be open to the clinician's help in identifying resources. In rare cases, there may be a respectful way to interface the traditional Native resources with the conventional interventions of Western medicine. The situations where such collaboration has been successful have usually emerged after a lengthy period of trust-building between practitioners, in which roles, information sharing, confidentiality, compensation, and other key issues were clearly delineated (Manson 1994).

Conventional health systems have successfully integrated some long-held tribal traditions, to the benefit of Indian/Native consumers. Examples are the use of adults in the extended family as nonparental disciplinarians in a Northwest tribe's group home for youth in foster care (Shore and Nicholls 1975), the use of the Plains Indian medicine wheel as a tool for self-analysis (Robbins 1994), and the use of the "talking circle" as a way to process psychological, social, and spiritual issues in a group format. Some health programs have sweat lodges for use by Indian and Native patients. The ceremony itself can be conducted by a health staff person or a community member, and in either case, the ceremony leader or "water pourer" is recognized by the Indian community as prepared to help others in the sweat lodge.

C. Cultural Factors Related to Psychosocial Environment and Levels of Functioning

> Susie's mother moved the family in with relatives who lived in an old Bureau of Indian Affairs house in the agency town. There were six adults and four children in a two-bedroom house. Overcrowding in substandard housing is very common on this reservation. Susie's mother was excited about being a college student for the first time, and awareness of the time that had passed between high school and her Associate of Arts college program created much anxiety for her. Susie had been coddled in her previous household, and there

were greater expectations in the new household for Susie to complete tasks around the home. Susie's mother did not have much time to prepare Susie for these new expectations, and tensions developed between Susie and other household members when Susie did not perform as expected.

Social Stressors

Indian communities are marked by great economic disadvantage; unemployment, underemployment, and housing shortages, among others, are indicators of widespread stress. From 1997 to 1999, about 26% of Indians and Natives lived in poverty; this percentage compared with 13% for the United States as a whole and 8% for white Americans (U.S. Census Bureau 1999). Asking about daily life in the patient's community provides the patient an opportunity to describe stressors common to many.

Social Supports

Most Indian communities, rural and urban, hold expectations based on cultural beliefs that the family will provide instrumental and emotional support for its members. The *tiospaye,* a Lakota expression of traditional lifestyle based on extended family, shared responsibility, and reciprocity (Mohatt and Blue 1982), is being revitalized in many northern Plains Indian communities. Contemporary stresses on Indian families often work against smooth provision of support. When the expectations do not match the actual behaviors, tensions can develop among family members, leading to many possible negative emotions and behaviors.

Intergenerational Relationships

The value of a strong extended family whose members from each generation actively support one another is very robust in American Indian and Alaska Natives. Children are considered sacred gifts to be nurtured and protected. Children are also considered teachers within the family and tribal nation. Similarly, elders are carriers of valuable indigenous knowledge and wisdom. Each phase of life holds tasks and blessings for the individual that will benefit the family and tribe. These teachings about intergenerational harmony and support are being articulated more clearly now as tribal nations revitalize the ways culture is celebrated and practiced. Families that have been challenged over the last three to four generations by the negative effects of boarding schools, out-of-home placements of the children, substance abuse, extreme poverty, and other devastating outcomes of colonialism are not in tune with these teachings about the strengths of the extended family. Thus, conflicts between generations often present concern at behavioral health clinics. Family-centered approaches are considered to be promising and consistent with the values of most Indian and Native communities.

Levels of Functioning and Disability

Culture very much defines the parameters of "normal" functioning and the assessment of abilities. In Indian cultures where belonging to and contributing to the larger group are highly valued, a child with severe developmental disabilities might be described as functioning highly because he brings wood into the house for the daily fire. In this case, the contribution to the household, however simple, overshadows what might be called disabilities by other standards.

D. Cultural Elements of the Relationship Between the Individual and the Clinician

> The clinician who evaluated Susie for poor school performance was a new behavioral health consultant to that public school's new medical clinic, which targeted diabetes prevention in the school population. She had not served Indian children before but was able to connect with Susie through drawing. Susie didn't want to talk about her cousin and did not bring up the voices; however, she did say that she missed her family from her former home. The clinician sought the guidance of the school's home-school coordinator, a Lakota woman who knew many families on the reservation. The home-school coordinator believed that Susie's extended family had many resources to give, and she urged the clinician to ask Susie to have other family members participate in the evaluation if she wished. Two older aunts came with Susie's mother for the intake interview at the new school. They listened carefully to the observations of the school staff and provided background information when Susie's mother indicated she wanted their input. They also made it clear what issues would be addressed by the family in their ceremonies. Together, they came up with ways the school staff could support Susie and her mother through the challenging circumstances.

Just as the clinician has questions about the patient and his or her situation, the patient has questions and expectations about the provider and about the processes called diagnosis, assessment, and therapeutic intervention. A focus

Table 5–2.   Native American patient's expectations of a non-Native healer

- I expect the healer not to know much about Indians in general, let alone the history of my tribe, its traditional beliefs and values, current tribal organization, and its problems and resources.
- I expect that the healer will not value healing rituals.
- I expect the healer to consider only the deficits and to ignore the strengths of myself, my family, and my community.
- I expect that the healer will understand reluctance to talk about my strengths and resources, since it could be interpreted as boasting.
- I expect that the healer will not understand how hard it is to honor Native traditions and survive in the host culture.
- I expect to question the trustworthiness of the healer.
- I expect to present a concrete problem before I talk about other kinds of problems.
- I expect not to trust the mental health system because I believe it is likely to be patronizing (based on experiences with the Bureau of Indian Affairs and Indian Health Service) and nonsupportive of self-determination.
- I expect that the healer will not talk about the mutual responsibilities of the healer and myself.

on counselor characteristics and considerations is prominent in the publications by counselors, clinicians, and scholars regarding mental health interventions with Native American Indians (Trimble and Thurman 2002).

Indians and Natives have ideas about—if not experience with—providers of mental health services from a Western health care system, and also about helpers from indigenous healing systems (Tables 5–2 and 5–3). The latter group are variously called *medicine men and women, shamans, spiritual leaders,* and *healers,* among other terms specific to certain tribes (e.g., the *hand trembler* of the Diné/Navajo). The non-Indian clinician may have difficulty with the belief systems associated with indigenous ceremonies and herbal medicines. However, because many Indians and Natives hold great respect for indigenous healing ways, the non-Native clinician is exhorted to suspend disbelief and to listen to and hear whatever the Indian patient shares (Trimble and Thurman 2002).

Although it is natural to focus on the differences in theory, belief, and approach between Western and indigenous healers, Torrey (1986) has described commonalities. Indian and Native healers often exemplify empathy, genuine-

Table 5–3.   Native American patient's expectations of an indigenous healer

- I expect that the healer/diagnostician will identify my problems without prying too deeply into my personal life or asking many intimate questions.
- I expect that family members will be involved.
- I expect that improvement will occur quickly.
- I expect the healer to "take charge" and solve the problem. I will be hopeful, but the healer is the active one.
- I expect the healer to consider all of myself: physical, mental, emotional, spiritual, and interpersonal domains.
- I expect to be understood within the context of my relationship to Nature.
- I expect that my individual hurt is also a community hurt.
- I expect that "harmony and balance" will be considered important in understanding my situation.
- I expect that the healer will understand how breaking a taboo or ignoring a tradition can result in my circumstance.

ness, availability, respect, warmth, congruence, and concreteness; correspondingly, most Western mental health theories and styles predicate their interventions on a basic therapeutic relationship in which the provider communicates these characteristics to the patient.

Reimer (1999) asked Inupiat villagers in Alaska to state the characteristics they found desirable in a healer. Their replies (described in Table 5–4) included expectations for community, cultural, and spiritual involvement, as well as attributes and behavior conventionally expected to be a major part of the clinical encounter.

If domains other than mental health are the purview of the respected healer, it stands to reason that Indians and Natives might meet a Western-trained provider of mental health services and expect assistance with medical concerns, spirituality, financial issues, or the problems of persons important to the patient (Helms and Cook 1999).

Empirical research, case studies, and clinical experience also identify the following clinician characteristics associated with effective therapeutic relationships: 1) is trustworthy (LaFromboise and Dixon 1981), 2) uses self-disclosure to show warmth and genuineness (Lockhart 1981), 3) provides practical advice and is flexible about the location of service (LaFromboise et

Table 5–4.   Native patients' desired characteristics of therapists

- Virtuous, kind, respectful, trustworthy, friendly, gentle, loving, clean, giving, helpful, not a gossip, and not one who wallows in self-pity
- Strong physically, mentally, spiritually, personally, socially, and emotionally
- Works well with others by becoming familiar with people in the community
- Has good communication skills, achieved by taking time to talk, visit, and listen
- Respected because of his or her knowledge, disciplined in thought and action, wise and understanding, and willing to share knowledge by teaching and serving as an inspiration
- Substance free
- One who knows and follows the culture
- One who has faith and a strong relationship with the Creator

Source.   Reimer 1999.

al. 1980), and 4) dresses and presents him- or herself in a way that reflects the community's beliefs about leadership and authority figures (Littrell and Littrell 1983) (see Table 5–5).

A number of researchers say that the best match for an Indian or Native patient is an Indian or Native provider (Darou 1987; Uhlemann et al. 1988). This seems to be particularly true of patients who are involved with their Indian/Native heritage (Johnson and Lashley 1989). In a study by Bennett and Big Foot-Sipes (1991), Indians said that being matched with counselors whose attitudes and beliefs are similar to theirs is more important than shared ethnicity. Dinges and colleagues (1981) acknowledged that ethnic match might support rapport-building but asserted that perceived effectiveness (e.g., warmth, genuineness, respect, and empathy) is more likely than ethnic match to sustain the therapeutic relationship. Herring (1999) pointed out that because very few Indians and Natives are mental health professionals, non-Indians will serve Indian and Native patients for quite a long time to come. Thus, although shared ethnicity is important, all clinicians need to be knowledgeable and skilled in assessing and treating Indians and Natives. Using a cultural consultant, clinician, or community member who is familiar with the patient's reference group is helpful in determining normative and non-normative behavior and symptoms. In addition, there are specific techniques that are likely to be helpful in engaging the patient (Table 5–6).

Table 5–5. Developing trust

Therapists who gained their patient's trust…

- Were attentive and responsive to patient
- Gave structure and direction to the interview
- Displayed respect for patient's cultural identity
- Used eye contact similar to that of patient
- Sat erect in their chair
- Avoided references to time until end of session

Source. Adapted from LaFromboise and Dixon 1981.

E. Overall Cultural Assessment for Diagnosis and Care

Susie and her mother are clearly identified with their clan and greater tribal community. At the time of referral for behavioral health services, the family had been separated from their extended family for a brief period and had not yet developed ties with their new community and its resources. Clearly, it was wise to mobilize the extended family in support of Susie and her mother during the assessment of Susie's needs. This was fairly easy to accomplish because of the home-school coordinator's wide knowledge of the several reservation communities and the ease with which family elders could travel the distance to the agency town and participate in sessions at the school. The consequence of this collaboration with the family's natural helping system was greater understanding of the severity of the illness experience (academic problems and worry) from the cultural point of view and clear expectations for appropriate intervention at the school.

The task of synthesizing the information gleaned from assessment that contains the culture context of the Indian patient is one that will likely result in a formulation that is balanced with the identification of problem areas and strengths. A key in the assessment process is to identify the Indian or Native's level of affiliation with non-Indian and Indian cultures. Another is to learn about the historical issues that affect the individual, and the family and community. Several recommendations for establishing a "culturally affirmative environment" (Herring 1999) for Indians and Natives have been identified. These suggestions (detailed in Table 5–7) call for candor, flexibility, patience, openness to family involvement, development of trust, respect for culture, and maintenance of confidentiality (Herring 1999).

Table 5–6.   Building effective relationships

- Explain to the patient that you will have plenty of time to get to know each other before discussing any concerns the patient may have.
- Communicate that there are no demands to behave a certain way or talk a certain amount.
- Avoid lengthy intake forms or questionnaires.
- Accept the presence of a friend or family member.
- Atmosphere should be relaxed, casual, and nonthreatening.
- Use informal, conversational verbal style.
- Talk about practical issues of daily life before talking about intimate issues.
- Use self-disclosure as a way to prompt self-disclosure on part of patient.
- Avoid direct questioning for a while.
- Communicate warmth, caring, genuineness, and respect.

Finally, certain therapeutic approaches may be more effective, such as a more direct, present-focused therapy that prioritizes problem-solving techniques. One should avoid techniques such as explorative psychotherapy, promotion of catharsis, and a permissive approach.

Conclusion

As time goes on, American Indian and Alaska Native populations will increasingly become consumers in health systems that are not yet prepared for them. The scenario that began this chapter can become a reality if certain developments occur to address the many knowledge and skill gaps that exist in mental health services for Indian and Native people. Clinical training programs can include curricula and access to clinical sites specific to this population. Researchers and clinicians can carefully document interventions that are effective not only globally with Indians and Natives but also with specific tribes. Health systems can institute in-service training on a regular basis to providers, can hire Indian/Native providers whenever possible, and can develop linkages with the Indian community or communities within the region. As Indian and Native communities continue on their journey of revitalization, they are becoming more active in designing health systems that work for them. There is an increased awareness that behavioral health services are vital to bettering the overall health of Indians and Natives. In *Mental Health: Cul-*

Table 5–7. Suggestions for working with Native American patients

- Address openly the issue of dissimilar ethnic relationships rather than pretending that no differences exist.
- Schedule appointments to allow for flexibility in ending the session.
- Be open to allowing the extended family to participate in the session.
- Allow time for trust to develop before focusing on problems.
- Respect the uses of silence.
- Demonstrate honor and respect for the patient's culture.
- Maintain the highest level of confidentiality.

Source. Herring 1999.

ture, Race, and Ethnicity. A Supplement to Mental Health: A Report of the Surgeon General (U.S. Department of Health and Human Services 2001), the take-home message was that "culture counts." The opportunity is ripe for establishing partnerships between the service provider sector and the Indian community. The efforts of each of us can count significantly in this important venture.

References

American Psychiatric Association: Appendix I: Outline for cultural formulation and glossary of culture-bound syndromes, in Diagnostic and Statistical Manual of Mental Disorders, 4th Edition, Text Revision. Washington, DC, American Psychiatric Association, 2000, pp 897–903

Balsam KF, Huang B, Fieland KC, et al: Culture, Trauma, and Wellness: A Comparison of Heterosexual and Lesbian, Gay, Bisexual, and Two-Spirit Native Americans. Cultur Divers Ethnic Minor Psychol 10:287–301, 2004

Beals J, Novins DK, Mitchell CM, et al: Comorbidity between alcohol abuse/dependence and psychiatric disorders: prevalence, treatment implications, and new directions for research among American Indian populations, in Alcohol Use Among American Indians and Alaska Natives: Multiple Perspectives on a Complex Problem (NIAAA Monograph, No 37). Edited by Mail PD, Heurtin-Roberts S, Martin SE, et al. Bethesda, MD, National Institute on Alcohol Abuse and Alcoholism, 2002, pp 317–410

Beals J, Manson SM, Whitesell NR, et al: Prevalence of DSM-IV disorders and attendant help-seeking in two American Indian reservation populations. Arch Gen Psychiatry 62:99–108, 2005a

Beals J, Manson SM, Whitesell NR, et al: Prevalence of major depressive episode in two American indian reservation populations: unexpected findings with a structured interview. Am J Psychiatry 162:1713–17222, 2005b

Bennett S, Bigfoot-Sipes D: American Indian and white college students' preferences for counselor characteristics. J Couns Psychol 38:440–445, 1991

Blue A, Blue M: The strain of stress. White Cloud Journal 3(1):15–22, 1983

Blum RW, Harmon B, Harris L, et al: American Indian-Alaska Native youth health. JAMA 267:1637–1644, 1992

Brown ER, Ojeda VD, Wyn R, et al: Racial and Ethnic Disparities in Access to Health Insurance and Health Care. Los Angeles, CA, UCLA Center for Health Policy Research and the Henry J. Kaiser Family Foundation, 2000

Buchwald DS, Beals J, Manson SM: Use of traditional healing among Native Americans in a primary care setting. Med Care 38:1191–1199, 2000

Cross TA, Earle KA, Simmons D: Child abuse and neglect in Indian country: policy issues. Fam Soc 81:49–58, 2000

Darou WG: Counseling and the northern Native. Canadian Journal of Counseling 32:33–41, 1987

Dinges N, Trimble JE, Manson S, et al: Counseling and psychotherapy with American Indians and Alaska Natives, in Cross-Cultural Counseling and Psychotherapy: Foundations, Evaluation, and Cultural Considerations. Edited by Marsella AJ and Pedersen PB. Elmsford, NY, Pergamon, 1981, pp 243–276

Dixon M, Mather DT, Shelton BL, et al: Economic and organizational changes in health care systems, in Promises to Keep: Public Health Policy for American Indians and Alaska Natives in the 21st Century. Edited by Dixon M, Roubideaux Y. Washington, DC, American Public Health Association, 2001, pp 89–12

Duran E, Duran B: Native American Postcolonial Psychology. Albany, State University of New York Press, 1995

Escobar JI, Vega WA: Mental health and immigration's AAAs: where are we and where do we go from here? J Nerv Ment Dis 188:736–740, 2000

Fleming W: The Complete Idiot's Guide to Native American History. Indianapolis, IN, Alpha Books, 2003

Gessner BD: Temporal trends and geographic patterns of teen suicide in Alaska, 1979–1993. Suicide Life Threat Behav 27:264–273, 1997

Gurley D, Novins DK, Jones MC, et al: Comparative use of biomedical services and traditional health options by American Indian veterans. Psychiatr Serv 52:68–74, 2001

Helms JE, Cook DA: Using Race and Culture in Counseling and Psychotherapy: Theory and Process. Boston, MA, Allyn & Bacon, 1999

Herring RD: Counseling With Native American Indians and Alaska Natives: Strategies for Helping Professionals. Thousand Oaks, CA, Sage, 1999

Horejsi C, Craig BHR, Pablo J: Reactions by Native American parents to child protection agencies: cultural and community factors. Child Welfare 71:329–342, 1992

Jilek-Aall L: The Western psychiatrist and his non-Western clientele: transcultural experiences of relevance to psychotherapy with Canadian Indian patients. Can Psychiatr Assoc J 21:353–359, 1976

Johnson M, Lashley K: Influence of Native Americans' cultural commitment on preferences for counselor ethnicity and expectations about counseling. J Multicult Couns Devel 17:115–122, 1989

Kettle PA, Bixler EO: Suicide in Alaskan Natives, 1979–1984. Psychiatry 54:55–63, 1991

Kim C, Kwok TS: Navajo use of native healers. Arch Intern Med 158:2245–2249, 1998

Kinzie JD, Manson SM: The use of self-rating scales in cross-cultural psychiatry. Hosp Community Psychiatry 38:190–196, 1987

Kleinfeld J: A Long Way From Home: Effects of Public High Schools on Village Children Away From Home. Fairbanks, AK, Center for Northern Educational Research and Institute of Social, Economic, and Government Research, 1973

Kleinfeld J, Bloom J: Boarding schools: effects on the mental health of Eskimo adolescents. Am J Psychiatry 134:411–417, 1977

LaFromboise T, Dixon D: American Indian perceptions of trustworthiness in a counseling interview. J Couns Psychol 28:135–139, 1981

LaFromboise T, Dauphinais P, Rowe W: Indian students' perceptions of positive helper attributes. Journal of American Indian Education 19:11–16, 1980

Littrell MA, Littrell JM: Counselor dress cues: Evaluations by American Indians and Caucasians. J Cross Cult Psychol 14:109–121, 1983

LNF Workgroup: Level of Need Funded Study (LNF Workgroup Report II). Rockville, MD, Indian Health Service, 1999

Lockhart B: Historic distrust and the counseling of American Indians and Alaskan Natives. White Cloud Journal 2(3):31–43, 1981

Manson SM: Culture and depression: discovering variations in the experience of illness, in Psychology and Culture. Edited by Lonner WJ, Malpass RS. Needham, MA, Allyn & Bacon, 1994, pp 285–290

Manson SM, Shore JH, Bloom JD: The depressive experience in American Indian communities: a challenge for psychiatric theory and diagnosis, in Culture and Depression. Edited by Kleinman A, Good B. Berkeley, University of California Press, 1985, pp 331–368

Marano L: *Windigo* psychosis: the anatomy of an emic-etic confusion, in The Culture-Bound Syndromes: Folk Illnesses of Psychiatric and Anthropological Interest. Edited by Simons RC, Hughes CC. Boston, MA, D. Reidel, 1985, pp 411–448

Marbella AM, Harris MC, Diehr S, et al: Use of Native American healers among Native American patients in an urban Native American health center. Arch Fam Med 7:182–185, 1998

May PA: A bibliography on suicide and suicide attempts among American Indians and Alaska Natives. Omega 21:199–214, 1990

Mock CN, Grossman DC, Mulder D, et al: Health care utilization as a marker for suicidal behavior on an American Indian reservation. J Gen Intern Med 11:519–524, 1996

Mohatt G, Blue AW: Primary prevention as it relates to traditionality and empirical measures of social deviance, in New Directions in Prevention Among American Indian and Alaska Native Communities. Edited by Manson SM. Portland, Oregon Health Sciences University, 1982, pp 91–116

National Congress of American Indians: Federal recognition. 2004. Available at: http://www.ncai.org/Federal_Recognition.70.0.html. Accessed January 27, 2006.

Nelson K, Cross T, Landsman M, et al: Native American families and child neglect. Child Youth Serv Rev 18:505–522, 1996

Nelson S, Manson SM: Mental health and mental disorder, in The Health of American Indians and Alaska Natives. Edited by Rhoades ER. Baltimore, MD, Johns Hopkins University Press, 2000, pp 311–327

Reimer CS: Counseling the Inupiat Eskimo. Westport, CT, Greenwood, 1999

Robbins ML: Native American perspective, in Managing Multiculturalism in Substance Abuse Services. Edited by Gordon JU. Thousand Oaks, CA, Sage, 1994, pp 148–176

Robin RW, Chester B, Rasmussen JK, et al: Prevalence, characteristics, and impact of childhood sexual abuse in a southwestern American Indian tribe. Child Abuse Negl 231:769–787, 1997

Roll S: Cross-cultural considerations in custody and parenting plans. Child Adolesc Psychiatr Clin N Am 7:445–454, 1998

Rural Policy Research Institute: Rural by the numbers: information about rural America. 1997. Available at: http://www.rupri.org/resources/rnumbers/demopop/demo.html. Accessed June 14, 2004.

Shore JH, Nicholls WW: Indian children and tribal group homes: New interpretations of the whipper man. Am J Psychiatry 132:454–456, 1975

Somervell PD, Beals J, Kinzie JD, et al: Use of the CES-D in an American Indian village. Cult Med Psychiatry 16:503–517, 1993

Special Subcommittee on Indian Education, Senate Committee on Labor and Public Welfare: Indian Education: A National Tragedy, a National Challenge (Senate Report No 91–501). Washington, DC, U.S. Senate, 1969

Tafoya T: Native gay and lesbian issues: The two-spirited, in Psychological Perspectives on Lesbian, Gay, and Bisexual Experiences, 2nd Edition. Edited by Garnets LD, Kimmel DC. New York, Columbia University Press, 2003, pp 401–409

Thornton R: American Indian Holocaust and Survival: A Population History Since 1492. Norman, University of Oklahoma Press, 1987

Torrey EF: Witch Doctors and Psychiatrists: The Common Roots of Psychotherapy and Its Future. New York, Harper & Row, 1986

Trimble J, Thurman PJ: Ethnocultural considerations and strategies for providing counseling services to Native American Indians, in Counseling Across Cultures, 5th Edition. Edited by Pedersen PB, Draguns JG, Lonner WJ, et al. Thousand Oaks, CA, Sage, 2002, pp 53–91

Trimble JE, Manson SM, Dinges NG, et al: Towards an understanding of American Indian concepts of mental health: some reflections and directions, in Mental Health Services: The Cross/Cultural Context. Edited by Pedersen P, Sartorius N, Marsala A. Beverly Hills, CA, Sage, 1984, pp 199–220

Uhlemann M, Lee D, France H: Counselor ethnic differences and perceived counseling effectiveness. Int J Adv Couns 11:247–253, 1988

U.S. Census Bureau: We, the First Americans. Washington, DC, U.S. Census Bureau, 1993. Available at: http://www.census.gov/apsd/wepeople/we-5.pdf

U.S. Census Bureau Census: Statistical Abstract of the United States: The National Data Book. Washington, DC, U.S. Census Bureau, 1999

U.S. Census Bureau: Overview of Race and Hispanic origin (Census 2000 Brief No. C2KBR/01–1). Washington, DC, U.S. Census Bureau, 2001

U.S. Department of Health and Human Services: Mental Health: Culture, Race, and Ethnicity. A Supplement to Mental Health: A Report of the Surgeon General. Rockville, MD, U.S. Department of Health and Human Services, Public Health Service, Office of the Surgeon General, 2001. Available at: http://www.surgeon-general.gov/library/mentalhealth/cre

Westermeyer J: Alcoholism and services for ethnic populations, in Encyclopedic Handbook of Alcoholism. Edited by Pattison E, Kaufman E. New York, Gardner Press, 1982, pp 709–717

Westermeyer J, Peake E: A ten-year follow-up of alcoholic Native Americans in Minnesota. Am J Psychiatry 140:189–194, 1983

Whittaker JO: Alcohol and the Standing Rock Sioux Tribe: a twenty-year follow up study. J Stud Alcohol 43:191–200, 1982

Yellow Horse Brave Heart M, DeBruyn LM: The American Indian holocaust: healing historical unresolved grief. Am Indian Alsk Native Ment Health Res 5:56–78, 1998

PART III

Culture, Psychopharmacological
Treatment, and Case Formulation

6

Ethnopsychopharmacology

Michael W. Smith, M.D.

Ethnic variation in response to a large array of psychotropic medications has been reported over the past 30 years (Kalow 1992). Studies in the field of pharmacogenetics indicate that ethnic-specific polymorphic variability may be in large part responsible for these differences (Lin et al. 1993). These ethnic-specific mutations correspond to varying efficiencies in drug metabolism among members of different ethnic minority populations. The biotransformation systems that break down pharmacological agents also display environmental responsivity, such as inhibition or induction of enzyme activity due to certain dietary substances. Nonbiological factors such as age, gender, diet, and smoking (Figure 6–1) also play a role in determining differential response. Finally, misdiagnosis due to ethnic variation in symptomatology has led to the use of treatment that is ineffectual or possibly toxic (Lawson 1996). In this chapter I introduce the drug-metabolizing enzymes, briefly review clinical reports of ethnic variation with several different classes of psychotropics, and then closely examine the relationship of pharmacogenetics, ethnicity, and environmental factors.

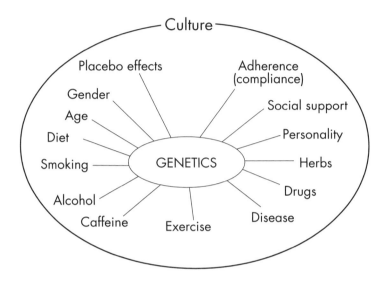

Figure 6–1.   Factors affecting drug metabolism.

Introduction to the Pharmacogenetics of Drug-Metabolizing Enzymes

A number of different xenobiotic-metabolizing enzymes have been identified in humans (Kalow 1992). Among these, the cytochrome P450 (CYP450) drug-metabolizing enzymes appear to be the most clinically relevant for the practice of psychiatry. They have also been the major focus of pharmacogenetic research (Gonzalez and Nebert 1990). The human CYP450 genes belong to a well-conserved gene family existing in all biological systems, including bacteria and plants. They perform other vital functions (e.g., biosynthesis) in addition to the biotransformation of xenobiotics (foreign substances). More than 20 human CYP450 enzymes have been identified and cloned. Of these, the following may be regarded as most important in terms of the metabolism of psychotropic medications: CYP2D6, CYP3A4, CYP1A2, CYP2C19, CYP2C9, CYP2E1, and CYP2A6. The first four have the most relevance to psychiatry and will be discussed in greater detail in this chapter. It is believed that the differences observed in ethnic minorities among patients who take psychotropics—such as the variations seen in efficacy, side effects, and plasma levels—are due to varying gene expression, and thus the amount of a particular enzyme present, among factors.

Ethnic Variation in Medication Response

Research on the variation in different ethnic groups' responses to psychiatric medications has been limited to several classes of medication, including antidepressants, antipsychotics, and benzodiazepines. Results for these medication classes are discussed in the following sections.

Antidepressants

Because of various factors including structural, linguistic, and cultural barriers to mental health care, depressed patients with ethnic minority backgrounds are infrequently seen by mental health professionals (Lin and Cheung 1999). When they do reach the system, many are misdiagnosed (Adebimpe 1984) and are not likely to receive treatment with antidepressants. Correspondingly, these facts verify that ethnic minority patients have rarely been included in most controlled clinical trials or other types of clinical studies on depression (Lawson 1996), thus limiting the amount of data that have been available to guide the use of these medications in ethnic minority populations.

Tricyclics

The paucity of objective data in regard to the use of antidepressants for ethnic minority patients is troubling, particularly because ethnic differences in the therapeutic range and side effect profiles of tricyclic antidepressants (TCAs) have been repeatedly reported (Silver et al. 1993). Among African Americans, depressed patients were less likely to receive antidepressants in comparison to whites, and those who did receive them were also significantly more likely to be treated with older antidepressants (e.g., tricyclics) rather than the newer, more developed antidepressants (e.g., selective serotonin reuptake inhibitors [SSRIs]) (Melfi et al. 2000). In studies with TCAs, African Americans displayed a faster and more favorable clinical response (Silver et al. 1993), as well as increased serious side effects such as delirium (Livingston et al. 1983). Reports of elevated TCA levels in African Americans in several studies suggest that pharmacogenetic factors may be responsible for the differential treatment response and the higher rate of TCA side effects (Silver et al. 1993). Studies involving Asians reported a substantially lower dose requirement of antidepressants for the treatment of depression (Silver et al. 1993). This difference may be due in part to the slower metabolism of TCAs reported in Asian subjects in several studies (Lin et al. 1993).

In a retrospective study of depressed Hispanic (predominantly Puerto Rican) female outpatients in New York, Hispanics responded to half the dosage given to non-Hispanic white patients and experienced more side effects (78% vs. 33%) and study dropout rates due to side effects (17% vs. 4.8%) (Marcos and Cancro 1982). In a prospective study of antidepressant response in patients from Colombia and the United States, the efficacy of trazodone was compared with that of imipramine and placebo in patients with depression (Escobar and Tuason 1980). The Colombian patients showed more improvement, regardless of the treatment selected, as well as significantly more anticholinergic side effects. No statistically significant differences between Hispanics (Mexican Americans) and non-Hispanic whites in pharmacokinetic studies of imipramine (K.M. Lin, R.E. Poland, I. Nuccio, et al.: "Ethnicity and Imipramine Response: Pharmacokinetic and Pharmacogenetic Influences," unpublished manuscript, 2003) or nortriptyline have been reported (Gaviria et al. 1986). The results of these studies are consistent with reports of CYP2D6 metabolism in Mexican Americans (Mendoza et al. 2001).

Newer Agents

Much less is known about ethnic variation with the newer antidepressant agents such as the SSRIs. For example, there have been only two reports comparing treatment response of SSRIs between African American and white depressed patients. In a small study of HIV-positive depressed patients, African Americans were more likely to be nonresponders to fluoxetine treatment than whites (Wagner et al. 1998). In contrast, a small study of paroxetine in treating elderly African American and white patients with DSM-IV major depression (Lesser et al. 1996) reported comparable response to medication and side effect rates in both groups. In a small open-label 6-week study of fluoxetine or paroxetine (20 mg/day) in the treatment of depression in Hispanic (Mexican descent) and white females (Alonso et al. 1997), similar improvement was noted; however, the white group reported significantly more side effects.

Antipsychotics

Ethnic variations in response include reports of higher blood levels of haloperidol (up to 50%) in Asian psychiatrically healthy volunteers (Lin et al. 1989) (Figure 6–2) and schizophrenic patients (Potkin et al. 1984) compared with their white counterparts. A series of studies (Jann et al. 1993) indicated that Asians have a lower rate of metabolism and consequently more prominent effects when given equivalent doses of medication. Greater prolactin responses to haloperidol in Asians have also been reported (Lin et al. 1989). In a multiethnic study of patients treated with therapeutic doses of haloperidol, a significantly different pharmacokinetic profile was noted in Chinese and African Americans compared with whites and Hispanics (Jann et al. 1993). Asian schizophrenic patients participating in a clinical treatment study responded optimally to a significantly lower plasma haloperidol concentration (Lin et al. 1989) than their white counterparts, suggesting that pharmacodynamic factors also contribute to ethnic differences in response to haloperidol.

In a study conducted in San Francisco, no ethnic variation in antipsychotic dosage or side effects was noted. However, immigrant Asian and Hispanic patients received significantly lower dosages than U.S.-born Asian and Hispanic patients (Lu et al. 1987). In a similar study conducted in New York with Anglo, Asian, and Hispanic (Puerto Rican and Dominican Republic) patients, the Hispanic and Asian patients received lower dosages and lower-potency antipsychotics (Collazo et al. 1996). As in Lu et al. 1987, the Hispanic and Asian subset (24 of 27 Hispanics and all the Asian patients) were foreign born. Environmental and cultural influences such as diet, alcohol, smoking, and exposure to toxins may explain the observed differences in drug response in these studies, suggesting that these two groups require lower doses than non-Hispanic white patients.

Although only limited information is available regarding the treatment and subsequent response to the newer generation of atypical antipsychotic agents among different ethnic groups, the existing data do suggest that there are ethnic variations in prescription rates (Kuno and Rothbard 2002) and in response to these new agents (Frackiewicz et al. 1999; Matsuda et al. 1996). Earlier-reported gaps between ethnic groups in the number of prescriptions of atypical agents have decreased over the past decade but continue to be apparent for African Americans (Daumit et al. 2003).

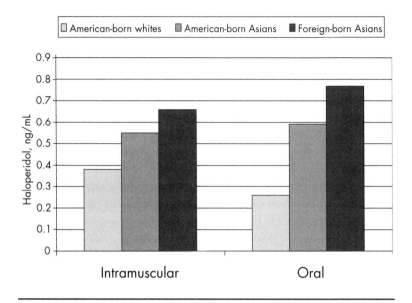

Figure 6–2. Haloperidol metabolism by route and ethnicity.

Source.   Lin et al. 1989.

Clozapine, the first atypical agent used in the United States, has shown variations by ethnicity in dosage, response, and side effects (Matsuda et al. 1996), as summarized in Table 6–1. Lower dosage requirements compared with white patients have been reported in Chinese patients (Chong et al. 2000), Korean American patients (Matsuda et al. 1996), and patients from Argentina and Chile (Ramirez 1996). In one study, a dosage requirement of 169 mg/day in Asian patients and 408 mg/day in white patients was reported (Chong et al. 2000). Lower blood levels in Korean Americans were associated with better response and more side effects than in whites (Matsuda et al. 1996). The reports of higher plasma concentrations of clozapine in Chinese patients suggest that ethnic variations in metabolism may be responsible for these dosage variations (Chong et al. 2000). Asian patients also appear to be at greater risk of developing the more serious side effect of agranulocytosis. Asian patients prescribed clozapine in the United Kingdom were found to have almost two and one half times the risk of developing agranulocytosis. Establishment of mandatory blood monitoring has proved essential in preven-

Table 6–1.   Ethnicity and atypical antipsychotics

Ethnicity	Clozapine	Risperidone	Olanzapine
African American	Benign neutropenia prevents selection for clozapine. Low white count may result in discontinuation.	N/A	No variation in dosage or side effects noted.[a] Increased rate of diabetic ketoacidosis with olanzapine and clozapine in case reports; 48% of cases were African American.[b]
Asian	Often excluded by selection criteria Lower dose given, resulting in higher plasma levels (30%–50%) Chinese: Lower dose given, with increased side effects Koreans: Lower dose given, 169 mg vs. 408 mg Southeast Asians: Higher risk of agranulocytosis (2.4×)	32% higher plasma concentration compared with white patients. Singapore: At average dose of 5.6 mg/day, 85% of treatment-resistant patients responded and showed improvement in EPS from baseline.	Japanese show increased plasma concentration. Asians responded to a lower dose than whites (11.3 mg vs. 17.1 mg)[c]
Hispanic	Argentina and Chile: Lower doses required.	Faster response: Puerto Rican and Dominican Republic patients.	N/A
Ashkenazi Jew	Increased risk of agranulocytosis	N/A	N/A

Note.   All dosages cited are mg/day. EPS=extrapyramidal side effects; N/A=not available.
Source.   [a]Lawson 1996. [b]Jin et al. 2002. [c]Leathart et al. 1998.

tion of agranulocytosis. However, these guidelines may also have prevented certain ethnic groups, such as African American patients, from receiving or continuing with clozapine because they have a significantly lower baseline white blood count than non–African American patients (Moeller et al. 1995).

For risperidone and olanzapine, ethnic variation has been found in metabolism, dosage requirements, and response (Table 6 –1). Asians were reported to have 30% higher plasma concentrations compared with whites (Lane et al. 1999a). A bimodal distribution of dosage requirement for risperidone has been reported in Hispanics in Latin America, with one group requiring dosages of up to 6 mg per day and another responding well to lower doses (Ramirez 1996). In a double-blind, parallel-group, inpatient multicenter study of patients treated with risperidone conducted in the United States, Hispanic (Puerto Rican and Dominican Republic) patients demonstrated a more rapid rate of symptom improvement and a higher rate of adverse effects, including extrapyramidal side effects (EPS), than non-Hispanic patients (Frackiewicz et al. 1999). Initial reviews of pharmacokinetic studies conducted in African Americans (Lawson 1996) and Chinese (Lane et al. 1999b) identified no important differences in the disposition of olanzapine compared with white subjects. A more recent study, however, found lower dosage requirements in Japanese patients (9.4±3.6 mg/day) (Ishigooka et al. 2001) compared with white patients (12.4 mg/day) (Conley and Mahmoud 2001). The potential of both clozapine and olanzapine for causing weight gain may be especially detrimental in ethnic minorities at increased risk for gaining weight and developing diabetes (Jin et al. 2002). In a review of published case reports, African Americans accounted for almost half of all cases of new-onset diabetes with atypical agents (Jin et al. 2002).

Benzodiazepines

Significant differences in the prescription rates, dosing, and side effects of benzodiazepines between Asians and whites have been reported both clinically (Lin et al. 1993) and in several pharmacokinetic studies (Ghoneim et al. 1981; Lin et al. 1988). Slower metabolism and higher plasma concentrations were noted for both diazepam (Ghoneim et al. 1981) and alprazolam (Lin et al. 1988). In a study of pharmacokinetics and pharmacodynamics of adinazolam, African Americans were found to have increased metabolism and notable drug effects on psychomotor performance (Lin et al. 1993).

Table 6–2. CYP2C19 psychiatric substrates

CYP2C19	• **Antidepressants:** amitriptyline, citalopram, clomipramine, L-deprenyl (selegiline), imipramine, moclobemide, sertraline, venlafaxine
	• **Antipsychotics:** clozapine,* perphenazine, zotepine*
	• **Benzodiazepines:** adinazolam, diazepam, flunitrazepam, temazepam, zolpidem*

*Partially metabolized by this enzyme.

The Pharmacogenetics of Drug-Metabolizing Enzymes

There are four CYP enzymes that are most important in terms of the metabolism of psychotropic medications: CYP2D6, CYP3A4, CYP1A2, and CYP2C19 (Table 6–2). Although the CYP enzymes are found in large quantities primarily in the liver and the gut, they have also been demonstrated to be present in other tissues including the brain, whose polymorphic expression (as described below) has been shown to be associated with specific personality traits, parkinsonism, and the risks of tardive dyskinesia, as well as substance abuse. For reasons that still are not completely understood (but are at least partially related to the ability of some of these enzymes to convert procarcinogens to carcinogens), some of these CYP enzymes (especially 1A2, 2E1, and 2D6) are implicated in increased risk for various kinds of malignancies and autoimmune conditions such as systemic lupus erythematosus.

CYP2D6

2D6 is one of the most important CYP enzymes in psychiatry for at least three reasons:

1. It is the major metabolic pathway for many psychotropics (Table 6–3), including most heterocyclic antidepressants (especially the secondary amine tricyclics, such as desipramine and nortriptyline), some of the SSRIs (e.g., paroxetine and fluoxetine), and many commonly used antipsychotics, morphine derivatives, and cardiac drugs (Kalow 1992; Lin et al. 1993; U.A. Meyer 1994).

Table 6–3. CYP2D6 substrates

- **Acetylcholinesterase inhibitors:** galantamine
- **Antidepressants:** amitriptyline,* desipramine, duloxetine, fluoxetine, imipramine,* nortriptyline, paroxetine, trazodone, venlafaxine
- **Antipsychotics:** haloperidol,* reduced haloperidol, olanzapine,* perphenazine, phenothiazines,* risperidone,* sertindole,* thioridazine*
- **Cardiovascular agents:** encainide, flecainide, propranolol,* metoprolol, timolol
- **Opiates:** codeine,* dextromethorphan, hydrocodone*

*Partially metabolized by this enzyme.

2. It is often responsible for drug-drug interactions because it is a low-capacity enzyme with high affinity (and thus is more easily saturated, leading to competitive inhibition).

3. It is highly polymorphic, with more than 30 functional mutations. Although most of these mutations are rare, seven of them are common but are variably distributed in different populations (as discussed below), and together these seven mutations capture more than 99% of the genetic variation (Gaedigk et al. 1999).

Because of the effects of these mutations, which range from inactivation to multiplication, individuals in any population can be classified into the following four groups (Table 6–4):

- Poor metabolizer (PM): the individual has no 2D6 enzyme activity.
- Intermediate metabolizer (IM): the individual has slower activity because he or she possesses alleles that encode less active forms of the enzyme.
- Extensive metabolizer (EM): the individual's genes are not affected by functional mutations ("wild type" allele; normal).
- Ultrarapid metabolizer (UM): the individual has duplication or multiplication (up to 13 copies) of the gene (Lundqvist et al. 1999).

Studies involving desipramine, venlafaxine, and a number of neuroleptics clearly suggest that 2D6 polymorphism is a major determinant of the pharmacokinetics of 2D6 substrates as well as of clinical response (Lessard et al. 1999). The gene-dose effects (corroborative of a cause-effect relationship between the genes and the disease) have also been clearly demonstrated (M.C. Meyer et al. 1996).

Table 6–4. CYP2D6 metabolic rates

Metabolic type	Metabolic rate	Plasma drug level	Clinical effects
Poor	None	Toxic	Side effects
Intermediate	Slow	High	Side effects at higher doses
Extensive	Normal	Normal	Normal response
Ultrarapid	Superfast	Low or none	No response at normal doses

As noted above, 2D6 is extremely polymorphic, and many of the identified mutations appear to be ethnic-specific. For example, the mutation responsible for the high rate of PM patients among whites (5%–9%), *CYP2D6*4* (expressed as CYP2D6B) is rarely found in any other ethnic group; similarly, alleles associated with lower enzyme activity and slower metabolism among those of African origins (*CYP2D6*17*) (Leathart et al. 1998; Masimirembwa and Hasler 1997) and Asian origins (*CYP2D6*10*) (Dahl et al. 1995) are rarely encountered in whites (Figure 6–3). Both of these latter two alleles may be partially responsible for previous findings of lower therapeutic dose ranges observed in Asians with antidepressants and antipsychotics and in African Americans with TCAs (Lin et al. 1993). In contrast, Mexican Americans display significantly *faster* overall 2D6 activity due to very low rates of any of these impairing mutations (Mendoza et al. 2001) (Figure 6–3).

Among individuals who possess duplicated genes and are ultrarapid metabolizers, ethnic variations have also been reported (Figure 6–4). Lower rates are noted in Swedes (1%), American whites (3.5%), and Spaniards (10%) (Agundez et al. 1995), and higher rates are found in Arabs (19%) (McLellan et al. 1997) and Ethiopians (29%) (Aklillu et al. 1996). Because of their extremely fast metabolism, UM patients are unlikely to respond to usual doses of medications that are biotransformed by 2D6, since they typically fail to achieve therapeutic levels. There have been reports of UM patients being regarded as noncompliant because they displayed no evidence of drug effects while being given seemingly adequate doses of medications (Aklillu et al. 1996; U.A. Meyer 1994). Clinicians should routinely inquire about adherence to medication and confirm by checking plasma levels if available, keeping in mind that absence of measurable blood levels may be explained by either noncompliance or ultrafast metabolism. In contrast, the report of excessive side effects at low dose may be indicative of toxic drug levels due to an inherited impairment in drug metabolism or a drug interaction with a 2D6 inhibitor (e.g., fluoxetine, paroxetine).

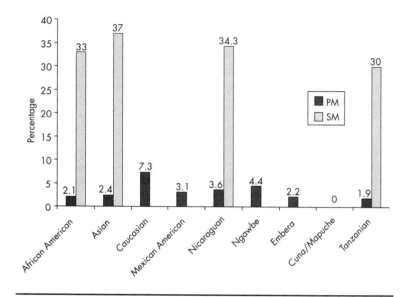

Figure 6–3.   CYP2D6 poor metabolizers (PM) and slow metabolizers (SM).

CYP3A4

3A4 is another important drug-metabolizing enzyme that is involved in the biotransformation of a large number of psychotropics, including most of the diazolo-benzodiazepines (e.g., alprazolam and clonazepam) and a number of newer antidepressants (e.g., nefazodone, mirtazapine, sertraline, reboxetine) and neuroleptics (e.g., aripiprazole, clozapine, quetiapine, ziprasidone) (Kalow 1992) (Table 6–5). It is the most abundant CYP enzyme expressed in the liver and is involved in the metabolism of many classes of drugs, including anticonvulsants, antihistamines (e.g., terfenadine), calcium channel blockers, macrolide antibiotics (e.g., erythromycin), steroid hormones, antiretrovirals, anticancer agents (e.g., ritonavir, cyclosporine), and antifungals (e.g., keto-conazole) (Table 6–6). 3A4 is often inhibited by its substrates, but drugs such as carbamazepine, phenobarbital, and rifampin can also induce it. A number of diet-drug and herb-drug interactions, such as the inhibitory effects of grapefruit juice and the inductive effects of St. John's wort on the metabolism of substrates of 3A4, have also been reported (Piscitelli et al. 2000).

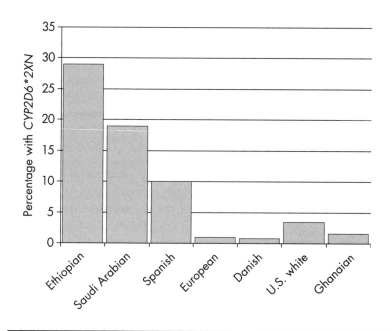

Figure 6–4. CYP2D6 ultrarapid metabolizers.

Substantial interindividual and cross-ethnic variations of 3A4 have been amply documented. Asian Indians (Kinirons et al. 1996), East Asians (Lin et al. 1988), and Mexicans (Palma-Aguirre et al. 1994) have been shown to have lower 3A4 activity, whereas African Americans (Johnson 2000) and Africans (Sowunmi et al. 1995) appear to possess higher 3A4 activity when compared with whites. Until recently, no genetic polymorphism was identified and the cause of these variations remained unknown. However, several polymorphisms have been reported recently. All three presented significant cross-ethnic variations. These include the *1B (66.7% in African Americans, 4.2% in whites, and 0% in Chinese), *2 (thus far found only in whites, at a low rate of 0.7%), and *3, *4, *5, and *6 (identified in Chinese) (Hsieh et al. 2001). In addition, there is a silent mutation (C682T) that has been found in 4.7% of African Americans, but not in other populations. Because these estimates were derived from limited sample sizes, the exact distribution of these alleles remains to be determined. It is still not yet clear if these silent mutations can explain some of

Table 6–5. CYP3A4 psychiatric substrates

- **Antidepressants, mood stabilizers, anticonvulsants:** carbamazepine, ethosuximide*, mirtazapine,* nefazodone, reboxetine, remoxipride, sertraline, tiagabine, trazodone,* zonisamide*
- **Antipsychotics:** aripiprazole, clozapine,* haloperidol,* pimozide, quetiapine, risperidone,* sertindole,* thioridazine,* ziprasidone
- **Benzodiazepines, sedative-hypnotics:** alprazolam, buspirone, clonazepam, diazepam,* midazolam, triazolam, zaleplon, zolpidem

*Partially metabolized by this enzyme.

the cross-ethnic variations in the activity of 3A4 reported earlier. The polymorphism of the 5' promoter region of 3A4 was not found in persons of Japanese ethnicity (Naoe et al. 2000). Although the clinical importance of genetic variation has yet to be determined, clinicians should be aware of the importance that environmental influences play in determining response (e.g., grapefruit juice may increase drug effects, and St. John's wort may decrease them).

CYP1A2

1A2 is involved in the metabolism of a large number of medications, including most of the commonly used psychotropics such as fluvoxamine, haloperidol, olanzapine, and clozapine. 1A2 is also responsible for the metabolism of important drugs and addictive substances, such as tacrine and caffeine (Carillo and Benitez 2000; Kalow 1992) (Table 6–7). 1A2 shows striking interindividual variability in the rate of the metabolism of substrates, which may be due to the inhibition and induction of these enzymes by an array of nongenetically determined factors (Carillo and Benitez 2000).

1A2 is also highly inducible. Its inducers include indoles contained in cruciferous vegetables (e.g., broccoli, Brussels sprouts, and cabbage), heterocyclic amines produced by char-broiling meat, constituents of tobacco, and high-protein diets (Ioannides 1999). Cigarette smoking has long been known to lower the steady-state concentrations of most psychotropics by up to 50% because of its ability to induce 1A2 (Schein 1995). Because this enzyme is highly inducible, it is reasonable to anticipate and predict its catalytic activity to vary substantially across ethnic/cultural demographic subgroups in association with cultural and socioeconomic divergent dietary habits (Smith and Mendoza 1996). A specific polymorphism in intron 1 of the 1A2 gene

Table 6–6. CYP3A4 nonpsychiatric substrates

- **Antibiotics, antifungals, immune modulators, chemotherapy agents:** clarithromycin, cyclosporine, erythromycin, dapsone, indinavir, ketoconazole, nelfinavir, paclitaxel,* ritonavir, saquinavir, tamoxifen, vincristine

- **Calcium channel blockers, cardiovascular agents:** amiodarone, amlodipine, atorvastatin, cerivastatin, diltiazem, felodipine, lercanidipine, lidocaine, lovastatin, nifedipine, nimodipine, nisoldipine, nitrendipine, quinidine, quinine, simvastatin, verapamil

- **Other:** alfentanil, astemizole, chlorpheniramine, cisapride, cocaine, codeine,* estrogens, fentanyl, hydrocortisone, methadone, progesterone, salmeterol, sildenafil, terfenadine, testosterone

*Partially metabolized by this enzyme.

(*C734A*) that markedly modulates the inducing productivity of the enzyme has been identified in whites (32% c allele frequency) (Sachse et al. 1999). Because no data are yet available for other ethnic groups in regard to the prevalence of this allele, it is unclear if ethnic variations in the polymorphism of this gene might explain ethnic differences in 1A2 activity (Masimirembwa et al. 1995; Relling et al. 1992).

Clinicians must be aware that concurrent smoking and consumption of 1A2 substrates (clozapine, haloperidol, and olanzapine) may result in decreased effectiveness of these medications compared with that seen in non-smoking or lower smoking environments (such as in inpatient environments or among nonsmokers). Similarly, abrupt changes in 1A2-inducing factors (smoking cessation or changing from a high-protein to a low-protein diet) may result in an increase in side effects due to increases in drug levels resulting from decreased drug metabolism. Appropriate dose adjustment will be needed to ensure effectiveness and avoid unnecessary side effects.

CYP2C19

Although the role of 2C19 in psychotropic metabolism does not appear as extensive as the ones discussed above, it does significantly influence the biotransformation of some of the commonly used medications, including diazepam, tertiary tricyclics, Proguanil (agent used for the treatment of malaria), and omeprazole. Most recently, 2C19 has also been found to be partly responsible for the metabolism of three SSRI antidepressants: citalopram, escitalopram (Kobayashi et al. 1997), and sertraline (Wang et al. 2001). 2C19

Table 6–7. CYP1A2 substrates

- **Antidepressants:** amitriptyline, fluvoxamine, imipramine
- **Antipsychotics:** clozapine,* fluphenazine,* haloperidol,* olanzapine,* thiothixine
- **Other:** acetaminophen, caffeine, cyclobenzaprine, estradiol, mexiletine, naproxen,* ondansetron,* propranolol,* riluzole, ropivacaine, tacrine, theophylline, zileuton, zolmitriptan

*Partially metabolized by this enzyme.

also represents a dramatic example of the existence of both cross-ethnic and interindividual variations in drug metabolism. With *S*-mephenytoin used as the probe, studies have demonstrated that 13%–23% of East Asians (Chinese, Japanese, and Koreans) (Blaisdell et al. 2002) are PMs, as opposed to only 3%–5% of whites. Although a small study in Pittsburgh, Pennsylvania, indicated a high rate of PM patients (19%) among older African American depressed patients (Pollock et al. 1991), several recent studies reveal PM rates similar to those of whites (Bradford 2005).

Identification and sequencing of the gene for the enzyme reveals that enzyme deficiency (the PM category) is caused by two unique mutations (*CYP2C19*2* and *CYP2C19*3*). Whereas *2* can be found in all ethnic groups, *3* appears to be specific to those of Eastern Asian origin. The presence of *3* and of a higher rate of *2* are together responsible for the higher rate of PMs among Asians and the resultant increased sensitivity to 2C19 substrates like diazepam (Goldstein et al. 1997) (Figure 6–5). Clinicians considering the use of diazepam in Asian populations should use the lowest possible starting dose and dose titration to avoid excessive sedation.

CYP450 Enzymes and Environmental Factors

A number of mechanisms are involved in the mediation of CYP450 environmental interactions, including competitive inhibition and induction (Kalow 1992). Of these, competitive inhibition probably occurs most often at specific times, and this could lead to serious clinical consequences. For example, as mentioned above, many psychotropics are substrates of 2D6 (e.g., SSRIs, TCAs, and neuroleptics) and each can competitively inhibit the other's metabolism when administered together, leading to serious consequences (Brosen

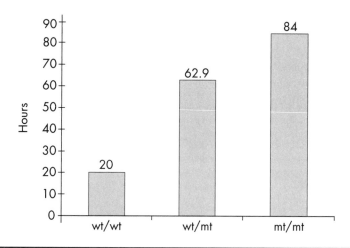

Figure 6–5. CYP2C19 activity and half-life of diazepam in Chinese.

wt=wild type (normal); mt=mutant type.

Source. Qin et al. 1999.

1995) (Table 6–8). Even for a high-capacity enzyme like 3A4, similar clinically significant interactions could occur; this was exemplified by the withdrawal of terfenadine from the market, due in particular to cases indicating its potential for serious interactions with ketoconazole (Jurima-Romet et al. 1994). Such interactions are not limited to pharmaceutical agents. They are clearly demonstrated by the observation that grapefruit juice significantly inhibits the metabolism of a number of antiviral and anticancer drugs, as well as psychotropics such as nefazodone and alprazolam (Oesterheld and Kallepalli 1997), even after 96 hours (Takanaga et al. 2000). Similarly, consumption of a corn diet that consisted of tortillas and *pozole* resulted in an increased rate of side effects with nifedipine compared with the lower rate observed with a non-corn diet (Palma-Aguirre et al. 1994) (Figure 6–6).

Both 3A4 and 1A2 are highly inducible by specific pharmaceutical agents and by certain natural substances. The effect of smoking and dietary changes on 1A2 has been described earlier. There is a body of literature showing that ethnic differences in dietary practices (i.e., a high-carbohydrate vs. a high-

Table 6–8.   CYP2D6 inhibitors

- **Antidepressants:** fluoxetine, moclobemide, norfluoxetine, paroxetine
- **Antipsychotics:** clozapine, fluphenazine, haloperidol, perphenazine, pimozide, thioridazine
- **Antihistamines:** chlorpheniramine, cimetidine, clemastine, diphenhydramine, hydroxyzine, loratadine, terfenadine, tripelennamine
- **Other:** astemizole, celecoxib, methadone, promethazine, quinidine, ritonavir

Source.   Hamelin BA, Bouayad A, Drolet B, et al: "In Vitro Characterization of Cytochrome P450 2D6 Inhibition by Classic Histamine H1 Receptor Antagonists." *Drug Metabolism and Disposition* 26:536–539, 1998; Nicolas JM, Whomsley R, Collart P, et al: "In vitro inhibition of human liver drug metabolizing enzymes by second generation antihistamines." *Chemico-Biological Interactions* 123:63–79, 1999.

protein diet) have contributed to variations in the metabolism of a number of drugs, including theophylline, antipyrine, and clomipramine (Anderson et al. 1991), presumably because of changes in 1A2 capacity. Some of these reports also showed that the dietary changes associated with acculturation have led to the amelioration of such ethnic differences.

Until recently (Eisenberg et al. 1993), very little attention had been paid to the potential of herbal medicines that affect drug-metabolizing enzymes (Table 6–9), even though it is self-evident that the natural targets of these enzymes are not pharmaceuticals, but potentially life-threatening products from the biological world. Herbs have always been extensively used in all human societies, and many have been found to have "real" biological effects. It is estimated that approximately one-third of modern medicines originated from herbal sources. People routinely and extensively use herbal medicines worldwide. There is a theoretical basis supported by empirical data for assuming that many of the herbs significantly modify the expression of drug-metabolizing enzymes, either by inhibition or induction (Gurley et al. 2002) (Table 6–10). Because patients typically are not aware of the potential of herb-drug interactions, they often combine the use of herbs and Western medicines. When severe toxic effects subsequently emerge, they usually blame them on the drugs prescribed by clinicians, rather than on herbal preparations obtained over the counter or from traditional/alternative practitioners (Smith et al. 1993). The potential for interaction between herbs and modern pharmaceutical agents is endless and remains largely unexplored. In this regard, it is likely that the reports of St. John's wort (*Hypericum*) producing drastic reduc-

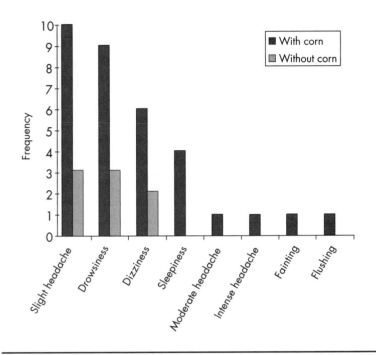

Figure 6–6. Nifedipine side effects and corn.

Source. Palma-Aguirre 1999.

tions in concentrations of indinavir (Piscitelli et al. 2000) and digoxin (Johne et al. 1999) may represent just the tip of the iceberg in terms of the magnitude of the impact of herbal preparations on ethnopsychopharmacology.

Similarly, many substances of abuse are of plant origin or are plant derivatives (e.g., ethanol, nicotine, morphine, and marijuana), and they too are metabolized through "drug-metabolizing" enzymes (Howard et al. 2002). Consequently, they have the potential to affect or to be affected by the status of particular enzymes. Many may interact with other substrates of these enzymes, including many psychotropics that are often prescribed for substance-abuse and dual-diagnosis patients. There also is evidence indicating that the genotypes of some of these enzymes (i.e., 2D6 and others) are significantly associated with the risk and severity of dependence (Howard et al. 2002). Together, the evi-

Table 6–9.   Herb–CYP450 drug interactions

Drug (A)	Herbal (B)	CYP450	Interaction
Ciprofloxin Enoxacin Pipemidic acid Fluvoxamine	*Coffea arabica* llex paullina yerba mate	1A2	inhibition ↑ concentration B caffeine toxicity
Theophylline Phenytoin	*Piper longum* *Piper nigrum*	1A2	inhibition ↑ concentration A
Quinidine Haloperidol Moclobemide	sparteine in *Cytisus scoparius*	2D6	inhibition ↑ concentration B circulatory collapse
Nifedipine Terfenadine, alprazolam	grapefruit, corn	3A4	inhibition ↑ concentration A ↑ effects
Cyclosporine Digoxin, indinavir Amitriptyline	St. John's wort	1A2, 2D6 3A4, pGPT	induction ↓ concentration A decreased effects

Note.   ↑=increased; ↓=decreased.

dence suggests that the field of pharmacogenetics represents a promising direction for substance-abuse and dual-diagnosis research in the future.

Xenobiotics (i.e., micronutrients, macronutrients, substances of abuse, and herbs) are natural substrates of the drug-metabolizing enzymes and are likely to have the potential to interact significantly with pharmaceutical agents. However, our knowledge base regarding such interactions is seriously deficient. Fortunately, with progress in the methodologies in pharmacogenetics, it is now possible to systematically assess such effects. With the resultant information, clinicians and patients will be able to make better-informed decisions with regard to herbal medications, at least in terms of their safety when combined with "modern" medicines. Clinicians should routinely ask about the use of food supplements, herbals, and teas at the initial visit and at follow-up visits. Patients should be asked to bring in their bottles so that the clinician can examine the individual ingredients contained in combination products.

Table 6–10. Herbal medications and cytochrome P450 enzymes

Herbal	Action	Type of study
Black pepper (*Piper nigrum*)[a]	Inhibits CYP1A2, 3A4	In vitro
Garlic (*Allium sativum*)[b]	Inhibits CYP2E1	In vitro
Green tea (*Camellia sinensis*)[c]	Inhibits CYP1A2, 3A4	In vitro
Kava (*Piper methysticum*)[d]	Inhibits CYP1A2, 2C9, 2C19, 2D6, 3A4	In vitro
St. John's wort (*Hypericum perforatum*)[b]	Induces CYP2E1 and CYP3A4	In vivo

*Partially metabolized by this substrate.
[a]Bhardwaj et al. 2002.
[b]Gurley et al. 2002.
[c]Muto et al. 2001.
[d]Mathews et al. 2002.

A number of reference Internet sites are available for consultation, including http://www.naturalmedicinedatabase.com and http://altmedicine.about.com.

Importance of Nonpharmacological Factors

Lastly, it should be emphasized that regardless of specificity and potency of any given pharmacological intervention, treatment effects are invariably even more powerfully determined by factors that are primarily nonbiological (Smith et al. 1993). These include issues related to expectations, adherence (compliance), placebo response, and clinician-patient relationships. Because they are largely mediated through symbolic and interactive processes, culture plays an important role in shaping these responses—which in turn powerfully determine whether a particular patient will respond to a particular treatment regimen. These issues have received little systematic research attention, so the literature covering this important area is meager. However, data from various sources, including clinical reports, anthropological observations, and utilization studies, converge to support the thesis that cultural factors are extremely important in influencing patients' attitude, adherence, and ultimate response to pharmacological treatment. For example, among Asians and Asian Americans, there is a widespread belief in the danger of the long-term use of "Western" medications, and this belief may contribute significantly to problems of noncompliance (Smith et al. 1993). However, without systematic research data, it remains unclear to what extent this may indeed be the case.

The therapeutic relationship is a two-way process, and the outcome of the therapeutic interaction is influenced not only by the patient but also by the clinician. In a cross-cultural situation, the clinician's ability to accurately assess a patient's symptoms, as well as responses to treatment, may be hampered by misperceptions and inadequate understanding of the patient's cultural norms (Lin et al. 1993). These deficiencies of understanding are the likely reason for the higher doses of neuroleptics that are prescribed for African American patients in comparison to their white counterparts (Strickland et al. 1991). In several studies, African Americans also have been shown to experience a higher rate of tardive dyskinesia (Glazer et al. 1994; Lawson 1996), which likely is related to their exposure to higher doses of neuroleptics over time. This is not an innocuous condition, and it also deserves more careful and systematic exploration in the future.

Conclusion

Culture and ethnicity are powerful determinants of an individual's response to psychopharmacotherapy. Knowledge of these factors will augment our current practice in using medications—as long as we also appreciate that these factors are superimposed on usually very substantial *interindividual* variations. For this reason, it is important that any findings regarding ethnic variations in pharmacological responses not be interpreted stereotypically. However, there are a few generalizations that may be helpful, as outlined below and in Table 6–11.

1. *Assessment:* Use the DSM-IV-TR Outline for Cultural Formulation (American Psychiatric Association 2000) for diagnosis and treatment planning to assess the patient's health beliefs, health practices, and family dynamics.
2. *Choice of medication:* With knowledge of enzyme activity in certain ethnic groups, take into consideration the patient's medical history, concurrent medications, and diet and food supplements or herbals.
3. *Monitoring:* Start with a low dose and proceed slowly. If side effects are

Table 6–11. Five tips for working with ethnic minority patients

When working with ethnic minority patients…

- Start at a slow dose and move up slowly.
- Ask about diet and smoking.
  When evaluating a patient for noncompliance, versus treatment resistance, always inquire about smoking, diet, and use of herbal medications.
- Check plasma levels.
  Although therapeutic plasma levels have yet to be established for many of the atypical antipsychotics, levels can be utilized to check for compliance.
- Involve the family.
  This is also helpful in improvement of treatment adherence.
- Use a different formulation.
  A number of medications are now available in either liquid or "quick dissolve" formulations.

intolerable, lower the dosage or choose a drug metabolized through a different route. When there is no response to the medication, check adherence, raise the dose, and monitor levels. Consider adding inhibitors (e.g., paroxetine to risperidone, or grapefruit juice to various agents) or switching drugs. Finally, consider alternative preparations, such as liquid, "quick dissolve," or depot formulations.

4. *Systems issues:* Involve the patient's family to improve treatment adherence.

It is to be hoped that many of the new technologies will become clinically available to allow for the individualization of medication intervention. Progress in this field of investigation is crucial for the provision of rational and appropriate care for patients of all ethnic and cultural backgrounds.

References

Adebimpe V: Overview: American blacks and psychiatry. Transcultural Psychiatric Research Review 21:83–111, 1984

Agundez JA, Ledesma MC, Ladero JM, et al: Prevalence of CYP2D6 gene duplication and its repercussion on the oxidative phenotype in a white population. Clin Pharmacol Ther 57:265–269, 1995

Aklillu E, Persson I, Bertilsson L, et al: Frequent distribution of ultrarapid metabolizers of debrisoquine in an Ethiopian population carrying duplicated and multiduplicated functional CYP2D6 alleles. J Pharmacol Exp Ther 278:441–446, 1996

Alonso M, Val E, Rapaport MH: An open-label study of SSRI treatment in depressed Hispanic and non-Hispanic women (letter). J Clin Psychiatry 58:31, 1997

American Psychiatric Association: Appendix I: Outline for cultural formulation and glossary of culture-bound syndromes, in Diagnostic and Statistical Manual of Mental Disorders, 4th Edition, Text Revision. Washington, DC, American Psychiatric Association, 2000, pp 897–903

Anderson KE, McCleery RB, Vesell ES, et al: Diet and cimetidine induce comparable changes in theophylline metabolism in normal subjects. Hepatology 13:941–946, 1991

Bhardwaj RK, Glaeser H, Becquemont L, et al: Piperine, a major constituent of black pepper, inhibits human P-glycoprotein and CYP3A4. J Pharmacol Exp Ther 302:645–650, 2002

Blaisdell J, Mohrenweiser H, Jackson J, et al: Identification and functional characterization of new potentially defective alleles of human CYP2C19. Pharmacogenetics 12:703–711, 2002

Bradford LD: The ethnopharmacology of atypical antipsychotics. CNS Spectr 10 (3, suppl 2):6–12, 2005

Brosen K: Drug interactions and the cytochrome P450 system. The role of cytochrome P450 1A2. Clin Pharmacokinet 29(suppl)1:20–25, 1995

Carrillo JA, Benitez J: Clinically significant pharmacokinetic interactions between dietary caffeine and medications. Clin Pharmacokinet 39:127–153, 2000

Chong SA, Remington GJ, Lee N, et al: Contrasting clozapine prescribing patterns in the east and west? Ann Acad Med Singapore 29:75–78, 2000

Collazo Y, Tam R, Sramek J, et al: Neuroleptic dosing in Hispanic and Asian inpatients with schizophrenia. Mt Sinai J Med 63:310–313, 1996

Conley RR, Mahmoud R: A randomized double-blind study of risperidone and olanzapine in the treatment of schizophrenia or schizoaffective disorder. Am J Psychiatry 158:765–774, 2001 [erratum, 158:1759, 2001]

Dahl ML, Yue QY, Roh HK, et al: Genetic analysis of the CYP2D locus in relation to debrisoquine hydroxylation capacity in Korean, Japanese and Chinese subjects. Pharmacogenetics 5:159–164, 1995

Daumit GL, Crum RM, Gualla E, et al: Outpatient prescriptions for atypical antipsychotics for African Americans, Hispanics, and whites in the United States. Arch Gen Psychiatry 60:121–128, 2003

Eisenberg DM, Kessler RC, Foster C, et al: Unconventional medicine in the United States: prevalence, costs, and patterns of use. N Engl J Med 328:246–252, 1993

Escobar JI, Tuason VB: Antidepressant agents: a cross cultural study. Psychopharmacol Bull 16:49–52, 1980

Frackiewicz E, Sramek J, Collazo Y, et al: Risperidone in the treatment of Hispanic schizophrenic inpatients, in Cross Cultural Psychiatry. Edited by Herrera JM, Lawson WB, Sramek JJ. Chichester, UK, Wiley, 1999, pp 183–192

Gaedigk A, Gotschall RR, Forbes NS, et al: Optimization of cytochrome P4502D6 (CYP2D6) phenotype assignment using a genotyping algorithm based on allele frequency data. Pharmacogenetics 9:669–682, 1999

Gaviria M, Gil AA, Javaid JI: Nortriptyline kinetics in Hispanic and Anglo subjects. J Clin Psychopharmacol 6:227–231, 1986

Ghoneim MM, Korttila K, Chiang CK, et al: Diazepam effects and kinetics in Caucasians and Orientals. Clin Pharmacol Ther 29:749–756, 1981

Glazer WM, Morgenstern H, Doucette J: Race and tardive dyskinesia among outpatients at a CMHC. Hosp Community Psychiatry 45:38–42, 1994

Goldstein JA, Ishizaki T, Chiba K, et al: Frequencies of the defective CYP2C19 alleles responsible for the mephenytoin poor metabolizer phenotype in various Oriental, Caucasian, Saudi Arabian and American black populations. Pharmacogenetics 7:59–64, 1997

Gonzalez F, Nebert D: Evolution of the P450 gene superfamily: animal plant "warfare" molecular drive and human genetic differences in drug oxidation. Trends Genet 6:182–186, 1990

Gurley BJ, Gardner SF, Hubbard MA, et al: Cytochrome P450 phenotypic ratios for predicting herb-drug interactions in humans. Clin Pharmacol Ther 72:276–287, 2002

Howard LA, Sellers EM, Tyndale RF: The role of pharmacogenetically variable cytochrome P450 enzymes in drug abuse and dependence. Pharmacogenomics 3:185–199, 2002

Hsieh KP, Lin YY, Cheng CL, et al: Novel mutations of CYP3A4 in Chinese. Drug Metab Dispos 29:268–273, 2001

Ioannides C: Effect of diet and nutrition on the expression of cytochromes P450. Xenobiotica 29:109–154, 1999

Ishigooka J, Murasaki M, Miura S: Efficacy and safety of olanzapine, an atypical antipsychotic, in patients with schizophrenia: results of an open-label multicenter study in Japan. Olanzapine Early Phase II Study Group. Psychiatry Clin Neurosci 55:353–363, 2001

Jann MW, Lam YWF, Chang WH: Haloperidol and reduced haloperidol plasma concentrations in different ethnic populations and interindividual variabilities in haloperidol metabolism, in Psychopharmacology and Psychobiology of Ethnicity. Edited by Lin KM, Poland RE, Nakasaki G. Washington, DC, American Psychiatric Press, 1993, pp 133–152

Jin H, Meyer, JM, Jeste DV: Phenomenology of and risk factors for new-onset diabetes mellitus and diabetic ketoacidosis associated with atypical antipsychotics: an analysis of 45 published cases. Ann Clin Psychiatry 14:59–64, 2002

Johne A, Brockmoller J, Bauer S, et al: Pharmacokinetic interaction of digoxin with an herbal extract from St John's wort (*Hypericum perforatum*). Clin Pharmacol Ther 66:338–345, 1999

Johnson JA: Predictability of the effects of race or ethnicity on pharmacokinetics of drugs. Int J Clin Pharmacol Ther 38:53–60, 2000

Juarez-Reyes MG, Shumway M, Battle C, et al: Clozapine eligibility: the effect of stringent criteria on ethnic, gender and age subgroups of schizophrenic patients. Prog Neuropsychopharmacol Biol Psychiatry 20:1341–1352, 1996

Jurima-Romet M, Crawford K, Cyr T, et al: Terfenadine metabolism in human liver: in vitro inhibition by macrolide antibiotics and azole antifungals. Drug Metab Dispos 22:849–857, 1994

Kalow W (ed): Pharmacogenetics of Drug Metabolism. New York, Pergamon, 1992

Kinirons MT, Lang CC, He HB, et al: Triazolam pharmacokinetics and pharmacodynamics in Caucasians and Southern Asians: ethnicity and CYP3A activity. Br J Clin Pharmacol 41:69–72, 1996

Kobayashi K, Chiba K, Yagi T, et al: Identification of cytochrome P450 isoforms involved in citalopram *N*-demethylation by human liver microsomes. J Pharmacol Exp Ther 280:927–933, 1997

Kuno E, Rothbard AB: Racial disparities in antipsychotic prescription patterns for patients with schizophrenia. Am J Psychiatry 159:567–572, 2002

Lane H, Chiu W, Chen C, et al: Risperidone dosing in acutely exacerbated schizophrenia: higher plasma levels in Chinese. Presented at Pacific Rim Association for Clinical Pharmacogenetics Meeting, Taipei City, Taiwan, April 13–15, 1999a

Lane H, Jann M, Liu H, et al: Olanzapine pharmacokinetics in Chinese schizophrenic patients: comparable with Caucasians. Presented at Pacific Rim Association for Clinical Pharmacogenetics Meeting, Taipei City, Taiwan, April 13–15, 1999b

Lawson WB: Clinical issues in the pharmacotherapy of African-Americans. Psychopharmacol Bull 32:275–281, 1996

Leathart JB, London SJ, Steward A, et al: CYP2D6 phenotype-genotype relationships in African-Americans and Caucasians in Los Angeles. Pharmacogenetics 8:529–541, 1998

Lessard E, Yessine MA, Hamelin BA, O'Hara, et al: Influence of CYP2D6 activity on the disposition and cardiovascular toxicity of the antidepressant agent venlafaxine in humans. Pharmacogenetics 9:435–443, 1999

Lesser IM, Smith MW, Whol M, et al: Brain imaging, antidepressants, and ethnicity: preliminary observations. Psychopharmacol Bull 32:235–242, 1996

Lin KM, Cheung F: Mental health issues for Asian Americans. Psychiatr Serv 50:774–780, 1999

Lin KM, Lau JK, Smith R, et al: Comparison of alprazolam plasma levels and behavioral effects in normal Asian and Caucasian male volunteers. Psychopharmacology (Berl) 96:365–369, 1988

Lin KM, Poland RE, Nuccio I, et al: A longitudinal assessment of haloperidol doses and serum concentrations in Asian and Caucasian schizophrenic patients. Am J Psychiatry 146:1307–1311, 1989

Lin KM, Poland RE, Nakasaki G (eds): Psychopharmacology and Psychobiology of Ethnicity, Washington, DC, American Psychiatric Press, 1993

Livingston R, Zucker D, Isenberg K, et al: Tricyclic antidepressants and delirium. J Clin Psychiatry 44:173–176, 1983

Lu FG, Chien CP, Heming G, et al: Ethnicity and neuroleptic drug dosage. Poster presentation, annual meeting of the American Psychiatric Association, Chicago, IL, May 12, 1987

Lundqvist E, Johansson I, Ingelman-Sundberg M: Genetic mechanisms for duplication and multiduplication of the human CYP2D6 gene and methods for detection of duplicated CYP2D6 genes. Gene 226:327–338, 1999

Marcos LR, Cancro R: Pharmacotherapy of Hispanic depressed patients: clinical observations. Am J Psychother 36:505–513, 1982

Masimirembwa CM, Hasler JA: Genetic polymorphism of drug metabolizing enzymes in African populations: implications for the use of neuroleptics and antidepressants. Brain Res Bull 44:561–571, 1997

Masimirembwa CM, Bertilsson L, Johansson I, et al: Diminished enzyme activity and lack of metabolic correlation of CYP2D6 probe drugs in a black Zimbabwean (Shona) population, in Pharmacogenetics of Drug Metabolizing Enzymes in a Black African Population. Edited by Masimirembwa CM. Stockholm, Kongl, Carolinska Medico Chirurgiska Institute, 1995, pp 1–21

Matsuda KT, Cho MC, Lin KM, et al: Clozapine dosage, serum levels, efficacy, and side effect profiles: a comparison of Korean American and Caucasian patients. Psychopharmacol Bull 32:253–257, 1996

Mathews JM, Etheridge AS, Black SR: Inhibition of human cytochrome P450 activities by kava extract and kavalactones. Drug Metab Dispos 30:1153–1157, 2002

McLellan RA, Oscarson M, Seidegard J, et al: Frequent occurrence of CYP2D6 gene duplication in Saudi Arabians. Pharmacogenetics 7:187–191, 1997

Melfi CA, Croghan TW, Hanna MP, et al: Racial variation in antidepressant treatment in a Medicaid population. J Clin Psychiatry 61:16–21, 2000

Mendoza R, Wan YJ, Poland RE, et al: CYP2D6 polymorphism in a Mexican American population. Clin Pharmacol Ther 70:552–560, 2001

Meyer MC, Baldessarini RJ, Goff DC, et al: Clinically significant interactions of psychotropic agents with antipsychotic drugs. Drug Safety 15:333–346, 1996

Meyer UA: Pharmacogenetics: the slow, the rapid, and the ultrarapid. Proc Natl Acad Sci U S A 91:1983–1984, 1994

Moeller FG, Chen YW, Steinberg JL, et al: Risk factors for clozapine discontinuation among 805 patients in the VA hospital system. Ann Clin Psychiatry 7:167–73, 1995

Muto S, Fujita K, Yamazaki Y, et al: Inhibition by green tea catechins of metabolic activation of procarcinogens by human cytochrome P450. Mutat Res 479:197–206, 2001

Naoe T, Takeyama K, Yokozawa T, et al: Analysis of genetic polymorphism in NQO1, GST-M1, GST-T1, and CYP3A4 in 469 Japanese patients with therapy-related leukemia/myelodysplastic syndrome and de novo acute myeloid leukemia. Clin Cancer Res 6:4091–4095, 2000

Oesterheld J, Kallepalli BR: Grapefruit juice and clomipramine: shifting metabolic ratios. J Clin Psychopharmacol 17:62–63, 1997

Palma-Aguirre JA, Nava RJ, Hoyo-Vadillo C, et al: Influence of Mexican diet on nifedipine pharmacodynamics in healthy volunteers. Proc West Pharmacol Soc 37:85–86, 1994

Piscitelli SC, Burstein AH, Chaitt D, et al: Indinavir concentrations and St John's wort. Lancet 355:547–548, 2000

Pollock BG, Perel JM, Kirshner M, et al: S-mephenytoin 4-hydroxylation in older Americans. Eur J Clin Pharmacol 40:609–611, 1991

Potkin SG, Shen Y, Pardes H, et al: Haloperidol concentrations elevated in Chinese patients. Psychiatry Res 12:167–172, 1984

Ramirez L: Ethnicity and psychopharmacology in Latin America. Mt Sinai J Med 63:330–331, 1996

Relling MV, Lin JS, Ayers GD, et al: Racial and gender differences in N-acetyltransferase, xanthine oxidase, and CYP1A2 activities. Clin Pharmacol Ther 52:643–658, 1992

Sachse C, Brockmoller J, Bauer S, et al: Functional significance of a C—>A polymorphism in intron 1 of the cytochrome P450 CYP1A2 gene tested with caffeine. Br J Clin Pharmacol 47:445–449, 1999

Schein JR: Cigarette smoking and clinically significant drug interactions. Ann Pharmacother 29:1139–1148, 1995

Silver B, Poland RE, Lin KM: Ethnicity and the pharmacology of tricyclic antidepressants, in Psychopharmacology and Psychobiology of Ethnicity. Edited by Lin KM, Poland RE, Nakasaki G. Washington, DC, American Psychiatric Press, 1993, pp 61–89

Smith M, Mendoza R: Ethnicity and pharmacogenetics. Mt Sinai J Med 63:285–290, 1996

Smith M, Lin K, Mendoza RL: "Non-biological" issues affecting psychopharmacotherapy: cultural considerations, in Psychopharmacology and Psychobiology of Ethnicity. Edited by Lin KM, Poland RE, Nakasaki G. Washington, DC, American Psychiatric Press, 1993, pp 37–58

Sowunmi A, Rashid TJ, Akinyinka OO, et al: Ethnic differences in nifedipine kinetics: comparisons between Nigerians, Caucasians and South Asians. Br J Clin Pharmacol 40:489–493, 1995

Strickland T, Ranganath V, Lin K, et al: Psychopharmacologic considerations in the treatment of black American populations. Psychopharmacol Bull 27, 441–448, 1991

Takanaga H, Ohnishi A, Murakami H, et al: Relationship between time after intake of grapefruit juice and the effect on pharmacokinetics and pharmacodynamics of nisoldipine in healthy subjects. Clin Pharmacol Ther 67:201–214, 2000

Wagner GJ, Maguen S, Rabkin JG: Ethnic differences in response to fluoxetine in a controlled trial with depressed HIV-positive patients. Psychiatr Serv 49:239–240, 1998

Wang JH, Liu ZQ, Wang W, et al: Pharmacokinetics of sertraline in relation to genetic polymorphism of CYP2C19. Clin Pharmacol Ther 70:42–47, 2001

7

Conclusions

Applying the DSM-IV-TR Outline for Cultural Formulation

Russell F. Lim, M.D.

The culturally appropriate psychiatric assessment is complex and challenging. However, some general themes emerge after reviewing chapters on the four major ethnic groups, and they can be organized by using the cultural formulation, beginning with a section on general principles.

The most useful generalization is that not all patients fit a profile or syndrome as the rest of DSM-IV-TR would have us believe. However, psychiatric assessment is often taught as if everyone had the same general background and the major differences were socioeconomic. Every group has a history that will color interactions with clinicians belonging to particular ethnic groups, such as Native Americans and African Americans interacting with whites. Identifying with and belonging to a particular ethnic group brings with it a set of values, health beliefs, and expectations of the individual and the family that are usually different from

237

the Western norms of rapid individuation by the age of 18. Therefore, the information in this handbook has been presented to the clinician to provide a normative starting point from which it becomes possible to see how that individual patient differs from other members of his or her cultural reference group.

A. Cultural Identity of the Individual

Understanding cultural identity is like hearing someone say "I'm depressed" and then asking the person, "What do you mean?" The important thing is not which group a patient *says* he or she belongs to, but what membership in that group *means* to the patient. This individual relationship to the group can affect the patient's relationship with you and can help you ask clarifying questions and rule in or rule out the relevance of group-based generalizations.

Cultural identity can be understood as a multifaceted core set of identities that contributes to how an individual understands his or her environment. Ethnic identity is often a crucial facet of an individual's overall cultural identity, but many other facets may contribute to identity as well. The greater the amount of detail a clinician is able to gather about the individual's cultural identity, the better understanding he or she will have of the individual's perspectives on health, illness, and the mental health system. Moreover, the clinician will more readily anticipate issues regarding cultural and identity conflicts that may arise during the course of evaluation and treatment. Two commonalities that have emerged among the four groups discussed in this volume are a divergence from the Western value of individualism and a convergence on the family as the central unit, its needs coming before those of the individual.

B. Cultural Explanations of the Individual's Illness

Again, knowing a patient's cultural group provides only a starting point for exploring their cultural beliefs about their illness. Exploring these beliefs requires sensitivity to subtle nuances of the patient's culture of origin and acceptance of differing points of view. We have learned about the significance of rootwork and hoodoo for African Americans, the various Asian belief systems such as the concepts of yin and yang, alternative healing practices such as coining and acupuncture, and herbal medicine. In addition, we have become aware of folk healers such as the Latino *curanderos* and conditions such as *ataques de nervios* and *mal de ojo*. African Americans believe strongly in the central role of religion in their lives and also feel that one should be able to fix one's own problems. "I'll put it in the Lord's hands," was cited as an expression of these beliefs. One set of beliefs common to some Latinos and African Americans is reflected in *santería,* as seen in Cuba, and *espiritismo,* as seen in Puerto Rico and elsewhere.

A cultural consultant or broker can be invaluable in helping the clinician identify normative behaviors and beliefs in patients whose ethnicity differs from the clinician's. We have also seen that many ethnic minority groups express their symptoms somatically, perhaps to avoid the stigma of a mental illness or to express their illness holistically, given that most believe that psyche, soma, and spirit are one. In fact, it is only Western biomedicine that artificially separates body and mind.

C. Cultural Factors Related to Psychosocial Environment and Levels of Functioning

We have seen throughout the four chapters the central importance of the family, in contrast to the Western ideal of individuation and independence. All four groups share a respect for the elders and act in accordance to family wishes and needs. In some groups, there is a hierarchical structure with clearly defined roles for each individual according to age and gender. For example, Asian cultures tend to be patriarchal, in contrast to African American cultural groups, which tend to be matriarchal. We have also seen specific gender roles in Latinos, with some male Latino patients displaying aspects of *machismo* and some Latino women displaying aspects of *marianismo.* The consequences of intergenerational conflicts were also discussed. Such conflict is most often seen in second-generation children who live in an environment steeped in old-world values yet go to school or work in a setting of Western values; this type of dissonance can often lead to involvement in gang activities.

D. Cultural Elements of the Relationship Between the Individual and the Clinician

Each patient and each clinician brings his or her own cultural identity, beliefs, and values system into the clinical encounter, and the preceding chapters have outlined various approaches to bridging the gap between them. The clinician needs to develop an awareness of his or her own cultural identity, prejudices, and biases. The clinician can then explore in a nonjudgmental manner the meaning of the patient's symptoms and of the behavior displayed between clinician and patient.

We have seen how historical and personal experience with racism can lead to distance between non–ethnically matched therapists and clients, just as we see idealization and denial between ethnically matched therapists and clients. Patients from disparate ethnic groups have a wide variety of communication styles. Clinicians need to be aware of the range of normative styles for an ethnic group so that they can best choose their interview style and assess the patient's thought processes and cognitive status. Other factors that may influence the relationship between the therapist and patient include religion, skin color, gender, age, language, and level of acculturation. Differing expectations can also play a role, in that the patient may expect the clinician to be authoritarian and directive, whereas the clinician may consider his or her role to be that of a consultant and may adopt a collaborative mode, thus creating a mismatch. Expectations that the clinician will be more directive are most often seen in Native Americans, Asian Americans, and less acculturated immigrants from various groups. Other patients, such as many Latinos, expect their clinician to be warm and friendly (*personalismo*), not detached and clinical.

We also have seen that much attention should be paid to the language in which the interview is conducted and to who does the interpreting. In addition, the similarities and differences in ethnicity between the therapist and the patient create patterns of relating through transference and countertransference reactions, which allows the clinician to modify the therapeutic approach accordingly.

E. Overall Cultural Assessment for Diagnosis and Care

Developing a culturally appropriate treatment plan for an ethnic minority patient requires the integration of Western values and ethnic and cultural beliefs. After the appropriate data have been gathered, consultation with family and cultural consultants can help to bridge the gap between the clinician's and the patient's cultures. Medication doses may be adjusted downward on the basis of the patient's ethnicity and clinical response. Regarding psychotherapy with ethnic minority patients, a common suggestion was that the clinician use a directive, problem-solving approach as opposed to the Western consultative/ collaborative model. A key element of the treatment plan is for the clinician to take an accepting attitude toward the patient's explanatory models and to use them in discussing the treatment with the patient. In addition, medication dosage must be adjusted to reflect the patient's diet, smoking habits, and ethnicity. As treatment progresses, the plan must remain dynamic to incorporate newly found clinical information and to monitor the patient's adherence with the treatment regimen. Only through repeated experience can we hope to master the subtleties of culturally appropriate diagnosis and treatment.

A Resident's Guide to the Cultural Formulation

Angel Caraballo, M.D.; Hamada Hamid, D.O.;
Jennifer Robin Lee, M.D.; Joy D. McQuery, M.D.;
Yanni Rho, M.D., M.P.H.; Elizabeth J. Kramer, Sc.M.;
Russell F. Lim, M.D.; Francis G. Lu, M.D.

Everyone brings his or her own personal and professional culture to an interaction; culture influences many aspects of psychiatric illness, including illness manifestation, coping, and help-seeking behavior. The DSM-IV-TR Outline for Cultural Formulation (American Psychiatric Association 2000b) is a critical framework for evaluation that belongs in the standard psychiatric evaluation. As noted in Chapter 1 of this volume, "Factual knowledge about cultural groups, while essential, can have limited utility without a framework to organize and to make sense of the information. Further, the clinician will encounter many patients who are affiliated with one or more cultural groups of which the clinician may have inadequate knowledge. In these instances, an organizing framework is helpful to guide the clinician to areas of potentially important inquiry."

This appendix was written by psychiatry residents for psychiatrists in training, and for others who may not be as familiar with cultural implications in mental health, in the hope that it will be helpful in the assessment and treatment of culturally diverse patients. The cultural formulation is a hypothesis-generating tool and is just one part of the overall assessment that can help the clinician sort out the patient's problems in cultural context. It is important to note that conclusions drawn at the first visit may be tentative and are subject to change as more information is obtained.

How does one apply the Outline practically to a clinical encounter? What factors does the clinician consider when thinking about how to apply the cultural formulation to a standard psychiatric evaluation? Here are some tips to consider in working with patients/clients from diverse cultural backgrounds.

- Building rapport is critical. Allow the patient to guide the process of getting to know him or her better. As a general rule, ask the least intrusive questions first.

- Explain the process of the interview and evaluation, and elicit questions and concerns along the way to help build trust. Normalize the line of questioning and respond appropriately to discomfort and doubt. Trust will be especially important when working with undocumented migrants and patients with long legacies of distrust of the medical profession.

- A critical part of the evaluation is respecting patients "where they are." Don't assume anything about patients' cultural identity; be curious and sensitive in determining their reference group, what terms they feel sensitive about or shamed by, and what types of experiences they have had with mental health professionals or others of your cultural background. Also, allow for curiosity that the patient may have about *your* cultural background.

- Clinicians should not be afraid to use interpreter/translator services, even if the clinician thinks the patients and their families understand English (or your language) well. Language is incredibly nuanced. If you do not have translators at your facility, use national translation phone services such as languagefon.com, certifiedlanguages.com, 1-800-translate.com, and languageline.com. All or most of these services will charge a fee.

- Family members should be used as interpreters only as a last resort. In addition to the issues surrounding patient confidentiality, a patient may withhold information when a family member is interpreting for a number of reasons: finding the problem too difficult or too traumatic to discuss in the presence of family members and not wanting to share it, fear of repercussions (e.g., in cases of domestic violence), or wanting to "save face." In addition, there may simply be a misunderstanding of what is reported, especially when children are used as the interpreters.

- Be very sensitive to the fact that for many people, there is great stigma attached to seeking help for mental illness. Be aware of discomfort, fear, and your reactions to what you might perceive as resistance (Lu 2005).

- It is important to get releases to speak to family, friends, community leaders, and others in your patient's life if the patient wants to have these people involved in care. Be aware that all may minimize reports of symptoms because of their fears of stigmatizing the patient and their fears of mental illness (Lu et al. 1995).

- Be aware of cultural dissonance and divergence in beliefs between the clinician, the patient, and friends and family (Henderson and Nguyen 2004). Remember, the clinician also brings his or her own cultural biases and belief systems to the interaction.

- Consider culturally and linguistically appropriate diagnostic screening questions, interviews, and schedules to help determine a differential diagnosis.

- Remember, there is not a 1:1 correspondence between culture-bound syndromes and DSM-IV-TR diagnostic criteria. Focus on symptoms that need to be addressed and collaborate on their alleviation (Guarnaccia and Rogler 1999).

- Do not overattribute or underattribute symptoms to culture. Check with others (such as family, reference group community members, and cultural consultants) to get a better sense of cultural norms.

- There may be situations in which you feel limited in your knowledge and skills in successfully performing and integrating a cultural formulation into your assessment. In such instances, consultation with an individual who is knowledgeable about the patient's culture may be helpful. One should never hesitate to use a culture broker or cultural consultant, someone who knows the culture well and can discuss it with the clinician.

- There are well-known mnemonics such as LEARN, ETHNIC, TRANSLATE, and BATHE that can help the clinician decide which questions to ask to obtain a quick, culturally appropriate evaluation regarding what aspects of the patient's presentation are cultural and what aspects are psychopathological. These mnemonics appear in Table A-1. (We have created other mnemonics to aid in an extended evaluation. These are listed throughout the appendix.)

A note: The questions presented in this appendix are only suggestions, not a formal checklist. They should not be construed as the definitive protocol for performing a cultural formulation. Additional questions may be important and relevant for any particular clinical encounter. Ultimately, the clinician

Table A–1.   Useful general mnemonics for cultural formulation

LEARN	ETHNIC	TRANSLATE	BATHE
Listen with sympathy	Explanation (of symptoms)	Trust	Background
Explain your perceptions of the problem	Treatment	Roles (of interpreter)	Affect (feeling state of patient)
Acknowledge and discuss differences and similarities in explanation of illness	Healers (previous use)	Advocacy (how will this occur?)	Trouble (what situation troubles you most?)
Recommend treatment	Negotiation of treatment	Nonjudgmental attitude	Handling (how are you handling this?)
Negotiate treatment	Intervention	Setting	Empathy
	Collaboration	Language (what methods of communication will occur?)	
		Accuracy (of information collected)	
		Time (how will this be managed in the encounter?)	
		Ethical issues (such as confidentiality)	

Source.   Chachkes 1999.

will tailor his or her use of the Outline according to the type and setting of the evaluation (one-time emergency department visit or ongoing therapy).

A. Cultural Identity of the Individual

Cultural identity is many-faceted (see Table 1–3 in Chapter 1). The role of the clinician is to encourage the patient to describe the cultural identity factors that are important to him or her (Lu 2005).

The way in which questions about cultural identity are asked is not trivial, but crucial; it will set the tone for the rest of the interview. For example, if the patient feels judged from the beginning of the interview, it will be very difficult to have him or her open up and cooperate during the rest of the interview.

Language

Language is an extremely important aspect of cultural identity.

- The patient's preferred language should be assessed first to facilitate communication between patient and therapist.
- Knowing how to speak a different language from that of the host country is a source of pride and acceptance for some, but it can be a source of embarrassment for others. Therefore, it is very important to assess the patient's level of comfort and to determine his or her preference regarding the language in which sessions are to be conducted.

Assessment of spoken language early in the interview is important for several reasons:

- It can give the clinician a rough approximation of level of acculturation and ensure that the diagnostic assessment is accurate. For example, psychotic symptoms may not be apparent until an assessment is done in the native language, in which the patient may be able to express the full complexity of his or her thought.
- It will also help the clinician determine whether an interpreter is needed for the session.

Questions to consider and how to ask them:

- *Primary questions:* What language(s) do you speak? Which language do you prefer? Do you know how to write or read in any language other than English?
- *Secondary questions:* What languages did you speak while growing up? Do you speak to your family in a language(s) other than English? What language(s) do you speak at work?

Chief Complaint

Having established the language of communication, the official interview should start with an assessment of the chief complaint. (Part B below discusses how to incorporate the Outline into the history of present illness.)

- *An appropriate question* would be: "What is the reason you are here today?"

Basic Information

For those patients who cannot formulate a chief complaint, you can start with three basic questions. This will allow the clinician to create rapport with the client and start the flow of the interview naturally:

- *Basics:* Where are you from? Who lives with you? How do you support yourself?

With these three questions, you can obtain information about socioeconomic status, relationships and sexual orientation, and place of origin and get a sense of severity of illness (for instance, the person might be socially isolated and living on psychiatric disability).

Questions to consider and how to ask them:

- *Place of origin:* Where were you born? If the patient's answer indicates he or she is from another country: How much contact do you have with family or friends who still live in that country? How often do you visit your country of origin?
- *Socioeconomic status:* How do you support yourself? To what extent do you have trouble affording the basics of life like housing and food? How does your current financial status affect your life? Has your lifestyle changed since you came to the United States (if the patient is an immigrant)?
- *Sexual orientation/relationship status:* Are you currently in a relationship?
  · If yes, is your partner a man or a woman? This area of inquiry may be very sensitive for persons from some cultures.
  · If the patient has *not* been involved in a relationship, you should inquire about sexual orientation gently and nondirectively.

Ethnicity and Race

The same principles that apply to language also apply to ethnicity and race, which are crucial components of an individual's cultural identity

Questions to consider and how to ask them:

- *Ethnicity:* Do you consider yourself part of any specific ethnic group? If so, which ethnic group do you identify with the most? Are you bicultural, "all American," or do you identify primarily with your culture of origin? It is important to keep in mind that identifying with a specific ethnic group does not imply that everyone is the same. For example, there are multiple subgroups included in the term *Latino* or *Hispanic*. Identification with subgroups can also have an impact on the way patients explain their illness. Inquiring about these other components will also facilitate the development of rapport because patients will feel that the clinician is interested in them as individuals and not just in their illnesses (Rohluf et al. 2001).

- *Race:* How do you identify yourself in terms of race?

Other Aspects of Cultural Identity

Some of the other aspects of cultural identity are already incorporated into a general psychiatric evaluation. Examples include age, religion/spirituality, and country of origin. However, more detailed questions will help the clinician better understand the importance that these aspects play for patients and how they identify culturally.

In particular, education and religion/spirituality are very important aspects of one's cultural identity. These aspects will also play a major role in how a patient explains the stressors and the supports in his or her life.

Questions to consider and how to ask them:

- *Age:* How old are you? Age is very important for some people but not for others. What role does age play in your life?

- *Education:* How far did you go in school? How important is education for you and for your family members?

- *Religion/spirituality:* An excellent religious/spiritual screening tool is FICA (Puchalski and Romer 2000), which asks four questions:

    F—Is religious **Faith** an important part of your day-to-day life? This question could be followed by associated questions about formal religious identity and level of spirituality.

    I—How has faith **Influenced** your life, past and present? This question may uncover important spiritual experiences.

    C—Are you currently part of a religious or spiritual **Community**? This question helps clarify the role a spiritual community might play in treatment interventions.

A—What are the spiritual needs that you would like me to **Address**? This question allows the clinician to identify spiritual areas that may become part of a treatment plan.

Immigration History

It is helpful to use the mnemonic "**Who, What, Where, When, Why, How**" (Cultural Consultation Service, Sir Mortimer Davis–Jewish General Hospital 2000).

WHO did you leave?
—It is common for families to be separated during migration, sometimes involuntarily.

- **How to ask:** Who came with you, and who are the important people in your life who weren't able to come? Do you have plans to be reunited?

WHAT did you leave?
—It is important to find out whether your patient wanted to immigrate or not. If the patient did not want to move, he or she will have a more difficult time adjusting.

- **How to ask:** What was the economic and political situation in your country when you left?

(Through) WHERE did you leave?
—This can be a sensitive question. Sometimes the immigration journey itself can be a traumatic experience. Be particularly attuned to this if your patient is a refugee or has an undocumented status. Entering the United States without legal paperwork can be both traumatizing and expensive (people may pay a "coyote" or "snakehead," a professional people smuggler, to transport them across the border or into this country).

- **How to ask:** The clinician may want to ask first, "What was your immigration journey like?" to find out if he or she is touching on a traumatizing topic, and then, "What was your immigration route?"

WHEN did you leave?
—Refugees, in particular, may have been displaced from their country of origin for years in refugee camps.

- **How to ask:** When did you leave home, and how long was your journey to this country?

  WHY did you leave?
  —Did the patient immigrate for economic reasons, or is he or she the fleeing the country of origin as a refugee? Immigrants who have no possibility of returning to their country of origin are more likely to find the process of acculturation more stressful, and hence to be more symptomatic. Immigrants who can frequently visit their home country or who are not planning to stay permanently in the United States are not faced with the full task of abruptly adjusting to a new culture and may have a less stressful experience (Tseng 2001).

- **How to ask:** Why did you leave your country? Was it your choice? Do you have a possibility of returning home?

  HOW [legally] did you leave (immigration status)?
  —This can be a sensitive question, especially if your patient has an undocumented status. It also can be a tremendous source of fear and point of vulnerability. People who do not have legal status may be afraid of deportation and afraid of accessing services, which greatly impedes their acculturation.

- **How to ask:** Is your legal status a source of stress for you? I know that many people are afraid to get the services they need because they do not have a documented legal status. This places them in a stressful situation that affects their health. This is why I ask. It is helpful for me to understand the obstacles you are facing.

Cultural Identity and Level of Acculturation

Cultural identity can be a source of distress or of support for an individual. For example, for some people, having to identify with a specific group can be a source of distress because this sets them apart from the majority, while others have a great fear of becoming acculturated with the majority. Further, people may have intrapsychic conflicts about their cultural identity. It is important to properly assess the level of acculturation of a patient.

Inquiring about cultural identity and level of acculturation will aid in establishing the proper diagnosis; the diagnosis may otherwise be influenced by erroneous assumptions and lead to the establishment of a treatment plan that is not well thought out.

Questions to consider and how to ask them:

- How do you feel about your culture of origin? How involved are you with your culture of origin? Which community organizations are you involved with and what role do you play in them? Do you belong to any group where there are people from your culture of origin (e.g., a religious organization or leisure setting) or groups with people mostly from the United States? Do you have any friends from your culture of origin or a culture other than yours? How do you relate to these people? How do you socialize with members of your extended family?
- How do you view the way you are treated by people from other cultures? What type of discrimination have you experienced? Have you ever experienced racism? Have any of these experiences transformed your life in any way?

B. Cultural Explanations of the Individual's Illness

Remember the mnemonic SPESial TEsT. (Symptoms, Precipitators and Explanation, Severity, Treatment history, Experiences with help-seeking, what patient Thinks about course of illness and treatment options). Most of the information in this section can be incorporated into the standard history of present illness or review of systems.

SPESial TEsT

Symptoms? What are your worst symptoms or most distressing experiences? (Elicit idioms of distress and culture-bound syndromes; see Table A–2 for examples of the latter.)

- **How to ask:** What kinds of things are you experiencing? How has this affected your life? What are your worst symptoms? What do you call these? — *Point to note:* Some of these experiences are self-limited and may not require treatment.

Precipitators and Explanation for symptoms and distress? Course of illness, symptoms, or distressing experiences?

• **How to ask:** How do you explain what is happening? When did it start, and what started it? How do your friends, family, and community, or those who know you best and/or are most like you (reference group such as specific ethnic or cultural affiliation, race, religious affiliation, sex, age, or acculturative stage) explain what is happening?

— *Points to note:*

· These explanations can include religious beliefs, magical explanations, exhaustion, perceived discrimination, disabilities, character weakness and moral judgment, and biological explanations.

· Explanations can also include beliefs related to specific subcultures, witchcraft/voodoo, spirits/demons, family legacy, migration histories, humoral explanations, and others.

It will be important to remember how the patient self-identifies and with which cultural group(s) he or she identifies. For example, level of acculturation may be very important, because a second-generation Chinese American male might have more Western belief influences in his or her explanations than a recent immigrant.

Severity? What are the level of dysfunction and the meaning of the symptoms and distressing experiences in reference to the host culture or culture of origin?

• **How to ask:** What does it mean that you are experiencing these symptoms? How serious are these symptoms for you, and does that have any meaning? Do you worry about what your symptoms might mean (Kleinman et al. 1978)?

— *Points to note:*

· The clinician should inquire about level of function, as is done in a typical psychiatric evaluation, because this will help guide the treatment decisions.

· The clinician will be able to derive an implicit sense of how these symptoms interface with the culture of origin and the host culture, but one can ask additional questions to elicit how these symptoms are perceived in the host culture, such as: Are these symptoms affecting your work? Has your boss [if the boss is of the host or majority culture] made any comments or complaints?

The following questions can be asked as part of the past psychiatric history or past medical history portion of the assessment.

Treatment history? This is a question of actual treatments that have been tried in the past.

- **How to ask:** What kinds of treatments have you received up until now? How would someone from your [reference group such as friends, family, geographic location, and religion] be treated, or what advice have you gotten on how to deal with the symptoms?

  — *Point to note:* Treatments can come in any form, such as prayer, decreasing stress by stress-reduction exercises, having family and friends leave the person alone, or using doctors, faith healers, shamans, alternative and traditional medicines, homeopathy, Ayurveda, cupping/coining, diet, meditation, or supplements.

Experiences with help-seeking? This is a question of the patient's emotional and overall experience with trying to get help for his or her problems. These experiences will greatly influence how the patient will perceive future (and current) help-seeking attempts and treatment options.

- **How to ask:** What kinds of experience have you had with previous types of treatment? What types of experiences have others that you know had (for example, did anyone in your family or friends see a psychiatrist)? What has helped the most? In your culture, is there shame associated with seeking psychiatric help? Who experiences the shame?

  — *Point to note:* EVERYONE has some emotional response to help-seeking attempts. Additional questions can include, What did it feel like for you when you previously sought help? How would you have wanted it to be different? People will refer to the experiences of their family and friends as well as to their own experiences, so it is important to ask about both.

What do you *Think* the course of your presentation is, and what type of *Treatment* would you like now? What do you fear most about your symptoms?

- **How to ask:** What do you think will happen now? What do you fear or worry about most regarding your symptoms and your treatment? What do you think will be most helpful at this point? (Choices can include discussing past and present experiences, receiving advice, exercise, medications, alternative treatments, psychoeducation, etc.)

— *Points to note:*

· It is important to remember that many treatment options can coexist at the same time. Thought must be given to what makes the most sense and what is the most helpful for the patient.

· The relationship between the patient and clinician is important to consider: it will be important to elicit expectations about you and your role in treatment, such as authoritarian figure or cooperative figure.

· Remember to be aware of the differences between the clinician and the patient regarding illness beliefs and treatment beliefs. It will be important to recognize when the clinician's specific beliefs are influencing patient care.

· It is important to remember that many people regard mental illness as greatly stigmatized. Stress that seeking help does not mean that they are "crazy" (Lewis-Fernandez et al. 2000).

Culture-Bound Syndromes and Idioms of Distress

Some specific culture-bound syndromes are listed in Table A–2. Many of these syndromes and idioms exist across and within cultural distinctions, and some cross-utilization of terms is indicated here. See Appendix C for definitions of these terms.

C. Cultural Factors Related to Psychosocial Environment and Levels of Functioning

When assessing the psychosocial environment, direct your inquiry in widening social circles. Begin with the individual, then move out to the partner, the family (including extended family), and the community. It is particularly important to move beyond the nuclear family for patients from communal cultures. With each social sphere, assess for supports as well as stressors.

Stressors and Supports

When considering this section, it is useful to begin thinking about the types of stressors that are commonly included in Axis IV, the Psychosocial and Environmental Problems axis in the standard DSM-IV-TR multiaxial diagnostic

Table A–2.   Culture-bound syndromes

Cultural groups (by locale)	Syndrome
Asian	
China	Qi-gong psychotic reaction
	Shenjing shuairuo ("neurasthenia")
	Shenkui
Japan	Taijin kyofusho
	Shinkeishitsu
Korea	Hwa-byung
	Shin-byung
India	Dhat (similar to sukra prameha in Sri Lanka and shenkuei in China)
Malaysia	Amok (similar experiences found in Laos, Papua New Guinea, the Philippines, Polynesia, and Puerto Rico, and among the Navajo)
	Koro (similar phenomenon found in parts of South Asia and East Asia)
	Latah (also found in other parts of Asia)
Latin American	
General	Locura (also found among Latinos in the United States)
	Susto (also found among Latino groups in the United States, Mexico, Central America, and South America)
	Nervios (also found among Latinos in the United States)
	Cólera (bilis, muina)
Puerto Rico	Ataque de nervios (also found in Latin and Mediterranean areas)
	Empacho (also found in Cuba)
Nicaragua	Gris siknis (noted in the Miskito group)

Table A–2. Culture-bound syndromes *(continued)*

Cultural groups (by locale)	Syndrome
Industrialized countries	
General	Anorexia nervosa and other eating disorders (found particularly in North America)
	Dissociative identity disorder
Germany	Involutional paraphrenia (also found in Spain)
United States	Spells (found in the southern United States)
Mediterranean cultures	Mal de ojo (also found in some Latin countries)
African and Caribbean	
General (Caribbean)	Falling out or blacking out (also found in the southern United States)
	Rootwork (also found in the southern United States in both African American and European American populations)
Haiti	Boufée delirante (also found in West Africa and France)
	Fright illness, among Native West Indians (also found in Africa and Brazil)
Trinidad	Tabanka
North Africa	Zar (also found in the Middle East)
West Africa	Brain fag
Sub-Saharan Africa	Amafufanyane (sleep paralysis), found among Zulu in southern Africa
Native American	
General	Ghost sickness
Mohave	Hi-wa itck
Algonquian	Wihtigo (windigo)
Eskimo (Arctic and Subarctic)	Pibloktoq
Inuit	Uqamairineq

Note. See Appendix C for definitions of the syndromes except where otherwise noted.
Source. American Psychiatric Association 2000b; Henderson and Nguyen 2004; Kaplan and Sadock 1998.

system (American Psychiatric Association 2000a). These would typically include stressors such as interpersonal, familial, economic, occupational, educational, and legal difficulties. To be able to assess how distressed an individual might be by the stressors that he or she faces, it is also important to examine his or her psychological context. The patient's context can either mitigate or exacerbate the impact of stressors (Harvey 1996). Aspects of context that may exacerbate problems include difficulties with acculturation and discrimination. Difficulty with systems (educational, health care, legal) as well as discord with representatives from these systems (teachers, counselors, social workers, physicians, lawyers) can be exacerbating factors. The context may also be one of poor resources and insufficient buffering, as when there is a sparse network of social supports or a lack of community resources.

Strength and support may come from several culturally related sources:

- **Individual**-based culturally related strengths and supports include pride in one's culture, religious faith or spirituality, artistic abilities, bilingual and multilingual skills, group-specific social skills, sense of humor, culturally related knowledge and practical skills, culture-specific social skills, culture-specific beliefs that help one cope, respectful attitude toward the natural environment, commitment to helping one's own group, and wisdom based on experience.

- **Family/community**-based culturally related strengths and supports include extended families, including non-blood-related kin, cultural or group-specific networks, religious communities, traditional celebrations and rituals, recreational playful activities, storytelling activities that make meaning and pass on the history of the group, and involvement in political or social action groups.

- **Environment**-based culturally related strengths and supports include an altar in one's home or room to honor deceased family members and ancestors, a space for prayer and meditation, foods related to cultural preferences (cooking and eating), pets, a gardening area, and access to outdoors for subsistence or recreation (Hayes 2001).

Assessing Psychosocial Environment and Functioning

The following is a basic schema for assessing psychosocial environment and functioning. The schema can be further elaborated based on the particular circumstances of your patient.

Stressors and supports: The basic questions are: What are the major sources of support in your life? What are the major stressors in your life?

Partner support

• **How to ask:** Is your partner a source of support for you?

Partner stressors (domestic violence)

• **How to ask:** Does your partner make you feel bad about yourself? Have you been hit, kicked, punched, or otherwise physically hurt by someone in the past year? If so, by whom? (Questions are from Feldhaus et al. 1997.)

— *Points to note:* When exploring the relationship with the partner, it is important to screen for domestic violence, because one out of eight cohabiting relationships are violent (American Medical Association Council of Scientific Affairs 1992). Because many women do not self-identify as abused, it is better to describe the specific behaviors that would constitute abuse. The above questions concerning physical abuse will detect 64% to 71% of abuse, including abuse by previous partners or other family members.

Family support

• **How to ask:** Which family members are major sources of support for you? Are there family members you are close to who are still in your home country?

Family stressors

• **How to ask:** What are some of the family problems that affect you? What are some of the family conflicts you've been having since moving to the United States?

— *Point to note:* Particularly in immigrant families, each family member may be at a different level of acculturation, with correspondingly different values, expectations, and behaviors; this can be a significant source of stress for the family.

Community support

- **How to ask:** Is it important to you to find a community that fits with your cultural background (Barrett 2005)? If so, have you been able to find it? Is it a major source of support? Does it meet your needs?

  — *Point to note:* The clinician may also have developed a sense of whether or not the patient is part of a cultural community from the acculturation assessment earlier.

Community stressors

- **How to ask:**
  - Have you and your family felt accepted in this country? Why or why not?
  - How respected are your values and traditions by mainstream society (Barrett 2005)? Do you feel that you are discriminated against in the community or at work?
  - Are you having other problems at work or in the community?

  — *Point to note:* The above questions are purposely broad enough to include racial as well as religious, gender-based, and sexual identity–based discrimination. The patient's awareness of racism is tied to the level of racial identity development and may be related to the level of acculturation. Also, the ability to cope with the stress of discrimination is improved if the patient has found a community that is supportive of his or her cultural identity.

Religion/spirituality: Screen for whether religion is important in your patient's life (see Section A above). If screening reveals that religion is important to the patient, perform the remainder of the spiritual assessment (Kehoe 1997; Richards and Bergin 1997). A helpful mnemonic for conducting the following assessment is **A HOLY** (are you **A**ctive in religion now, has religion **H**urt you, could it help you **O**vercome your problems, could a spiritual **L**eader be helpful, what were your beliefs when **Y**oung).

- Are you **Actively** involved in your religion, currently?

  — *Point to note:* Understanding how and why the patient is involved in his or her religion will help the clinician distinguish if their patient has an *intrinsic orientation* (internalized and lived beliefs regardless of consequences), which is associated with improved mental health, or an *extrinsic orientation* (using religion as a means of obtaining status, security, self-justification or sociability), which is associated with increased anxiety and difficulties with social and emotional adjustment.

- Do you believe that religious or spiritual influences have **Hurt** you or contributed to your problem?
  — *Points to note:*
  - Incongruence between spiritual values and lifestyle can be a source of guilt and anxiety.
  - Patients may believe that their problems have a spiritual source. Although they may not feel comfortable divulging this to the clinician, a representative of the Western scientific model, one may be able to get a sense of their beliefs and practices by speaking to the family.
- Are there religious or spiritual resources that could help you **Overcome** your problem?
  — *Point to note:* Patients may have a *self-directing,* a *deferring,* or a *collaborative problem-solving* relationship with God or with their faith. This pattern may affect how they interact with the person who is treating them.
- Would it be helpful if we consulted a religious **Leader** or a traditional healer?
  — *Points to note:*
  - Religious patients who have lost a sense of a *positive spiritual identity* and no longer feel that they have a divine worth or potential may benefit from interventions such as counsel from a spiritual leader to help them reconnect with their spiritual identity and worth.
  - At times, religion can have a negative impact because patients may have a misunderstanding of the doctrines of their religion (i.e., may not have critically examined understandings they developed as children).
- What were your religious beliefs when you were **Young**?
  — *Point to note:* Often the patient's core spiritual belief system was formed during childhood.

Functioning: It can be difficult to assess functioning when the clinician does not know the norm for functioning in the patient's culture. The following questions can be helpful because they harness the community's values and norms to judge functioning. It can also be helpful to consult with a cultural broker such as the interpreter.

- **How to ask:** Each community has certain images of a successful person. Would your community judge you to be successful or unsuccessful (Berg-Cross and Chinen 1995)? Before you came to this country, would your community have judged you to be successful or unsuccessful?

D. Cultural Elements of the Relationship Between the Individual and the Clinician

Taking the time to examine the interactions between the cultural identities of the clinician and the patient is essential for the conduct of the clinical interview. The following are some suggestions for gathering this information.

1. Consider your own cultural background.

- Self-reflection, awareness, and understanding of one's own personal and professional identity development is essential for maintaining objectivity with the patient.
- Be aware of their own biases and limitations of knowledge and skills that might affect the clinical encounter.

2. Consider the patient's cultural identity compared with the clinician's, and compare similarities and differences.

3. Move from a categorical approach to an understanding of the patient's self-construal of identity. Factor in the context of the clinical encounter, assessment, and treatment that might arise from similarities and differences.

4. Maintain ongoing assessment of the cultural elements of the relationship.

- Factors to consider include rapport and respect, dealing with stigma and shame, empathy, verbal and nonverbal communication, and involvement with significant others and community organizations. What is the history of the relationships between the patient's culture of origin and the clinician's (e.g., colonization, sociopolitical conflict, local history and conflict, racism)? What is the relationship of the patient's culture of origin and the host/adopted country? Are there any value conflicts between the clinician and the patient?

5. **Be aware of transference and countertransference issues,** which may be interethnic (when patient and client are from different ethnic backgrounds) and intraethnic (when therapist and client share the same ethnicity).

- Common interethnic transference themes include patients distrusting the authority figure (whether it be therapist or institution), being overcompliant or friendly to please the authority figure, denial of cultural factors, and ambivalence. Interethnic countertransference may include the "clinical anthropologist" syndrome of pursuing cultural differences that are not necessarily clinically relevant. Therapists may have feelings of guilt or pity toward clients of differing ethnicities, resulting in a more timid approach when interviewing the patient.

- Examples of intraethnic transference: The patient may overidentify with the therapist, which may result in idealizing the therapist. Conversely, minority patients, for instance, may assume that an "ethnic" therapist is less competent than the therapist from the dominant culture. Patients who have different levels of acculturation from their therapists may also feel the therapist has "sold out" to the dominant culture. Examples of intraethnic countertransference include overidentification, guilt arising from the therapist's sociocultural and economic circumstances, anger because of increased demands from the patient, and defensive distancing due to feeling too close to the patient (Comas-Diaz and Jacobsen 1991).

6. **Consider the need for cultural consultation.** Do you have any specific knowledge about the patient's culture or ethnic group? If not, you may need to ask a person familiar with the patient's culture, known as a cultural broker or cultural consultant.

   —*Tip:* The U.S. Department of State Web site (http://www.state.gov) has "Country Background Notes" for independent states and regions of special sovereignty. These notes include information on the history, politics, religion, and minority populations, and are useful for a quick review before you see a patient from another country or culture.

7. **Consider the patient's motivation for seeking treatment.** Is the patient coming to see the clinician of his or her own accord? Is the patient being forced to see the clinician by family? A school? A community? The law? What does the clinician expect the patient's attitude will be when they meet? The assessment

of attitudes toward medical personnel may be most helpful in a psychotherapy assessment. Working with a cultural consultant can be beneficial in this regard.

Questions to consider and how to ask them:

- What are your expectations of your doctors? How is mental illness viewed in your country of origin? Is there stigma against mentally ill people? How are they treated (institutionalized, ignored, supported by the community)? How are psychiatrists portrayed in the media in your country? Do you think those portrayals are accurate? In your country, have psychiatrists ever been used to persecute people? Have psychiatrists ever taken part in human rights abuses? Do you have fears about your treatment? Can you talk about them?

- Do you feel that you can speak freely with doctors? Are you comfortable telling them when you don't agree with something they say? If not, would you be able to express these feelings to an intermediary, such as a translator or social worker?

- When medical staff advises something or prescribe medicines, do you feel that you must take the advice or use the medicines? Have you ever told a doctor you would do something you didn't want to, simply because you didn't want to openly disagree with him or her? Do you feel free to ask questions about alternatives to medications?

- Before you came here, did you have any expectations about what your psychiatrist would be like (young, old, male, female)? How do I fit or not fit with those expectations? How do you think these differences will affect our work together?

- Do you have a preference for male or female psychiatrist/therapist? If so, why [possible choices to offer: trust, shame, greater likelihood that they will understand, easier to express yourself....]?

- Do you have a preference for a psychiatrist/therapist with a cultural background that is similar to yours, or of a different background, or don't you think this matters? Why [see choices above]?

- Would you like sessions to be conducted in your own language? Would it help you feel that you were being understood properly?

- Do you ever have difficulty understanding what your therapist is saying?

- Do you feel comfortable with your therapist?

E. Overall Cultural Assessment for Diagnosis and Care

Part E of the cultural formulation entails integrating the previous four sections to inform a culturally competent differential diagnosis and a culturally congruent treatment plan. Therefore we must have an adequate description of the patient's cultural identity, his or her cultural explanations of the illness, his or her stressors and supports, and the relationship between the clinician and the patient. Factors such as the role of family members and ethnic community, cultural, and religious institutions should be integrated into the formulation. The experiences of immigration, acculturation, and discrimination may be relevant. Understanding the patient's expectations regarding outcome of treatment is often helpful in negotiating a treatment plan.

1. **Make the differential diagnosis:** What is psychopathological and what is cultural? Does the clinician feel comfortable with his or her knowledge of the normative practices and values of the patient's culture?

Many psychiatric disorder, such as conduct, adjustment, anxiety, mood, somatoform, dissociative, personality, and dysthymic disorders are most likely to present differently across cultures (Kleinman 1988), whereas psychotic, bipolar, and substance abuse disorders vary less across cultures (Johnson 1988). For instance, some cultures believe that hearing the voice of a lost loved one is a natural rite of the mourning process. Be aware that a delusion, by definition, must be incongruent with culturally held values.

During this part of the cultural formulation, using a cultural consultant is critical (Lu et al. 1995). The clinician is advised to read the narrative introductions to each section of DSM-IV-TR, specifically the paragraphs on age, gender, and cultural features, and see if any of them apply to the patient. Also, consider Other Conditions That May be a Focus of Clinical Attention as a source of other, more appropriate diagnoses, such as an acculturation problem, a religious or spiritual problem, or an identity problem.

2. **Formulate a narrative of the patient's case incorporating the cultural factors.** When putting together the patient's story, bring in his or her cultural perspective, explanatory model, and mental health concept. The clinical narrative should reflect the patient's worldview, model of causality and illness,

and expectations. The degree to which historical, political, and environmental factors affecting the patient are understood by the clinician may reflect the degree to which the clinician can empathize with the patient.

3. Consider how the cultural formulation will affect management. The type of treatment recommended for the patient should be congruent with the patient's cultural experience. A large percentage of patients are nonadherent to their medications. Possible explanations for nonadherence may include a nonbiologically based explanatory model for symptoms, mistrust of medical institutions and authorities, fear of side effects, and resistance to addressing interpsychic conflicts.

Psychotherapeutic approaches should also be selected to fit the patient's needs. People who come from collectivist cultures may not be as amenable to individual psychotherapy and may be more receptive to family therapy and to involvement of individuals outside their immediate family. Conversely, people who come from societies that value individualism and autonomy may benefit more from more expressive psychodynamic psychotherapy.

Culture affects our choice of medications as well (Gaw 2001). We may choose a medication that has a combination of effects to avoid giving patients "too many" pills. The physician also has to prepare the patient for side effects and for the duration of therapy. Many patients believe that the medications work immediately and that they are very powerful. Therefore they will take only half the prescribed dose. Checking drug levels and having the patient bring in his or her pill bottles are useful strategies. Finally, the adage of "start low, go slow" warns clinicians that patients may inherit different forms of the CYP450 enzymes that metabolize medications, resulting in medication side effects or nonrespose.

Culture also affects the patient's social system, which often includes extended family and religious groups and their leaders. Part of the treatment plan should involve the family and religious groups if relevant. Appropriate interventions include family meetings, gathering collateral history, and asking patients to seek support from their church. Not involving all parts of the patient's social system can derail the treatment plan by giving the patient mixed messages about his or her treatment. For instance, an individual who plays a central role in the patient's decisionmaking process may discourage the patient from adhering to the treatment. Addressing the concerns of all parties involved may increase the likelihood of adherence.

To ensure that the clinician has provided comprehensive and culturally competent care, he or she may consider the useful mnemonic **LEARN**: Listen with sympathy, Explain your perceptions of the problem, Acknowledge and discuss differences and similarities in explanation of illness, Recommend treatment, and Negotiate treatment. The first guideline is good for developing the therapeutic alliance, and the other four pertain to Part E of the Outline for Cultural Formulation. We have to tell the patient that we understand his or her situation, note the cultural differences, and then act as a bridge between the differing belief systems to negotiate an acceptable treatment plan. Only then can we be satisfied that we have used the Outline to its fullest advantage. Of course, the formulation will evolve over time as we see the patient more often, but it offers a helpful framework for beginning to understand patients from culturally diverse backgrounds that might differ from that of the clinician.

References

American Medical Association Council of Scientific Affairs: Violence against women: relevance for medical practitioners. JAMA 267:3184–3189, 1992

American Psychiatric Association: Diagnostic and Statistical Manual of Mental Disorders, 4th Edition, Text Revision. Washington, DC, American Psychiatric Association, 2000a

American Psychiatric Association: Appendix I: Outline for cultural formulation and glossary of culture-bound syndromes, in Diagnostic and Statistical Manual of Mental Disorders, 4th Edition, Text Revision. Washington, DC, American Psychiatric Association, 2000b, pp 897–903

Barrett H: Guidelines and suggestions for conducting successful cross-cultural evaluations for the courts, in Race, Culture, Psychology, and Law. Edited by Barrett KH, George WH. Thousand Oaks, CA, Sage, 2005, pp 107–123

Berg-Cross L, Chinen RT: Multicultural training models and the Person-in-Culture Interview, in Handbook of Multicultural Counseling. Edited by Ponterotto JG, Casas JM, Suzuki LA, et al. Thousand Oaks, CA, Sage, 1995, pp 333–356

Chachkes E: Multiculturalism: patient and provider diversity, in Patient and Family Education in Managed Care and Beyond. Edited by Bateman WB, Kramer EJ, Glassman KS. New York, Springer, 1999, pp 84–86

Comas-Diaz L, Jacobsen FM: Ethnocultural transference and countertransference in the therapeutic dyad. Am J Orthopsychiatry 61:392–402, 1991

Cultural Consultation Service, Sir Mortimer Davis–Jewish General Hospital: Cultural Assessment Outline: Version A, in Report: Cultural Consultation Service in Mental Health, appendices. Montreal, QC, Canada, McGill University, Division of Social and Transcultural Psychiatry, 2000. Available at: http://www.mcgill.ca/tcpsych/publications/report/appendices/handbook/assessment. Accessed Oct. 2, 2005.

Feldhaus KL, Koziol-McLain J, Amsbury HL: Accuracy of 3 brief screening questions for detecting partner violence in the emergency department. JAMA 277:1357–1361, 1997

Gaw AC: Cultural context of nonadherence to psychotropic medications in psychiatric patients, in Concise Guide to Cross-Cultural Psychiatry. Washington, DC, American Psychiatric Publishing, 2001, pp 141–164

Guarnaccia PJ, Rogler LH: Research on culture-bound syndromes: new directions. Am J Psychiatry 156:1322–1327, 1999

Harvey M: An ecological view of psychological trauma and trauma recovery. J Trauma Stress 9:3–23, 1996

Hayes PA: Addressing Cultural Complexities in Practice. Washington, DC, American Psychological Association, 2001

Henderson DC, Nguyen DD: Culture and psychiatry, in Massachusetts General Hospital: Psychiatry Update and Board Preparation, 2nd Edition. Edited by Stern TA, Herman JB. New York, McGraw-Hill, 2004, pp 551–561

Johnson FA: Contributions of anthropology in psychiatry, in Review of Psychiatry, 2nd Edition. Edited by Goldman H. Norwalk, CT, Appleton & Lange, 1988, pp 167–181

Kaplan HI, Sadock BJ: Synopsis of Psychiatry, 8th Edition. Baltimore, MD, Lippincott Williams & Wilkins, 1998, p 499

Kehoe N: Religious/Spiritual History Questionnaire. Cambridge, MA, Harvard University Press, 1997

Kleinman A: Rethinking Psychiatry. New York, Free Press, 1988

Kleinman A, Eisenberg L, Good B: Culture illness and care: clinical lessons from cross cultural research. Ann Intern Med 88:251–258, 1978

Koenig HG: Spirituality in Patient Care: Why, How, When, and What. Philadelphia, PA, Templeton Foundation Press, 2002

Lewis-Fernandez R, Diaz N: The cultural formulation: a method for assessing cultural factors affecting the clinical encounter. Psychiatr Q 73:271–295, 2000

Lu FG: Cultural assessment in clinical psychiatry: DSM-IV-TR Outline for Cultural Formulation. Grand Rounds, Yale Medical School, June 3, 2005

Lu FG, Lim RF, Mezzich JE: Issues in the assessment and diagnosis of culturally diverse individuals, in American Psychiatric Press Review of Psychiatry, Vol 14. Edited by Oldham JM, Riba MB. Washington, DC, American Psychiatric Press, 1995, pp 477–510

Puchalski C, Romer AL: Taking a spiritual history allows clinicians to understand patients more fully. J Palliat Med 3:129–137, 2000

Richards PS, Bergin AE: Religious and spiritual assessment, in A Spiritual Strategy for Counseling and Psychotherapy. Washington, DC, American Psychological Association, 1997, pp 171–199

Rohlof H, Loevy N, Sassen L, et al: The cultural interview in the Netherlands: the Cultural Formulation in your pocket. Foundation Centrum '45 Web site, 2000. Available at: http://www.centrum45.nl/lectures/ukhrny05.htm. Accessed Oct. 2, 2005.

Tseng WS: Migration, refuge, and adjustment, in Handbook of Cultural Psychiatry. Edited by Tseng WS. San Diego, CA, Academic Press, 2001, pp 695–728

Annotated Bibliography of Cultural Psychiatry and Other Topics

Francis G. Lu, M.D.

*Highly recommended. **Top ten.

Books

*Adams N, Grieder DM: Treatment Planning for Person-Centered Care: The Road to Mental Health and Addiction Recovery. Burlington, MA, Elsevier Academic, 2005

*Akhtar S: Immigration and Identity. Northvale, NJ, Jason Aronson, 1999 — *A psychodynamic perspective on an important cultural identity issue.*

Akhtar S, Kramer S (eds): The Colors of Childhood: Separation–Individuation Across Cultural, Racial and Ethnic Diversity. Northvale, NJ, Jason Aronson, 1998

*Alarcon RD, Foulks EF, Vakkur M: Personality Disorders and Culture: Clinical and Conceptual Interactions. New York, Wiley, 1998 —*An immediate classic on culture and personality disorders.*

*Al-Issa I (ed): Mental Illness in the Islamic World. Madison, CT, International Universities Press, 1999 —*One of the few books on this timely topic.*

American Medical Association: Cultural Competence Compendium. Chicago, IL, American Medical Association, 1999

Aponte JF, Wohl J (eds): Psychological Intervention and Cultural Diversity. Boston, MA, Allyn & Bacon, 2000

*Association of American Medical Colleges: Medical School Objectives Project, Parts I–III. Washington, DC, Association of American Medical Colleges, 1998, 1999 —*Essential for medical student education.*
   • http://www.aamc.org

Axtell RE: Gestures: The Do's and Taboos of Body Language Around the World. New York, Wiley, 1997

Berzoff J, Flanagan LM, Hertz P: Inside Out and Outside In. Northvale, NJ, Jason Aronson, 1996 —*Discusses impact of cultural identity variables (race, gender, class, etc.) on psychotherapy.*

Boehnlein J (ed): Religion and Psychiatry. Washington, DC, American Psychiatric Association, 2001 —*An important update on issues at the interface of religion and psychiatry.*

Boorstein S: Clinical Studies in Transpersonal Psychotherapy. Albany, State University of New York Press, 1997 —*Case-based approach from a seasoned transpersonal psychiatrist.*

Boyd-Franklin N: Black Families in Therapy, 2nd Edition. New York, Guilford, 2003

Bronstein P, Quina K: Teaching Gender and Multicultural Awareness. Washington, DC, American Psychological Association, 2003

Brown DR, Keith VM (eds): In and Out of Our Right Minds: The Mental Health of African American Women. New York, Columbia University Press, 2003

Burt V, Hendrick V: Concise Guide to Women's Health, 2nd Edition. Washington, DC, American Psychiatric Press, 2001

*Burt V, Hendrick V: Clinical Manual of Women's Mental Health. Washington, DC, American Psychiatric Publishing, 2005

**Cabaj RP, Stein TS: Textbook of Homosexuality and Mental Health. Washington, DC, American Psychiatric Press, 1996 —*Very comprehensive. The standard essential textbook in this area.*

*California Endowment: A Manager's Guide to Cultural Competence Education for Health Care Professionals. Woodland Hills, CA, The California Endowment, 2003—*Essential for medical student education.*
- http://www.calendow.org/reference/publications/pdf/cultural/TCE0217-2003_A_Managers_Gui.pdf
**California Endowment: Principles and Recommended Standards for Cultural Competence Education of Health Care Professionals. Woodland Hills, CA, The California Endowment, 2003
- http://www.calendow.org/reference/publications/pdf/cultural/TCE0215-2003_Principles_and.pdf
*California Endowment: Resources in Cultural Competence Education for Health Care Professionals. Woodland Hills, CA, California Endowment, 2003
- http://www.calendow.org/reference/publications/pdf/cultural/TCE0218-2003_Resources_in_C.pdf
California Healthcare Interpreters Association: California Standards for Healthcare Interpreters. Woodland, CA, California Endowment, 2003
- http://www.calendow.org/reference/publications/pdf/cultural/TCE0701-2002_California_Sta.pdf
Canino I, Spurlock J: Culturally Diverse Children and Adolescents, 2nd Edition. New York, Guilford, 2000
Cardeña E, Lynn SJ, Krippner S (eds): Varieties of Anomalous Experience: Examining the Scientific Evidence. Washington, DC, American Psychological Association, 2000
**Carter RT (ed): Handbook of Racial-Cultural Psychology and Counseling. Hoboken, NJ, Wiley, 2005 —*A two-volume set that thoroughly explores racial identity and its implications on psychotherapy.*
Castillo RJ: Culture and Mental Illness: A Client-Centered Approach. Pacific Grove, CA, Brooks/Cole, 1997
Castillo RJ: Meanings of Madness. Pacific Grove, CA, Brooks/Cole, 1998
*Center for Mental Health Services (CMHS), Substance Abuse and Mental Health Services Administration (SAMHSA): Cultural Competence Standards in Managed Care Mental Health Services for Four Underserved/Underrepresented Racial/Ethnic Groups. Washington, DC, CMHS/SAMHSA, 1998 —*Essential for understanding systems cultural competence.*
- http://www.mentalhealth.samhsa.gov/media/Ken/pdf/Cc-stds.pdf

Center for Substance Abuse Treatment (CSAT)/Substance Abuse and Mental Health Services Administration (SAMHSA): Cultural Issues in Substance Abuse Treatment. Washington, DC, CSAT/SAMHSA, 1999 —*An outstanding monograph on substance abuse and cultural issues.*

*Chambers ED, Siegel C, Haugland G, et al: Cultural Competence Performance Measures for Managed Behavioral Healthcare Programs. Albany, New York State Office of Mental Health, 1998
- http://csipmh.rfmh.org

*Chin JL (ed): The Psychology of Prejudice and Discrimination. Westport, CT, Praeger, 2004 —*A landmark four-volume set provides the most comprehensive overview on this topic.*

Chin JL: Learning From My Mother's Voice. New York, Columbia Teachers College Press, 2005

Chin JL, Liem JH, Domokos-Cheng Ham MA, Hong GK: Transference and Empathy in Asian American Psychotherapy: Cultural Values and Treatment Needs. Westport, CT, Praeger, 1993

Chun KM, Organista PB, Marin G (eds): Acculturation: Advances in Theory, Measurement and Applied Research. Washington, DC, American Psychological Association, 2003

*Constantine MC, Sue DW (eds): Strategies for Building Multicultural Competence in Mental Health and Educational Settings. New York, Wiley, 2005

Culhane-Pera KA, Wawter DE, Phua Xiong, Babbitt B, Solberg MM (eds): Healing by Heart: Clinical and Ethical Case Stories of Hmong Families and Western Providers. Nashville, TN, Vanderbilt University Press, 2003

Dana RH: Understanding Cultural Identity in Intervention and Assessment. Thousand Oaks, CA, Sage, 1997

Davis-Russell E: California School of Professional Psychology Handbook of Multicultural Education, Research, Intervention, and Training. San Francisco, CA, Jossey-Bass, 2002

DeLoache J, Gottlieb A: A World of Babies. Cambridge, UK, Cambridge University Press, 2000 —*Imagined childcare guides for seven societies.*

*Fadiman A: The Spirit Catches You and You Fall Down. New York, Noonday Press, 1997 —*An extraordinary story about the importance of cultural competence in medical care.*

Fong R (ed): Culturally Competent Practice With Immigrant and Refugee Children and Families. New York, Guilford, 2003

Foster RP: The Power of Language in the Clinical Process: Assessing and Treating the Bilingual Person. Northvale, NJ, Jason Aronson, 1998

Foster RP, Moskowitz M, Javier RA: Reaching Across Boundaries of Culture and Class: Widening the Scope of Psychotherapy. Northvale, NJ, Jason Aronson, 1996

Friedman S (ed): Cultural Issues in the Treatment of Anxiety. New York, Guilford, 1997 —*Essential reading for those treating anxiety disorders.*

Fukuyama MA, Sevig TD: Integrating Spirituality Into Multicultural Counseling. Thousand Oaks, CA, Sage, 1999

*Galanter M: Spirituality and the Healthy Mind. New York, Oxford University Press, 2005

Gardiner H, Kosmitzki C: Lives Across Cultures: Cross-Cultural Human Development, 3rd Edition. Boston, MA, Allyn & Bacon, 2005

Garnets LD, Kimmel DC (eds): Psychological Perspectives on Lesbian, Gay, and Bisexual Experiences. New York, Columbia University Press, 2003

*Gaw AC: Concise Guide to Cross-Cultural Psychiatry. Washington, DC, American Psychiatric Publishing, 2001

Gibbs J, Huang L (eds): Children of Color: Psychological Interventions With Minority Youth. San Francisco, CA, Jossey-Bass, 2003

*Griffith J, Griffith M: Encountering the Sacred in Psychotherapy: How to Talk With People About Their Spiritual Lives. New York, Guilford, 2001

Group for the Advancement of Psychiatry: Alcoholism in the United States: Racial and Ethnic Considerations. Washington, DC, American Psychiatric Press, 1996

**Group for the Advancement of Psychiatry Committee on Cultural Psychiatry: Cultural Assessment in Clinical Psychiatry. Washington, DC, American Psychiatric Publishing, 2002 —*An outstanding companion reading with clinical cases concerning the DSM-IV-TR Outline for Cultural Formulation.*

Grumbach K, Munoz C, Coffman J, Rosenoff E, Gandara P, Sepulveda E: Strategies for Improving the Diversity of the Health Professions. Woodland Hills, CA, California Endowment, 2003

**Hays PA: Addressing Cultural Complexities in Practice. Washington, DC, American Psychological Association, 2001 —*Very highly recommended complement to the DSM-IV-TR Outline for Cultural Formulation.*

Hellman R, Drescher J (eds): Handbook of LGBT Issues in Community Mental Health. New York, Haworth, 2005

*Helms JE, Cook DA: Using Race and Culture in Counseling and Psychotherapy: Theory and Process. Boston, MA, Allyn & Bacon, 1999 —*An outstanding textbook on racial and cultural themes in psychotherapy.*

Herrera JM, Lawson WB, Sramek JJ (eds): Cross Cultural Psychiatry. Chichester, UK, Wiley, 1999

Hong GK, Ham MD: Psychotherapy and Counseling With Asian American Clients. Thousand Oaks, CA, Sage, 2001

Illovsky M: Mental Health Professionals: Minorities and the Poor. New York, Brunner Routledge, 2002

Institute of Medicine: Speaking of Health: Assessing Health Communication Strategies for Diverse Populations. Washington, DC, National Academies Press, 2002
   • http://www.iom.edu/CMS/3775/4471.aspx

Institute of Medicine: Health Literacy: A Prescription to End Confusion. Washington, DC, National Academies Press, 2004
   • http://www.iom.edu/CMS/375/3827/19723.aspx

Jackson LC, Greene B (eds): Psychotherapy With African American Women. New York, Guilford, 2000

Jaranson J, Popkin M (eds): Caring for Victims of Torture. Washington, DC, American Psychiatric Press, 1998

*Johnson-Powell G, Yamamoto J (eds): Transcultural Child Development: Psychological Assessment and Treatment. New York, Wiley, 1997 —*A comprehensive update of the 1983 classic* The Psychosocial Development of Minority Group Children.

Jones RL (ed): African American Mental Health. Hampton, VA, Cobb & Henry, 1998

Jones RL (ed): Black Psychology. Hampton, VA, Cobb & Henry, 2002

Jordan J, Walker M, Hartling L (eds): The Complexity of Connections: Writings From the Jean Baker Miller Training Institute. New York, Guilford, 2004 —*Innovative writing about women's issues.*

*Josephson AM, Peteet JR (eds): Handbook of Spirituality and Worldview in Clinical Practice. Washington, DC, American Psychiatric Publishing, 2004 —*An outstanding contribution on spirituality.*

Kiefer CW: Health Work With the Poor. New Brunswick, NJ, Rutgers University Press, 2000

**Kleinman A: Rethinking Psychiatry: From Cultural Category to Personal Experience. New York, Free Press, 1988 —*The most important conceptual work in cross-cultural psychiatry; a classic.*

Koenig HG (ed): Handbook of Religion and Mental Health. San Diego, CA, Academic Press, 1998

*Koenig HG: Spirituality in Patient Care: Why, How, When, and What. Philadelphia, PA, Templeton Foundation Press, 2002

*Koenig HG: Faith and Mental Health. Philadelphia, PA, Templeton Foundation Press, 2005

*Koenig HG, McCullough ME, Larson DB: Handbook of Religion and Health. Oxford, UK, Oxford University Press, 2001 —*An encyclopedic review of the research literature on religion and health and mental health.*

Kurasaki K, Okazaki S, Sue S (eds): Asian American Mental Health: Assessment Theories and Methods. New York, Plenum, 2002

Larson D, Lu F, Swyers J (eds): Model Curriculum for Psychiatry Residency Training Programs: Religion and Spirituality in Clinical Practice. Rockville, MD, National Institute for Healthcare Research, 1997

Larson DB, Swyers JP, McCullough ME (eds): Scientific Research on Spirituality: A Consensus Report. Rockville, MD, National Institute for Healthcare Research, 1998

*Lee E (ed): Working With Asian Americans: A Guide for Clinicians. New York, Guilford, 1997 —*One of the best clinical guides to working with Asian Americans.*

Lee LC, Zane NW (eds): Handbook of Asian American Psychology. Thousand Oaks, CA, Sage, 1997

Leininger M, McFarland M: Transcultural Nursing. New York, McGraw-Hill, 2002

Linde P (ed): Of Spirits and Madness: An American Psychiatrist in Africa. New York, McGraw-Hill, 2001

*Lipson JG, Dibble SL (eds): Culture and Clinical Care, 2nd Edition. San Francisco, CA, UCSF Nursing Press, 2005 —*Essential for care of culturally diverse patients.*

*Lopez A, Carrillo E (eds): The Latino Psychiatric Patient: Assessment and Treatment. Washington, DC, American Psychiatric Press, 2001 —*The only volume that reviews specific issues from specific Central and Latin American countries.*

Lynch EW, Hanson MJ: Developing Cross-Cultural Competence: A Guide for Working With Children and Their Families, 3rd Edition. Baltimore, MD, Paul H. Brookes, 2004—*On children's mental health and cultural competence.*

Marsella AJ, Friedman MJ, Gerrity ET, Scurfield R (eds): Ethnocultural Aspects of Posttraumatic Stress Disorder: Issues, Research and Clinical Applications. Washington, DC, American Psychological Association, 1996 —*Classic overview for those working in this area.*

McGoldrick M: Re-Visioning Family Therapy: Race, Culture, and Gender in Clinical Practice. New York, Guilford, 1998

**McGoldrick M, Giordano J, Garcia-Preto N (eds): Ethnicity and Family Therapy, 3rd Edition. New York, Guilford, 2005 —*Outstanding comprehensive review of cultures and family systems.*

Mezzich JE, Kleinman A, Fabrega H, Parron D (eds): Culture and Psychiatric Diagnosis: A DSM-IV Perspective. Washington, DC, American Psychiatric Press, 1996 —*Papers from the NIMH Workgroup on Culture, Diagnosis and Care submitted to the APA Task Force on DSM-IV.*

Miller WR (ed): Integrating Spirituality Into Treatment. Washington, DC, American Psychological Association, 1999 —*Well researched and practical.*

Miller WR, Delaney HD (eds): Judeo-Christian Perspectives on Psychology. Washington, DC, American Psychological Association, 2005

Moodley R, West W (eds): Integrating Traditional Healing Practices Into Counseling and Psychotherapy. Thousand Oaks, CA, Sage, 2005

Murphy-Shigematsu S: Multicultural Encounters. New York, Teachers College, Columbia University, 2002

Muskin PR (ed): Complementary and Alternative Medicine and Psychiatry (Review of Psychiatry Series, Vol 19; Oldman JM and Riba MB, series eds). Washington, DC, American Psychiatric Press, 2000

Mutha S, Allen C, Welch M: Toward Culturally Competent Care: A Toolbox for Teaching Communication Strategies. San Francisco, CA, UCSF Center for the Health Professions, 2002

Nader K, Dubrow N, Stamm BH (eds): Honoring Differences: Cultural Issues in the Treatment of Trauma and Loss. Philadelphia, PA, Brunner/Mazel, 1999 —*On posttraumatic stress disorder and culture.*

Nagayama-Hall GC, Okazaki S (eds): Asian American Psychology. Washington, DC, American Psychological Association, 2003

Nebelkopf E, Phillis M (eds): Healing and Mental Health for Native Americans. Walnut Creek, CA, Altamira Press, 2005

Okasha A, Arboleda-Florez J, Sartorius M (eds): Ethics, Culture and Psychiatry: International Perspectives. Washington, DC, American Psychiatric Press, 2000

*Okpaku SO (ed): Clinical Methods in Transcultural Psychiatry. Washington, DC, American Psychiatric Press, 1998

O'Nell TD: Disciplined Hearts: History, Identity and Depression in an American Indian Community. Berkeley, University of California Press, 1996 —*On Native American issues and depression.*

Paniagua F: Diagnosis in a Multicultural Context: A Casebook for Mental Health Professionals. Thousand Oaks, CA, Sage, 2001

Paniagua F: Assessing and Treating Culturally Diverse Individuals, 3rd Edition. Thousand Oaks, CA, Sage, 2005

Pargament K: The Psychology of Religion and Coping. New York, Guilford, 1997

Parham TA (ed): Counseling Persons of African Descent. Thousand Oaks, CA, Sage, 2002

Pedersen PB, Draguns JG, Lonner WJ, Trimble JE (eds): Counseling Across Cultures, 5th Edition. Thousand Oaks, CA, Sage, 2002 —*Cutting-edge chapters from a counseling psychology perspective.*

Perez R, Debord K, Bieschke K (eds): Handbook of Counseling and Psychotherapy With Lesbian, Gay, and Bisexual Clients. Washington, DC, American Psychological Association, 1999

**Pinderhughes E: Understanding Race, Ethnicity and Power. New York, Free Press, 1988 —*A classic on the impact of race, ethnicity, and power on the interpersonal dynamics in therapy. Experientially focused.*

*Ponterotto J, Casas J, Suzuki L, Alexander C (eds): Handbook of Multicultural Counseling, 2nd Edition. Thousand Oaks, CA, Sage, 2001

Pope-Davis D, Coleman H (eds): The Intersection of Race, Class and Gender: Implications for Multicultural Counseling. Thousand Oaks, CA, Sage, 2001

Pope-Davis DB, Coleman HLK, Ming Liu W, Toporek RL (eds): Handbook of Multicultural Competencies in Counseling and Psychology. Thousand Oaks, CA, Sage, 2003

*Richards PS, Bergin AE: Handbook of Psychotherapy and Religious Diversity. Washington, DC, American Psychological Association, 1999

Richards PS, Bergin AE (eds): Casebook for A Spiritual Strategy in Counseling and Psychotherapy. Washington, DC, American Psychological Association, 2003

*Richards PS, Bergin AE: A Spiritual Strategy for Counseling and Psychotherapy, 2nd Edition. Washington, DC, American Psychological Association, 2005 —*Extraordinary synthesis on the psychotherapy/spirituality interface.*

*Ridley C: Overcoming Unintentional Racism in Counseling and Therapy, 2nd Edition. Thousand Oaks, CA, Sage, 2005 —*Essential reading on an extraordinarily difficult topic.*

Romans S, Seeman M (eds): Women's Mental Health: A Life-Cycle Approach. Philadelphia, PA, Lippincott Williams & Wilkins, 2006

Root MP (ed): Filipino Americans. Thousand Oaks, CA, Sage, 1997

Roysircar G, Arredondo P, Fuertes JN, Ponterotto JG, Toporek RL: Multicultural Counseling Competencies 2003. Alexandria, VA, American Counseling Association, 2003 —*Important document from the American Counseling Association.*

Roysircar G, Sandhu DS, Bibbins VE (eds): Multicultural Competencies. Alexandria, VA, Association for Multicultural Counseling and Development, 2003

*Ruiz P (ed): Ethnicity and Psychopharmacology. Washington, DC, American Psychiatric Press, 2000

Samuda RJ: Psychological Testing of American Minorities: Issues and Consequences. Thousand Oaks, CA, Sage, 1998

*Sanchez-Hucles J: The First Session With African-Americans: A Step-by-Step Guide. San Francisco, CA, Jossey-Bass, 2000

Sandoval J, Geisinger KF, Frisby C (eds): Test Interpretation and Diversity: Achieving Equity in Assessment. Washington, DC, American Psychological Association, 1999

Santiago-Rivera A, Arredondo P, Gallardo-Cooper M: Counseling Latinos and La Familia: A Practical Guide. Thousand Oaks, CA, Sage, 2002

*Satcher D, Pamies R (eds): Multicultural Medicine and Health Disparities. New York, McGraw-Hill, 2006 —*A landmark work on this topic.*

Schumaker JF, Ward T (eds): Cultural Cognition and Psychopathology. Westport, CT, Praeger/Greenwood, 2001

*Scotton B, Chinen A (eds): Textbook of Transpersonal Psychiatry and Psychology. New York, Basic Books, 1996 —*Essential reading for those interested in spirituality/psychiatry.*

*Smedley BD, Stith AY, Nelson AR (eds): Unequal Treatment: Confronting Racial and Ethnic Disparities in Health Care. Institute of Medicine. Washington, DC, National Academies Press, 2003 —*Note chapter 4 on the clinical encounter: very important on bias.*
  • http://www.iom.edu/CMS/3740/4475.aspx

*Smedley BD, Butler AS, Breistow LR (eds): In the Nation's Compelling Interest: Ensuring Diversity in the Health Care Workforce. Institute of Medicine,. Washington, DC, National Academies Press, 2004
  • http://www.iom.edu/CMS/3740/4888/18287.aspx

Sperry L, Shafranske EP (eds): Spiritually Oriented Psychotherapy. Washington, DC, American Psychological Association, 2005

Spilka B, Hood RW Jr, Hunsberger B, Gorsuch R: The Psychology of Religion: An Empirical Approach, 3rd Edition. New York, Guilford, 2003

Spurlock J (ed): Black Psychiatrists and American Psychiatry. Washington, DC, American Psychiatric Association, 1999

Stone JH (ed): Culture and Disability. Thousand Oaks, CA, Sage, 2004

Stotland NL, Stewart DE: Psychological Aspects of Women's Health Care: The Interface Between Psychiatry and Obstetrics and Gynecology, 2nd Edition. Washington, DC, American Psychiatric Press, 2001

Straussner S, Ashenberg L: Ethnocultural Factors in Substance Abuse Treatment. New York, Guilford, 2001

Sue D, Ivey A, Pedersen P (eds): A Theory of Multicultural Counseling and Therapy. Pacific Grove, CA, Brooks/Cole, 1996 —*Analogous in scholarly importance for counseling psychology to Kleinman's* Rethinking Psychiatry *for psychiatry.*

*Sue DW: Overcoming Our Racism. San Francisco, CA, Jossey-Bass, 2003—*Essential reading in this area.*

*Sue DW, Sue D: Counseling the Culturally Diverse, 4th Edition. New York, Wiley, 2003 —*An update on a classic from counseling psychology.*

Suzuki LA, Meller PJ, Ponterotto JG (eds): Handbook of Multicultural Assessment. San Francisco, CA, Jossey-Bass, 2000

Ting-Toomey S: Communicating Across Cultures. New York, Guilford, 1999

Tribe R, Raval H: Working With Interpreters in Mental Health. New York, Brunner-Routledge, 2003

**Tseng W-S: Handbook of Cultural Psychiatry. San Diego, CA, Academic Press, 2001

*Tseng W-S: Clinician's Guide to Cultural Psychiatry. New York, Elsevier, 2003

Tseng W-S, Streltzer J (eds): Culture and Psychopathology: A Guide to Clinical Assessment. New York, Brunner/Mazel, 1997

Tseng W-S, Streltzer J (eds): Culture and Psychotherapy: A Guide to Clinical Practice. Washington, DC, American Psychiatric Press, 2001

Tseng W-S, Streltzer J (eds): Cultural Competence in Clinical Psychiatry. Washington, DC, American Psychiatric Publishing, 2004

Tseng W-S, Matthews D, Elwyn T: Cultural Competence in Forensic Mental Health. New York, Taylor & Francis, 2004

Tseng W-S, Chang SC, Nishizono M (eds): Asian Culture and Psychotherapy: Implications for East and West. Honolulu, University of Hawaii Press, 2005

**U.S. Department of Health and Human Services: Mental Health: Culture, Race, and Ethnicity. A Supplement to Mental Health: A Report of the Surgeon General. Rockville, MD, U.S. Department of Health and Human Services, Public Health Service, Office of the Surgeon General, 2001 *—A landmark essential reading on mental health disparities.*

- http://www.surgeongeneral.gov/library/mentalhealth/cre

Velásquez RJ, Arellano LM, McNeill BW (eds): The Handbook of Chicana/o Psychology and Mental Health. Northvale, NJ, Lawrence Erlbaum, 2004

Walsh F (ed): Spiritual Resources in Family Therapy. New York, Guilford, 1999

*Weinreich P, Saunderson W (eds): Analyzing Identity: Cross-Cultural, Societal and Clinical Contexts. New York, Routledge, 2002 *—A most important work on identity.*

Wilson JP, Drozdek B (eds): Broken Spirits. The Treatment of Traumatized Asylum Seekers, Refugees, War and Torture Victims. New York, Brunner-Routledge, 2004

Young-Bruehl E: The Anatomy of Prejudices. Cambridge, MA, Harvard University Press, 1996 *—A psychoanalytic perspective on many forms of prejudice.*

Journals

Four major journals explore mental health topics across cultures:

- *Culture, Medicine, and Psychiatry* (Kluwer)
- *Cultural Diversity and Ethnic Minority Psychology* (American Psychological Association)
- *Journal of Multicultural Counseling and Development* (Association for Multicultural Counseling and Development; a member association of the American Counseling Association).
- *Transcultural Psychiatry* (Sage)

Videotapes

The Culture of Emotions is a 58-minute training videotape (2002) that discusses the DSM-IV Outline for Cultural Formulation. It features 23 multidisciplinary experts in cultural psychiatry commenting on sections of the Outline. It was written, produced, and directed by Harriet Koskoff and is available through Fanlight Productions. A study guide and companion reading are available as downloads from the Web page describing the videotape. A DVD version was produced in 2005.)

- http://www.fanlight.com/catalog/films/361_coe.shtml

Harriet Koskoff and Francis Lu have also created two 17-minute videotapes, *A Visit With Irma Bland, M.D.: Discussing the DSM-IV Outline for Cultural Formulation* and *A Visit With Evelyn Lee, Ed.D.: Working With Asian-American Immigrants and Refugees.* Dr. Bland and Dr. Lee, two pioneers in cultural competence, both passed away in 2003.

Web Sites

Listed in order of significance.

1. *Mental Health: Culture, Race, and Ethnicity.* U.S. Surgeon General, 2001.
   - http://www.surgeongeneral.gov/library/mentalhealth/cre
2. *The Institute of Medicine (IOM) has published since 2001 a series of

important books that have made an impact on health care policy. Academic psychiatry can benefit from utilizing these perspectives.

• http://www.iom.edu

—*Crossing the Quality Chasm* (2001) focused on six aims for improving health care: safety, effectiveness, patient-centeredness, timeliness, efficiency and equity. The IOM issued a report entitled *Improving the Quality of Health Care for Mental and Substance-Use Conditions: Quality Chasm Series*, in November 2005, adapting this work to mental health and addictive disorders; input is welcome at their Web site.

• http://www.iom.edu/CMS/3089/19405/30836.aspx

—*Health Professions Education: A Bridge to Quality* (2003) suggested five core areas for education that would enhance quality.

• http://www.iom.edu/CMS/3089/4634/5914.aspx

—*Unequal Treatment: Confronting Racial and Ethnic Disparities in Health Care* (2002) has clearly established the importance of this area in health care policy.

• http://www.iom.edu/CMS/3740/4475.aspx

—*Speaking of Health: Assessing Health Communication Strategies for Diverse Populations* (2002) addressed the challenge of improving health communication in a culturally diverse society.

• http://www.iom.edu/CMS/3775/4471.aspx

—*Research Training in Psychiatry Residency: Strategies for Reform* (2003) has sparked efforts for change within the Association for Academic Psychiatry, the American Association of Directors of Psychiatric Residency Training, and the National Institute of Mental Health.

• http://www.iom.edu/CMS/3775/15646.aspx

—*Health Literacy: A Prescription to End Confusion* (2004) recommended that health care systems should develop programs sensitive to cultural and language preferences that reduce the negative effect of limited health literacy. If patients cannot comprehend needed health information, attempts to improve the quality of care and reduce health care costs and disparities may fail.

• http://www.iom.edu/CMS/3775/19723.aspx

—*Improving Medical Education: Enhancing the Behavioral and Social Science Content of Medical School Curricula* (2004) has relevance for our

teaching in medical school both within and outside psychiatry.
- http://www.iom.edu/CMS/3775/3891/19413.aspx

—*In the Nation's Compelling Interest: Ensuring Diversity in the Health Care Workforce* (2004) assesses the benefits of increased diversity in the health professions in five areas: 1) admissions policies at health professions education institutions; 2) public sources of financial support for health professions training; 3) diversity standards of health professions accreditation organizations; 4) the institutional climate for diversity at health professions education institutions; and 5) the relationship between community benefit principles and diversity. The report can be read online or purchased in PDF form or as hard-copy text at:
- http://iom.edu/CMS/3740/4888/18287.aspx

3. *Achieving the Promise: Transforming Mental Health Care.* President's New Freedom Commission on Mental Health. "Elimination of disparities" is one of six goals.
   - http://www.mentalhealthcommission.gov/reports/FinalReport/toc.html

4. *Cultural Competence Standards in Managed Care Mental Health Services: Four Underserved/Underrepresented Racial/Ethnic Groups.* Substance Abuse and Mental Health Services Administration, Center for Mental Health Services.
   - http://www.mentalhealth.samhsa.gov/publications/allpubs/SMA00-3457/default.asp

5. *Assuring Cultural Competence in Health Care: Recommendations for National Standards.* U.S. Department of Health and Human Services (HHS) Office of Minority Health.
   - http://www.omhrc.gov/clas

6. *A Family Physician's Practical Guide to Culturally Competent Care.* This is a Web-based continuing medical education training unit about the 14 Culturally and Linguistically Appropriate Services (CLAS) standards from the HHS Office of Minority Health. Although intended for practicing family physicians, it is useful for any health professional or trainee. Available on DVD. December 2004.
   - http://www.thinkculturalhealth.org

7. *Setting the Agenda for Research on Cultural Competence in Health Care.* This project looks at the question of what impact cultural competence

interventions have on the delivery of health care and health outcomes and investigates the opportunities and barriers that affect how further research in this area might be conducted. August 2004.

- http://www.omhrc.gov/cultural/cultural18.htm

8. *Developing a Self-Assessment Tool for Culturally and Linguistically Appropriate Services in Local Public Health Agencies: Final Report.* HHS Office of Minority Health. December 2003.

- http://www.omhrc.gov/cultural/LPHAs_FinalReport.pdf

9. *HHS Centers for Medicare and Medicaid Services provides information and downloads for three outstanding recent cultural competence guides from HHS:

—*Providing Oral Linguistic Services: A Guide for Managed Care Plans*

—*Planning Culturally and Linguistically Appropriate Services: A Guide For Managed Care Plans*

—*Best Practices for Culturally and Linguistically Appropriate Services in Managed Care Conference: June 3 and 4, 2002 in Research Triangle Park, North Carolina.*

- http://www.cms.gov/healthplans/quality/project03.asp

The first two items were the principal material for the handout at three national CLAS trainings given by the University of North Carolina School of Public Health in 2003. Information about the HHS CLAS standards can be obtained at:

- http://www.omhrc.gov/clas

10. *Indicators of Cultural Competence in Health Care Delivery Organizations: An Organizational Cultural Competence Assessment Profile.* The Lewin Group for the U.S. Department of Health and Human Services Health Resources and Services Administration (HRSA). April 2002.

- http://www.hrsa.gov/omh/cultural1.htm

"How do we know cultural competence when we see it?" is the central question that prompted the HRSA to sponsor a project to develop indicators of cultural competence in health care delivery organizations. The Assessment Profile builds on previous work in the field, such as the CLAS, and serves as a future building block that advances the conceptualization and practical understanding of how to assess cultural competence at the organizational level. The Assessment Profile is an analytic or organizing framework and set of specific indicators to be used as a tool for examining, demonstrating, and documenting cultural competence in organizations involved in the direct delivery of health care and services. At a general level, the Assessment Profile can help organizations frame and organize their perspectives and activities related to the assessment of cultural competence. More specifically, it can be used in routine performance monitoring, regular quality review and improvement activities, assessment of voluntary compliance with cultural competence standards or guidelines, and periodic evaluative studies.

11. *The Provider's Guide to Quality and Culture.* An outstanding Web-based training unit on clinical cultural competence from HRSA and others.
    - http://erc.msh.org/mainpage.cfm?file=1.0.htm&module= provider&language=English&ggroup&mgroup=

12. Many of the institutes of the National Institutes of Health have written strategic plans to reduce health disparities. Plans by the National Institute on Drug Abuse, National Institute on Alcohol Abuse and Alcoholism, Office of Behavioral and Social Sciences Research, and others can be found at:
    - http://healthdisparities.nih.gov/working/institutes.html

13. The National Center on Minority Health and Health Disparities.
    - http://www.ncmhd.nih.gov

14. The *National Healthcare Quality Report* and the *National Healthcare Disparities Report* present data on the quality of and disparities among services for seven clinical conditions and provide "a snapshot of the American health care system."
    - http://qualitytools.ahrq.gov

    In a February 10, 2004, hearing before the House Committee on Ways and Means, HHS Secretary Tommy Thompson admitted that his department made a mistake in revising a December 23, 2003, report from the Agency for Healthcare Research and Quality (AHRQ) on racial and ethnic disparities in health care. Secretary Thompson told the committee that HHS would release the original version of the National Healthcare Disparities Report, in its unaltered form, "without any changes whatsoever." On January 13, Representative Henry Waxman and seven other House members had complained to Secretary Thompson that the first publicly released version of the report was a "watered-down" version of the original findings and that "HHS substantially altered the conclusions of its scientists" in order to portray a less pervasive national health disparities problem.

15. *The California Endowment has three very important monographs:

—*Principles and Recommended Standards for Cultural Competence Education of Health Care Professionals*

—*A Manager's Guide to Cultural Competence Education for Health Care Professionals*

—*Resources in Cultural Competence Education for Health Care Professionals*. Other important monographs on interpreters can be found in the annotated bibliography *Multicultural Health 2002*, 2nd Edition, by Murray-García JL.

  • http://www.calendow.org/reference/publications/pdf/disparities/TCE0222-2002_Multicultural_.pdf

16. *The American Psychological Association (APA) *Guidelines on Multicultural Education, Training, Research, Practice, and Organizational Change for Psychology* is a landmark document, available at:

  • http://www.apa.org/pi/multiculturalguidelines.pdf

One can also search for the term "disparity" on the APA Web site:

  • http://search3.apa.org

17. The American Medical Association efforts on disparities can be seen at:

  • http://www.ama-assn.org. Also check:

  • http://www.ama-assn.org/ama/pub/category/7983.html

18. The Association of American Medical Colleges (AAMC) sponsors a campaign to reduce health care disparities. The Henry J. Kaiser and Robert Wood Johnson foundations, along with the AAMC and nine other co-sponsoring health care associations, have launched a $1 million campaign to reduce racial and ethnic disparities in health care. This national initiative includes an outreach effort to engage physicians in dialogue; an advertising campaign in major medical publications; and a review of the evidence on racial/ethnic disparities in health care. The campaign begins with a focus on cardiac care and, as part of the effort, the American College of Cardiology and the Kaiser Foundation recently released a report listing racial and ethnic disparities in cardiac care. For information, see:

  • http://www.kff.org/uninsured/20021009c-index.cfm.

For additional resources, see the AAMC site's "diversity" section at:

  • http://www.aamc.org

19. Massachusetts General Hospital Office of Multicultural Education has a search engine for updated literature:
    • http://www.mgh.harvard.edu
20. *McGill Department of Psychiatry Division of Transcultural Psychiatry Cultural Consultation Program.
    • http://www.mcgill.ca/ccs/report
21. *Ensuring Linguistic Access in Health Care-Settings: Legal Rights and Responsibilities, 2nd Edition.* August 2003. National Health Law Program.
    • http://www.calendow.org
22. *Reducing Disparity: Achieving Equity in Behavioral Health Services.* Proceedings of the 2003 Santa Fe Summit of the American College of Mental Health Administration
    • http://www.acmha.org/summit/summit_2003.cfm
23. *Strategies for Improving the Diversity of the Health Professions* (2003), funded by The California Endowment, focuses on California.
    • http://www.futurehealth.ucsf.edu/pdf_files/StrategiesforImproving FINAL.pdf
24. *Cultural Competency for California Public Health Staff.* September 2004. As part of the HHS Office of Minority Health's State Partnership Initiative, the University of California, San Francisco, Center for the Health Professions has completed a report that outlines a cultural competency curriculum specifically for public health staff. The report, *Cultural Competency for California Public Health Staff: Train-the-Trainer State Partnership Project,* was written for the California Department of Health Services Office of Multicultural Health.
    • http://futurehealth.ucsf.edu/pdf_files/Final%20OMH%20Report.pdf
25. *Multicultural Health Disparities: California 1990–1999.* April 2003.
    • http://www.dhs.ca.gov/hisp/chs/OHIR/reports/others/ multiculturalhealth.pdf
26. *Health for All: California's Strategic Approach to Eliminating Racial and Ethnic Health Disparities.* November 2003.
    • http://www.preventioninstitute.org/pdf/H4A_MAIN_1Scites_ 021304.pdf
27. State of California Department of Mental Health Office of Multicultural Affairs.
    • http://www.dmh.cahwnet.gov/multicultural

28. *Final Report to the Legislature Pursuant to AB 2394.* State of California Task Force on Culturally and Linguistically Competent Physicians and Dentists
    • http://www.dca.ca.gov/cltaskforce
29. San Francisco Department of Public Health Cultural and Linguistic Competency Policy.
    • http://www.dph.sf.ca.us/CLAS

Glossary of Culture-Bound Syndromes

The term *culture-bound syndrome* denotes recurrent, locality-specific patterns of aberrant behavior and troubling experience that may or may not be linked to a particular DSM-IV diagnostic category. Many of these patterns are indigenously considered to be "illnesses," or at least afflictions, and most have local names. Although presentations conforming to the major DSM-IV categories can be found throughout the world, the particular symptoms, course, and social response are very often influenced by local cultural factors. In contrast, culture-bound syndromes are generally limited to specific societies or culture areas and are localized, folk, diagnostic categories that frame coherent meanings for certain repetitive, patterned, and troubling sets of experiences and observations.

Reprinted from the *Diagnostic and Statistical Manual of Mental Disorders,* 4th Edition, Text Revision. Washington, DC, American Psychiatric Association, 2000, pp. 898–903. Copyright © 2000 American Psychiatric Association. Used with permission.

There is seldom a one-to-one equivalence of any culture-bound syndrome with a DSM diagnostic entity. Aberrant behavior that might be sorted by a diagnostician using DSM-IV into several categories may be included in a single folk category, and presentations that might be considered by a diagnostician using DSM-IV as belonging to a single category may be sorted into several by an indigenous clinician. Moreover, some conditions and disorders have been conceptualized as culture-bound syndromes specific to industrialized culture (e.g., anorexia nervosa, dissociative identity disorder), given their apparent rarity or absence in other cultures. It should also be noted that all industrialized societies include distinctive subcultures and widely diverse immigrant groups who may present with culture-bound syndromes.

This glossary lists some of the best-studied culture-bound syndromes and idioms of distress that may be encountered in clinical practice in North America and includes relevant DSM-IV categories when data suggest that they should be considered in a diagnostic formulation.

amok A dissociative episode characterized by a period of brooding followed by an outburst of violent, aggressive, or homicidal behavior directed at people and objects. The episode tends to be precipitated by a perceived slight or insult and seems to be prevalent only among males. The episode is often accompanied by persecutory ideas, automatism, amnesia, exhaustion, and a return to premorbid state following the episode. Some instances of amok may occur during a brief psychotic episode or constitute the onset or an exacerbation of a chronic psychotic process. The original reports that used this term were from Malaysia. A similar behavior pattern is found in Laos, Philippines, Polynesia (*cafard* or *cathard*), Papua New Guinea, and Puerto Rico (*mal de pelea*), and among the Navajo (*iich'aa*).

ataque de nervios An idiom of distress principally reported among Latinos from the Caribbean but recognized among many Latin American and Latin Mediterranean groups. Commonly reported symptoms include uncontrollable shouting, attacks of crying, trembling, heat in the chest rising into the head, and verbal or physical aggression. Dissociative experiences, seizurelike or fainting episodes, and suicidal gestures are prominent in some attacks but absent in others. A general feature of an ataque de nervios is a sense of being out of control. Ataques de nervios frequently occur as a direct result of a stressful event relating to the family (e.g., news of the death of a close relative, a separation or divorce from a spouse, conflicts with a spouse or children, or witnessing an accident involving a family member). People may experience amnesia for what occurred during the ataque de nervios, but they otherwise return rapidly to their usual level of functioning. Although descriptions of some ataques de nervios most closely fit with the DSM-IV description of panic attacks, the association of most ataques with a precipitating event and the frequent absence of the hallmark symptoms of acute fear or apprehension distinguish them from panic disorder. Ataques span the range from normal expressions of distress not associated with having a mental disorder to symptom presentations associated with the diagnoses of anxiety, mood, dissociative, or somatoform disorders.

bilis and colera (also referred to as *muina*) The underlying cause of these syndromes is thought to be strongly experienced anger or rage. Anger is viewed among many Latino groups as a particularly powerful emotion that can have direct effects on the body and can exacerbate existing symptoms. The major effect of anger is to disturb core body balances (which are understood as a balance between hot and cold valences in the body and between the material and spiritual aspects of the body). Symptoms can include acute nervous tension, headache, trembling, screaming, stomach disturbances, and, in more severe cases, loss of consciousness. Chronic fatigue may result from the acute episode.

boufée delirante A syndrome observed in West Africa and Haiti. This French term refers to a sudden outburst of agitated and aggressive behavior, marked confusion, and psychomotor excitement. It may sometimes be accompanied by visual and auditory hallucinations or paranoid ideation. These episodes may resemble an episode of brief psychotic disorder.

brain fag A term initially used in West Africa to refer to a condition experienced by high school or university students in response to the challenges of schooling. Symptoms include difficulties in concentrating, remembering, and thinking. Students often state that their brains are "fatigued." Additional somatic symptoms are usually centered around the head and neck and include pain, pressure or tightness, blurring of vision, heat, or burning. "Brain tiredness" or fatigue from "too much thinking" is an idiom of distress in many cultures, and resulting syndromes can resemble certain anxiety, depressive, and somatoform disorders.

dhat   A folk diagnostic term used in India to refer to severe anxiety and hypochondriacal concerns associated with the discharge of semen, whitish discoloration of the urine, and feelings of weakness and exhaustion. Similar to *jiryan* (India), *sukra prameha* (Sri Lanka), and *shen-k'uei* (China).

falling-out or blacking out   These episodes occur primarily in southern United States and Caribbean groups. They are characterized by a sudden collapse, which sometimes occurs without warning but sometimes is preceded by feelings of dizziness or "swimming" in the head. The individual's eyes are usually open but the person claims an inability to see. The person usually hears and understands what is occurring around him or her but feels powerless to move. This may correspond to a diagnosis of conversion disorder or a dissociative disorder.

ghost sickness   A preoccupation with death and the deceased (sometimes associated with witchcraft) frequently observed among members of many American Indian tribes. Various symptoms can be attributed to ghost sickness, including bad dreams, weakness, feelings of danger, loss of appetite, fainting, dizziness, fear, anxiety, hallucinations, loss of consciousness, confusion, feelings of futility, and a sense of suffocation.

hwa-byung (also known as *wool-hwa-byung*)   A Korean folk syndrome literally translated into English as "anger syndrome" and attributed to the suppression of anger. The symptoms include insomnia, fatigue, panic, fear of impending death, dysphoric affect, indigestion, anorexia, dyspnea, palpitations, generalized aches and pains, and a feeling of a mass in the epigastrium.

koro   A term, probably of Malaysian origin, that refers to an episode of sudden and intense anxiety that the penis (or, in females, the vulva and nipples) will recede into the body and possibly cause death. The syndrome is reported in south and east Asia, where it is known by a variety of local terms, such as *shuk yang, shook yong,* and *suo yang* (Chinese); *jinjinia bemar* (Assam); or *rok-joo* (Thailand). It is occasionally found in the West. Koro at times occurs in localized epidemic form in east Asian areas. This diagnosis is included in the *Chinese Classification of Mental Disorders,* Second Edition (CCMD-2).

latah   Hypersensitivity to sudden fright, often with echopraxia, echolalia, command obedience, and dissociative or trancelike behavior. The term *latah* is of Malaysian or Indonesian origin, but the syndrome has been found in many parts of the world. Other terms for this condition are *amurakh, irkunii, ikota, olan, myriachit,* and *menkeiti* (Siberian groups); *bah tschi, bah-tsi,* and *baah-ji* (Thailand); *imu* (Ainu, Sakhalin, Japan); and *mali-mali* and *silok* (Philippines). In Malaysia it is more frequent in middle-aged women.

locura   A term used by Latinos in the United States and Latin America to refer to a severe form of chronic psychosis. The condition is attributed to an inherited vulnerability, to the effect of multiple life difficulties, or to a combination of both factors. Symptoms exhibited by persons with locura include incoherence, agitation, auditory and visual hallucinations, inability to follow rules of social interaction, unpredictability, and possible violence.

mal de ojo   A concept widely found in Mediterranean cultures and else-where in the world. *Mal de ojo* is a Spanish phrase translated into English as "evil eye." Children are especially at risk. Symptoms include fitful sleep, crying without apparent cause, diarrhea, vomiting, and fever in a child or infant. Sometimes adults (especially females) have the condition.

nervios   A common idiom of distress among Latinos in the United States and Latin America. A number of other ethnic groups have related, though often somewhat distinctive, ideas of "nerves" (such as *nevra* among Greeks in North America). Nervios refers both to a general state of vulnerability to stressful life experiences and to a syndrome brought on by difficult life cir-cumstances. The term *nervios* includes a wide range of symptoms of emotional distress, somatic disturbance, and inability to function. Common symptoms include headaches and "brain aches," irritability, stomach disturbances, sleep difficulties, nervousness, easy tearfulness, inability to concentrate, trembling, tingling sensations, and *mareos* (dizziness with occasional vertigo-like exac-erbations). Nervios tends to be an ongoing problem, although variable in the degree of disability manifested. Nervios is a very broad syndrome that spans the range from cases free of a mental disorder to presentations resembling adjustment, anxiety, depressive, dissociative, somatoform, or psychotic dis-orders. Differential diagnosis will depend on the constellation of symptoms experienced, the kind of social events that are associated with the onset and progress of nervios, and the level of disability experienced.

pibloktoq An abrupt dissociative episode accompanied by extreme excitement of up to 30 minutes' duration and frequently followed by convulsive seizures and coma lasting up to 12 hours. This is observed primarily in arctic and subarctic Eskimo communities, although regional variations in name exist. The individual may be withdrawn or mildly irritable for a period of hours or days before the attack and will typically report complete amnesia for the attack. During the attack, the individual may tear off his or her clothing, break furniture, shout obscenities, eat feces, flee from protective shelters, or perform other irrational or dangerous acts.

qi-gong psychotic reaction A term describing an acute, time-limited episode characterized by dissociative, paranoid, or other psychotic or nonpsychotic symptoms that may occur after participation in the Chinese folk health-enhancing practice of qi-gong ("exercise of vital energy"). Especially vulnerable are individuals who become overly involved in the practice. This diagnosis is included in the *Chinese Classification of Mental Disorders,* Second Edition (CCMD-2).

rootwork A set of cultural interpretations that ascribe illness to hexing, witchcraft, sorcery, or the evil influence of another person. Symptoms may include generalized anxiety and gastrointestinal complaints (e.g., nausea, vomiting, diarrhea), weakness, dizziness, the fear of being poisoned, and sometimes fear of being killed ("voodoo death"). "Roots," "spells," or "hexes" can be "put" or placed on other persons, causing a variety of emotional and psychological problems. The "hexed" person may even fear death until the "root" has been "taken off" (eliminated), usually through the work of a "root doctor" (a healer in this tradition), who can also be called on to bewitch an enemy. "Rootwork" is found in the southern United States among both African American and European American populations and in Caribbean societies. It is also known as *mal puesto* or *brujeria* in Latino societies.

sangue dormido ("sleeping blood") This syndrome is found among Portuguese Cape Verde Islanders (and immigrants from there to the United States) and includes pain, numbness, tremor, paralysis, convulsions, stroke, blindness, heart attack, infection, and miscarriage.

shenjing shuairuo ("neurasthenia") In China, a condition characterized by physical and mental fatigue, dizziness, headaches, other pains, concentration difficulties, sleep disturbance, and memory loss. Other symptoms include gastrointestinal problems, sexual dysfunction, irritability, excitability, and various signs suggesting disturbance of the autonomic nervous system. In many cases, the symptoms would meet the criteria for a DSM-IV mood or anxiety disorder. This diagnosis is included in the *Chinese Classification of Mental Disorders*, Second Edition (CCMD-2).

shen-k'uei (Taiwan); shenkui (China)   A Chinese folk label describing marked anxiety or panic symptoms with accompanying somatic complaints for which no physical cause can be demonstrated. Symptoms include dizziness, backache, fatigability, general weakness, insomnia, frequent dreams, and complaints of sexual dysfunction (such as premature ejaculation and impotence). Symptoms are attributed to excessive semen loss from frequent intercourse, masturbation, nocturnal emission, or passing of "white turbid urine" believed to contain semen. Excessive semen loss is feared because of the belief that it represents the loss of one's vital essence and can thereby be life threatening.

shin-byung   A Korean folk label for a syndrome in which initial phases are characterized by anxiety and somatic complaints (general weakness, dizziness, fear, anorexia, insomnia, gastrointestinal problems), with subsequent dissociation and possession by ancestral spirits.

spell   A trance state in which individuals "communicate" with deceased relatives or with spirits. At times this state is associated with brief periods of personality change. This culture-specific syndrome is seen among African Americans and European Americans from the southern United States. Spells are not considered to be medical events in the folk tradition but may be misconstrued as psychotic episodes in clinical settings.

susto ("fright," or "soul loss")   A folk illness prevalent among some Latinos in the United States and among people in Mexico, Central America, and South America. Susto is also referred to as *espanto, pasmo, tripa ida, perdida del alma,* or *chibih*. Susto is an illness attributed to a frightening event that causes the soul to leave the body and results in unhappiness and sickness. Individuals with susto also experience significant strains in key social roles. Symptoms may appear any time from days to years after the fright is experienced. It is believed that in extreme cases, susto may result in death. Typical symptoms include appetite disturbances, inadequate or excessive sleep, troubled sleep or dreams, feeling of sadness, lack of motivation to do anything, and feelings of low self-worth or dirtiness. Somatic symptoms accompanying susto include muscle aches and pains, headache, stomachache, and diarrhea. Ritual healings are focused on calling the soul back to the body and cleansing the person to restore bodily and spiritual balance. Different experiences of susto may be related to major depressive disorder, posttraumatic stress disorder, and somatoform disorders. Similar etiological beliefs and symptom configurations are found in many parts of the world.

taijin kyofusho   A culturally distinctive phobia in Japan, in some ways resembling social phobia in DSM-IV. This syndrome refers to an individual's intense fear that his or her body, its parts or its functions, displease, embarrass, or are offensive to other people in appearance, odor, facial expressions, or movements. This syndrome is included in the official Japanese diagnostic system for mental disorders.

zar   A general term applied in Ethiopia, Somalia, Egypt, Sudan, Iran, and other North African and Middle Eastern societies to the experience of spirits possessing an individual. Persons possessed by a spirit may experience dissociative episodes that may include shouting, laughing, hitting the head against a wall, singing, or weeping. Individuals may show apathy and withdrawal, refusing to eat or carry out daily tasks, or may develop a long-term relationship with the possessing spirit. Such behavior is not considered pathological locally.

Index

*Page numbers printed in **boldface** type refer to tables or figures.*